Patient & Person

Fourth edition

Interpersonal skills in nursing

Jane Stein-Parbury

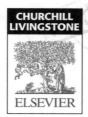

CHURCHILL
LIVINGSTONE

ELSEVIER

Sydney   Edinburgh   London   New York   Philadelphia   St Louis   Toronto

Churchill Livingstone
is an imprint of Elsevier

Elsevier Australia. ACN 001 002 357
(a division of Reed International Books Australia Pty Ltd)
Tower 1, 475 Victoria Avenue, Chatswood, NSW 2067

ELSEVIER

© 2009 Elsevier Australia
Third edition © 2005
Second edition © 2000
First edition © 1993

National Library of Australia Cataloguing-in-Publication entry

Stein-Parbury, Jane.
Patient and person : interpersonal skills in nursing.

4th ed.
Includes index.
Bibliography.
ISBN: 9780729538916 (pbk.)

1. Nurse and patient. 2. Interpersonal relations

610.730699

Publishing Editor: Luisa Cecotti
Developmental Editor: Sabrina Chew
Publishing Services Manager: Helena Klijn
Editorial Coordinator: Andreea Heriseanu
Edited and project managed by Ruth Matheson
Proofread by Brenda Hamilton
Cover and internal design by Darben Design
Index by Forsyth Publishing Services
Typeset by TNQ
Printed by Ligare

Contents

Preface

This book is for nurses who want to learn about establishing interpersonal contact with patients, not as patients but as people whose unique experiences as patients are significant to their nursing care. In caring for patients, nurses need to understand patients' experiences not simply on a theoretical level but also on a personal level. One way they can do this is through the effective use of the interpersonal skills described in this book. Through relating to and interacting with patients as people, nurses place themselves in a position to understand the experience of the person who is the patient. This understanding forms the basis of a therapeutic relationship that is central to good nursing.

Although the intended audience is undergraduate students of nursing and their educators, *Patient and Person* will also be useful to practising nurses, who will find the information beneficial in extending and refining their interpersonal skills, regardless of the extent of their nursing experience. In fact, many practising nurses have commented on the usefulness of the material. Although written from a nursing perspective, the material in this book is also applicable to any healthcare professional wanting to learn more about communicating effectively with patients.

The fourth edition of *Patient and Person* contains new, updated and restructured information. Chapter 2 now has a section about professional boundaries in relation to patient–nurse relationships. Chapter 3 has been renamed, as the skills in this book enable nurses to function as therapeutic agents when relating to patients. Its revision includes a full discussion of emotional intelligence and communication competence as necessary requisites for developing therapeutic agency in nursing. Also, this chapter introduces readers to the need for responsive and assertive interpersonal skills. Previous editions of the book emphasised the former, with little attention to the latter.

Chapter 4 contains information about culture that has been updated and moved to this earlier section of the book, as this material is essential from the outset. Also new to this edition is a complete revision of what was previously Chapter 8, which is now Chapter 9. Rather than focus on crisis, this chapter now uses the concept of transition to relate how people cope with illness.

Chapter 10 is completely revised and now includes a discussion of challenging contexts, including interpersonal conflicts and the need for assertive skills in their successful negotiation. Information regarding age-related factors, which was part of the original text, also is updated and contained within this chapter. The final chapter, previously Chapter 10, and now Chapter 11, focuses on the need for effective relationships with nursing colleagues. As such an endeavour requires a whole-of-systems approach, this chapter has been renamed.

The basic structure of the text remains intact. The first four chapters include background material for the 'skills', which are dissected and explained in Chapters 5 to 8. Experiential learning activities are incorporated throughout these chapters. These activities are designed to focus on the development of skills in a practical, workable manner. The 'skills' are then placed into particular contexts in Part III (Chs 9–11).

There are a few other changes to this edition. The research evidence has been updated and revised throughout the text. Selecting appropriate research findings for a book such as this proved somewhat challenging because of the type of evidence that is available on the topic of patient–nurse relationships. Much of the research evidence about patient–nurse relationships is descriptive and theoretical in nature. Those readers who are familiar with the evidence-based practice movement will appreciate that this is not the 'strongest' evidence possible, in the sense that cause–effect relationships between healthcare interventions and patient outcomes are not established. The type of evidence provided is appropriate because the material in this book is not concerned with the clinical interventions themselves. It is not a book about psychotherapy—that is, intervening in particular ways of talking to patients in order to alter their thoughts, feelings or behaviours. Rather, it is a book with information about how nurses can be therapeutic in their everyday interactions with patients.

Another challenging aspect of writing a book about interpersonal aspects of nursing is the tension between the need to capture the complexity of interpersonal connections and the need to present concrete guidelines and general rules for beginning nurses. Beginning nurses, like novices in any discipline, rely on guidelines and rules. In presenting rules and guidelines, there is an inherent danger of a 'cookbook' approach. Such an approach assumes that there is a rational, objective, 'right' way for nurses to interact with patients. Recipes such as 'Combine three open-ended questions with two empathic statements, add 1 large tablespoon of support and reassurance, then mix well for 10 minutes during an interaction with a patient' are simple to understand but inadequate in addressing the intricacy of patient–nurse interactions.

In meeting this challenge, I have tried to avoid an oversimplified approach to the use of interpersonal skills by including discussion of the contextual variables that need to be considered. I have done so in the hope that the guidelines and rules presented in this book will not be interpreted as prescriptions or recipes.

The use of the word patient is purposive. While I do not want to perpetuate the problems of treating patients as passive recipients of nursing care, this term is one that is most frequently recognised in nursing. The central point of the book, that patients should be treated as people, speaks for itself about the humanistic basis of my philosophical beliefs. The term nurse is used in the generic sense to refer to any level of nurse, from students of nursing to experienced registered nurses.

Finally, I want to emphasise that I realise that skills are not learnt simply by reading about them in a book. While this book offers guidelines and suggestions for the development of interpersonal skills in nursing, the best way to learn them is through interacting with patients. In listening to and understanding patients' experiences of health and illness, nurses will come to appreciate that their real teachers are the people who happen to be patients.

JS-P, Sydney, 2008

The author and publisher wish to thank the following for reviewing this text:

Alison Anderson RN, RM, FETC, BAppSci(Nurs), MEd(Leadership); Lecturer, School of Nursing and Health Studies, Waiariki Institute of Technology, NZ

Tony Bush DPH, MPHC (Palliative Care), BAppSc, Dip App Sc, RN, RPN, FRCNA; Senior Lecturer, Nursing & Midwifery, RMIT University, VIC

Jenny Day RN, ADCHN(Occupational Health Nursing), BHSc(Nursing), MEd(Adult Ed); Lecturer, School of Nursing & Midwifery, The University of Newcastle, NSW

Nel Glass RN, Dip Neuroscience Nsg, BA, MHPEd, PhD, FCN(NSW), FRCNA; Associate Professor, Research Director, School of Health & Human Sciences, Southern Cross University, NSW

Katrina Recoche RN, BA(SocSc), Grad Dip BM, MN; Lecturer, School of Nursing & Midwifery, Monash University (Peninsula Campus), VIC

Acknowledgments

A special note of appreciation is extended to all of the students of nursing whom I have had the pleasure of teaching over the years. Your questions, although often challenging, expanded my thinking, sharpened my focus and enriched my insights into the struggles of learning interpersonal skills. The many experiences that you shared in class helped in the development of the stories in this book. Also, your comments on the activities used in this book assisted in their development and refinement.

Thanks also to my colleagues and the numerous people who have provided feedback on the other editions. Your comments were encouraging and helpful in the production of the fourth edition. Special thanks to all the people who continue to make this book a success.

I am very grateful to the reviewers of the manuscript, especially Jenny Day from the University of Newcastle. Your suggestions were most helpful. I would also like to thank the additional reviewers, Nel Glass, Katrina Recoche, Alison Anderson and Tony Bush. Your feedback proved invaluable. Thanks so much.

I appreciate the ongoing assistance provided by staff at Elsevier, especially Sabrina Chew and Helena Klijn. Your patience has not gone unnoticed.

Finally, I would like to acknowledge my family. I am grateful to my mum, dad and sister who enabled me to understand the importance of caring for others. Thanks to my sons, Richard and Russell, who always find ways of keeping me from taking myself too seriously. My most enthusiastic applause goes to my husband, Charles, who continues to provide the support that was needed to sustain the effort in the preparation of the manuscript.

How to use this book

Patient and Person is a textbook about the practice and theory of developing interpersonal skills in nursing. Incorporated throughout Chapters 3–8 and 10 are various learning activities designed to provide a means by which skills can be developed and theoretical concepts understood. The text that precedes and follows each activity reinforces the point of that activity. For this reason, it is essential that the activities be used in their context (i.e. that they *not* be separated from the text).

Activities throughout the text adhere to a standard format. Importantly, this serves to develop a working pattern of reflection and enquiry. The activity structure comprises two major sections: *process* and *discussion*. The process includes detailed instructions for completing the activity, setting the parameters of the learning experience. The discussion contains exploratory statements and questions designed to encourage reflection on and dialogue about the learning experience, focusing attention on the theoretical concepts highlighted in the learning experience.

Defining learners as both *participants* and *members* in activities is an intended feature. 'Participants' denotes an entire learning group; 'members' specifically refers to people within a smaller group (i.e. participants who are part of a subdivided total group).

Some activities are identified with the symbol ➡ (followed by a page number), which indicates that there is further material in the appendix, primarily intended for those instructors who are facilitating learning through the use of the activity. (It is useful to note at this point that the appendix itself is organised on a chapter-by-chapter basis, preceded by some very useful information to assist facilitators conducting practical sessions.) When an activity in the text is identified with the symbol ➡, this should immediately alert the facilitator to read the additional information for that activity in the appendix, on the page indicated, before proceeding. Activities are characterised by symbols as follows:

indicates that the activity is to be completed in solitude.

 indicates that the activity requires group interaction and discussion.

 indicates that the activity can be completed in solitude, although learning is enhanced through group interaction.

The use of cross-referencing between chapters is of considerable value, due to the overlap between concept and skills. Readers can therefore refer back and forth between chapters, reinforcing and building their understanding of both theory and skills.

The book is not intended for use as a workbook. Therefore, it is recommended, finally, that readers record all written responses and notes to activity instructions on separate sheets of paper. These should be retained in a folder (or similar) for later revision and future reference, especially because some activities build on the results of previous activities.

Activities

Part I
Introduction

The four chapters in Part I reinforce each other by pursuing the same intention—to distil the overall significance of interpersonal relationships in nursing, especially in relation to the potential for nurses to realise their therapeutic agency in helping others. Although similar in intent, each chapter realises its aim through different means. The stories in Chapter 1 engage the reader through identification and serve as illustrations that reassert the subject of this book. The stories are reinforced with relevant research that provides evidence about the importance of interpersonal connections between nurses and patients. Chapter 2 presents theoretical evidence that reinforces the importance of interpersonal communication that builds and maintains therapeutic relationships between nurses and patients. The evidence is a synthesis of relevant and meaningful research into the nature of basic psychosocial care in nursing and healthcare. Of particular relevance is the variability in each relationship. Chapter 3 explores the nurses' therapeutic use of self and the development of therapeutic agency through reflective learning that promotes self-understanding and acceptance. The importance of culture is discussed in Chapter 4, with an emphasis on the promotion of culturally congruent care of patients. The presentation of stories juxtaposed with discussion of research sets a scene that is carried throughout the remaining chapters in this book.

CHAPTER 1

Why interpersonal skills?

INTRODUCTION

Throughout the course of their professional lives, nurses interact with a variety of people, in a variety of contexts and for a variety of reasons. During these social interactions they need to be able to effectively communicate with and relate to other people. As such, nursing is a social activity and nurses need to be socially competent. They must be skilled in the art of interpersonal communication and human relationship building.

The interpersonal skills of communicating and relating, described throughout this book, are central to developing the social competence nurses need to demonstrate in their professional role. This is especially true in relation to the people nurses call patients. For example, with this role comes a mandate for nurses to competently communicate with patients in order to gather relevant and useful data for clinical assessment (Australian Nursing and Midwifery Council (ANMC) 2005). Furthermore, nurses need to relate to patients as more than simply a source of data. Professional codes and standards of practice (ANMC 2003, 2002) dictate that nurses are capable of relating therapeutically with patients as more than passive recipients of care. That is, engaging the patient through communicating and relating are necessary to professional nursing practice.

Interpersonal relationships between patients and nurses humanise healthcare because they are the vehicles through which nurses are responsive to patients' subjective experiences. The relationship meshes the nurse's compassion and knowledge with the patient's experience of health events. Through their relationships with patients, nurses express concern, care and commitment. In the absence of interpersonal relationships with nurses, patients can be viewed as objects, clinical conditions or a set of problems to be solved. Nursing care that is offered without a human connection is impoverished. It lacks a caring connection.

The central premise of this book is that human connection, in the form of a patient–nurse relationship, is vital to nursing. Along with technical capability, the capacity to establish human connection is required for clinical competence in nursing practice. The connection is created by the way nurses and patients interact, and every interaction between nurse and patient is placed within the overall context of a relationship. For example, listening without judging and responding with understanding help to create a therapeutic relationship based on acceptance and respect.

The significance of interpersonal skills in nursing practice is sometimes difficult for beginning nurses to fully appreciate. The completion of skilled tasks often comes to the foreground, as technical proficiency is required for clinical competence. Interpersonal contact may seem like something that happens after tasks are completed. Focusing on interpersonal aspects of nursing does not mean that attention to task-related nursing functions is diminished. In fact, interpersonal contact increases the therapeutic effectiveness of nursing activities. For example, the restful state of feeling reassured by knowing what to expect, through explanations about details of an upcoming procedure, is of benefit to patients. Nurses are often in a prime position to establish interpersonal contact in order to provide such explanations. Nursing care involves making contact with the person who is the patient.

Chapter overview

This chapter contains a theoretical overview of the therapeutic patient–nurse relationship, because interpersonal skills live within a relational context in nursing practice. Emphasis is placed on the moral imperative to relate to patients in a caring manner. In addition, the importance of understanding the human health experience (Newman 2002) is highlighted as fundamental to the relationship. As the relationship is embedded into concepts of caring, this subject of nursing inquiry is reviewed. Interspersed with theory are stories that illustrate the importance of interpersonal aspects of nursing care. Theoretical concepts described throughout the chapter reinforce the significance and centrality of interpersonal contact in nursing.

THE NATURE OF THE PATIENT–NURSE RELATIONSHIP

Numerous other professions also involve the ability to interact with and relate to people. In fact, good interpersonal skills are needed for successful employment across a range of disciplines. In this respect, nursing is not unique. What differs in the nursing context is what qualifies as 'effective' within the context of patient interaction. 'Effective' in the nursing care context refers to interpersonal interactions between nurses and patients that are helpful to patients. In effective patient–nurse interactions, there is an orientation on the part of the nurse *to be* of benefit to the patient and, more importantly, the patient feels assisted in some way by the interaction.

The helpful nature of effective patient–nurse interactions is important to bear in mind because effective interaction in other contexts would have other meanings and orientations. For example, an effective interaction in the world of business sales is oriented towards company profit. While assisting the customer is important to successful ongoing interactions, the intention of the business sales interaction is the exchange of money for goods and services. Furthermore, customers in a sales transaction are not vulnerable; they are not dependent on the salesperson for their wellbeing. People in need of healthcare are often not in such a position—they are vulnerable. Nurses are in a prime position to reduce patient vulnerability.

Nurses are able to reduce patient vulnerability when they operate from a position of 'being for' the patient—that is, they need to function as a useful resource in reducing distress and suffering (Eriksson 2002). 'Being for' patients reflects an attitude and a value; it is a moral positioning on the part of the nurse, a commitment and a promise to embody caring. Such positioning is an imperative in nursing practice (Coffey 2006, Brilowski & Wendler 2005, Newman 2002, Bishop & Scudder 1999, Watson 1999, Watson 1985, Gadow 1980). An attitude of 'being for' patients is how nurses demonstrate that they care.

The act of aligning oneself alongside another person in an attempt to help or be of assistance—in this case, to nurse—helps to distinguish that interpersonal relationship from other social relationships such as friendships. True friends meet each other's needs on a regular basis and reciprocate in giving and receiving. In addition, they expect to remain friends for life. The patient–nurse relationship is usually time-limited and more one-way, with the nurse being there 'for' the patient. The focus of the nurse's interest in the person who is the patient is for the sake of the patient's wellbeing. While nursing can be an extremely rewarding profession, professional nurses do not use their relationships with patients to meet their own needs.

Making explicit the beneficial aspects of the interpersonal interventions (i.e. helping patients by talking and relating to them) is an attempt to move away from nursing care that is predominantly task-oriented to that which is holistic, personalised care. Such care is contingent on knowing more about a patient than simply a diagnostic category or an anticipated clinical pathway.

Sometimes, nurses become so accustomed to the routine of healthcare that they treat patients in a routine manner. They treat patients as objects and fail to demonstrate an appreciation that, to patients, illness and health are not routine matters—they are highly personal and often significant. When nurses demonstrate understanding of the personal and unique experiences of patients, they are therapeutically connecting on an interpersonal level.

Consider the following story, told by a patient:

As I awaited my coronary bypass surgery I was filled with mixed emotions. I was pleased that technological advances in healthcare enabled such surgery to be performed, but at the same time I was worried about the outcome. When the surgeons explained the surgical procedure, they did so with a detail that I appreciated. Everything I wanted to know had been covered and they answered each of my questions with patience and complete explanations. But I could still see that to them the procedure was routine. They had successfully completed hundreds, even thousands, of these procedures and approached the explanations with a matter-of-fact manner that would be expected with such familiarity. But, to me, the surgery could never be routine.

After they left my hospital room, the nurse who was caring for me that day, Jan, came in to see me. I had come to know and trust Jan during my stay in hospital. She had been present as the surgical team explained what was to happen during the bypass procedure. Jan also had many years of experience in caring for patients who were undergoing coronary bypass surgery.

I did have a few more questions that Jan answered with knowledge and detail. She then sat down next to my bed and explained that sometimes patients need more than factual details. Sometimes, they also have fears related to the surgery that cannot be allayed through information alone. She asked me if I had any fears.

Because I knew and trusted Jan, I told her my greatest fear was that of becoming a cripple, unable to care for myself and function as an independent person. Some of the possible complications that the surgeons reviewed led me to believe that this was a possibility. I was surprised at how freely the words came out, as I am not a person who discusses feelings easily, especially when these feelings are related to my fears. Obviously, I had some fears and Jan's concern and interest helped me to express them. I told her that I was not afraid of dying, only afraid of living half a life following the surgery.

She understood what I was telling her. She didn't try to alleviate my fears by offering me statistics about the probability of my becoming a cripple. The surgeons had already presented the statistics. There is not much consolation in knowing that there is a 10% chance of this complication or a 5% chance of that complication. Although I was somewhat reassured in hearing these facts, how was I to know whether I'd be the 90% or the 10%?

Instead of focusing on further details, Jan just listened to me. And she demonstrated to me that she understood. When my daughter came to visit me that evening I relayed my conversation with Jan to her. I told my daughter how impressed I was with the fact that Jan initiated this discussion with me. Talking about my interaction with Jan provided an opportunity for me to discuss my fears with my daughter, who also listened and understood. Without the trigger from Jan, I'm not sure I would have discussed my feelings with my daughter. My daughter demonstrated the same level of supportive understanding as Jan. We both felt relieved and a bit closer that evening.

Contrast the above story with the following, told by a patient:

When Therese entered my hospital room that morning I had the feeling the day wasn't going to be all that pleasant. She had the manner of an army drill sergeant, moving quickly from patient to patient, not asking how our night had been or how we were feeling. She was one of those nurses who was focused on what *she* was doing as if we, the patients in that room, were superfluous to her mission. Had she bothered to ask, or even notice the expression on my face, she would have realised how awful the previous night had been for me. I had not slept or even rested for that matter. I could not find a comfortable position in bed because the pain in my hip seemed to be getting worse.

My hip had been badly broken in a car accident 6 days earlier. When the surgeons described how they repaired my hip, it sounded like carpentry work to me. There were metal pins, screws and plates used to repair and strengthen what would now be a weak part of my body. The pain in my hip was excruciating. During the 21 years of my life, I had not experienced anything like it. In fact, I can hardly recall ever being sick.

The nurses in hospital seemed to come in two varieties—the ones who were sympathetic and understanding about my pain, and the ones who treated me like a sook when I complained. Therese seemed like the latter type. She briskly attended to the other patients in the room before coming to me. I had the feeling she was going to make a big deal about having a shower *right now*. She did. As she approached me she said, 'Now it's your turn, young man. Time to get up. Let's go.'

I tried to be pleasant when I asked her to let me have my shower after morning tea. I explained that the pain medication I had received earlier was starting to take effect and I wanted to relax and rest awhile before getting out of bed. But Therese was not open to any negotiation on the shower time. She told me that I had to get up and get going now. 'Part of the treatment,' she said. She offered no explanation about why the shower had to be now, only that *now* is what she expected. I felt angry and frustrated, but knew better than to try to talk her out of her plans for me. She was in control. She did not seem to care about me.

In the first story, Jan demonstrated that she understood what this man was experiencing in relation to his impending surgery. Jan demonstrated that she knew his impending surgery was more than just another statistic or a routine event. He was facing a major event in his life and she was there to understand what this event might mean to him. She was concerned about the patient as a person.

In the second story, Therese failed to take an individual patient's needs into account. Had Therese listened to this patient and explored his reasons for wanting to delay the shower, she might have understood his request. Instead she alienated him and gave the impression of only caring about what *she* believed was best. Not only did she fail to negotiate care with the patient, but she also contributed to his distress and suffering. In doing so, she increased his vulnerability.

An attitude of 'being for' the patient means that nurses will take time to listen and understand the patient's experience. A central aim of a helping relationship includes 'initiating supportive interpersonal communication in order to understand the perceptions and needs of the others' (Reynolds & Scott 1999 p 363). In addition to such empathic understanding, this type of relationship will reduce or resolve difficulties being experienced by those in need of help. Finally, a helping relationship will enable the person in need to cope with the demands placed on them by difficult situations.

As such, a helping relationship between nurse and patient is based on shared understanding—alignment that enables them to engage in mutual endeavours. In this sense, relating to patients assists nurses in their clinical decision making because of the importance of 'knowing the patient', a central aspect of sound clinical judgments that are *in the interest* of the patient.

Knowing the patient

In making clinical decisions about nursing care of patients, nurses take into account different sources of knowledge and different ways of knowing. For example, knowledge about pathophysiology assists nurses in knowing what to do when patients are recovering from abdominal surgery. In addition to knowledge such as anatomy and physiology, nurses need to take into account how individual patients are responding as they recover from abdominal surgery. In synthesising results of field studies in a variety of nursing care settings, Liaschenko and Fisher (1999) have differentiated three different types of knowledge that nurses use in their work. These knowledge types assist in understanding the importance of relating to patients.

The first of these knowledge types is referred to by Liaschenko and Fisher as *case knowledge*. This knowledge is generalised and objective, and includes areas such as the knowledge of anatomy, physiology, physical disease processes and pharmacology. Such knowledge is based on statistics and probabilities of the clinical situation. Nurses need not necessarily interact with patients in order to use this knowledge. They can understand the biomechanics of a myocardial infarction without ever seeing a patient who has experienced one.

The second type of knowledge in Liaschenko and Fisher's schema is central to nursing work. Referred to as *patient knowledge*, it is the knowledge of how individual patients are responding to their clinical situations. This knowledge enables nurses to negotiate the care of patients within a healthcare system. This type of knowing is based on understanding what individual patients are experiencing and therefore requires interaction between nurse and patient. That is, nurses need interpersonal skills to understand a patient's response to the clinical situation at hand.

A third type of knowledge identified by Liaschenko and Fisher involves an understanding of the unique individuality of the patient, knowing the patient's personal and private biography and understanding how that person's actions make sense for them. It is *person knowledge*.

Patient knowledge and person knowledge encompass what is currently identified in the nursing literature as the concept of 'knowing the patient' (Mok & Chui 2004, Wilkin & Slevin 2004, Luker et al 2000, Henderson 1997, Liaschenko 1997, Radwin 1995). This relates to what Carper (1978) referred to as 'personal knowing'—that is, knowledge gained through interacting with patients. Broadly speaking, the concept refers to a process whereby nurses are able to treat a patient as an individual person because they know something about them. 'Knowing the patient' is identified as a central caring behaviour (Swanson 1993), and associated with expert clinical nursing practice (Benner et al 1992).

There is also empirical evidence that 'knowing the patient' aids clinical decision making (Radwin 1995, Jenks 1993, Tanner et al 1993, Jenny & Logan 1992). Clinical decision making involves complex processes that are cognitive and experiential. Effective decisions require multiple ways of coming to know a situation and knowing the patient is one of those ways. For example, the critical care nurses in Jenny and Logan's study (1992) used individual patient responses in determining how to wean the patient from mechanical ventilation. The physiology of respiratory functioning and the mechanics of artificial ventilation provide nurses with 'case knowledge' (Liaschenko & Fisher 1999) based on standardised, statistical evidence, generalisable to a majority of patients. Nevertheless, nurses in this study also used knowledge of how an individual patient was responding to the gradual discontinuation of mechanical ventilation (Jenny & Logan 1992).

'Knowing the patient' reinforces strongly held beliefs and values in nursing that treating patients holistically as unique individuals is part of a professional identity. 'Knowing the patient' is a result of interacting with and relating to that person in some way; it does not mean that nurses have formed a long-term relationship with the patient, nor that they even have to talk with the patient. The patients whom nurses were discussing in Jenny and Logan's study (1992) could not speak during the weaning process because there were endotracheal tubes through their vocal cords. And yet nurses were able to 'know the patient' by observing their responses to nursing actions; in doing so, they were using *patient knowledge*.

The types of knowledge that are used in nursing will vary with clinical contexts. For example, therapeutic relationships formed in a palliative care setting will often bring *person knowledge* to the foreground. In an outpatient context where patients are being seen for a routine screening test, *person knowledge* might not be necessary. It is not always desirable or necessary for nurses to enter into the personal and intimate aspects of a patient's life (i.e. to have *person knowledge*). Such entry may even be intrusive (May 1992a) or coercive (Liaschenko 1997). However, knowing how individual patients are responding to their state of health and healthcare, *patient knowledge*, is essential in all clinical contexts of nursing.

There is recent evidence to suggest that nurses' ability to 'know the patient' is affected by more than clinical context. Speed and Luker (2004) found that 'knowing the patient' was diminished by healthcare policy that directed community nurses' attention to the technical side of care at the expense of the personal knowledge that comes through direct experience of interacting with patients. Likewise, McCabe (2004) found that nurses are thwarted in their attempts to personalise care by organisational systems that place more emphasis on task completion. That is, the sociopolitical context in which the nurses work has impact on their care that extends beyond the individual nurse's desire to know the patient and the patient's need to be known in this way (see Ch 11).

Patient participation in care

The notion of patients as active participants in healthcare challenges the traditional sick role (Parsons 1951/1987), which brings expectations of passivity, relinquishing of responsibilities, and following the advice of healthcare experts. Such a role prevents people from assuming responsibility for their own health and, more importantly, places decision-making authority in the hands of the healthcare practitioners. As such, the sick role can disempower patients, thus rendering them more vulnerable.

The contemporary movement towards patient participation in healthcare alters the power balance such that patients are encouraged to engage in partnerships with healthcare practitioners, with increased capacity to act on their own behalf as a result (Jonsdottir et al 2004, Gallant et al 2002). Partnership is a respectful, negotiated way of working that enables choice and participation in care (Bidmead & Cowley 2005). The negotiation aspect is essential as patients' desire and capacity to participate is quite variable (Sahlsten et al 2007, Florin et al 2006). Not all patients either want to or are able to participate in their own healthcare (see Ch 8).

No matter what term is used, patient or partner, therapeutic relationships between nurses and those entrusted to their care are characterised by respect for the dignity of each person and recognition that, at a human level, both are equal. The concept of human caring is useful in understanding these aspects of the relationship further.

Caring and the patient–nurse relationship

Much of what is said and written about the patient–nurse relationship rests on the assumption that the nature of the relationship is helpful—that is, patients are assisted in some way through their interpersonal interactions with nurses. One explication of the notion of 'being helpful' is found in nursing research investigating the concept of caring. Caring is a way of being rather than a way of doing (Smith 2004, Bishop & Scudder 1999).

Caring is often considered fundamental to nursing—that is, it is considered an essential ingredient in nursing. There are nursing leaders who have consistently asserted that caring is the most central concept to good nursing (most notably Benner & Wrubel 1989, Watson 1985, Leininger 1984). As such, the assertion suggests that understanding the theoretical construct of caring is akin to understanding nursing itself. Regardless of whether the claim is accepted or rejected, caring and nursing remain intrinsically linked (Hanson 2004, Tarlier 2004, Wilkin & Slevin 2004, Cheung 1998). This raises a number of questions, not the least of which is the meaning of the word *caring* in the context of nursing. Quite simply, caring means 'it matters' (Benner & Wrubel 1989).

If a person cares about their car, then what happens to the vehicle matters to them. In the process of caring *about* the vehicle, they will also care *for* the car (e.g. by keeping it tuned and running smoothly). To understand the person's care, it is useful to consider why they care (i.e. the motivation to care). The motivation to care may be because the machine is their sole means of transportation, or it may be because the car is a symbol that boosts the owner's sense of self and identity.

Attention to the motivation to care in nursing is also important to consider, especially in relation to the need for reflection and self-understanding (see Ch 3). Nurses who care because it helps them to increase their self-concept run the risk of harming others by confusing their own needs with the needs of patients. The self-awareness required to understand this motivation is considered a requisite for caring (Brilowski & Wendler 2005).

Although claims about the centrality of caring in nursing had been expressed previously, it was not until the early to mid-1980s that extensive nursing research into caring was undertaken when researchers were attempting to explicate a meaning of caring that was unique to nursing. Despite numerous research studies into caring, the concept continues to be reported as poorly defined and ambiguous (Brilowski & Wendler 2005, Swanson 1999, Sourial 1997, Kyle 1995, Morse et al 1990).

In a comprehensive, literary meta-analysis of 130 research articles published in nursing (mostly between 1980 and 1996), Swanson (1999) developed a schema that is useful in understanding how caring is conceptualised in nursing. Five levels of caring were identified in analysis. The levels are hierarchical in the sense that the conditions of each preceding level are assumed to be met before the next level is possible. The five levels are:

1 the capacity to care (compassion, empathy, knowledge, positive outlook)
2 values and beliefs about connecting with and building rapport with patients
3 conditions—personal, organisational and patient-related—which affect the capacity to care
4 caring actions (i.e. behaviours associated with therapeutic interventions), and
5 the consequences of caring, both positive and negative (absence of caring).

The majority of nursing studies have been undertaken to investigate level 4 (i.e. investigation of caring actions). In addition, most of the early studies relied on nurses' reports of their caring interventions.

In a recent concept analysis of the meaning of caring in nursing, the core dimensions, or defining attributes, of caring were identified as relationship, action, attitude, acceptance and variability (Brilowski & Wendler 2005). Relationship involves the mutual and reciprocal give and take of social interactions, while action refers to a voluntary act such as physical care and presence. The attitude of caring involves genuine concern and regard for patients. Acceptance of the patient includes recognising the intrinsic value and worth of each patient. Variability indicates that caring is fluid and ever-changing in response to the context. These are characteristics and actions that are indicative of nurses' perspectives about caring.

In an effort to measure caring from the patients' perspective, Duffy et al (2007) have developed an instrument that describes caring behaviours. These behaviours include:

- mutuality in problem solving, as nurses assist patients in understanding and dealing with illness
- attentive reassurance in relation to being available and interested, and instilling hope
- respect for and acceptance of me as a person
- encouragement and support; appreciation of my unique meanings
- creation of an environment for healing that includes my comfort and privacy; involving my family in my care, and
- meeting my basic needs like food and sleep.

From this list it can be seen that patients feel cared for when they are respected as an individual—a unique being who is worthy of attention, encouragement and support.

The common aspects of research into the meaning of caring in nursing, identified in Watson's theory (Watson 1985), were both instrumental or action-oriented, and expressive or feeling oriented. Instrumental actions include meeting basic needs and the provision of physical care, while expressive caring is related to the recognition and acknowledgment of the personhood of the patient. More importantly, the research demonstrates the importance of nurses being accessible and available to engage in a relationship characterised by respect and genuine regard by the nurse for the worth of the patient and built through interpersonal interaction.

An interesting finding in this body of research reveals divergent views of nurses and patients in their perceptions of what constitutes caring (summarised in Chang et al 2005). Nurses' responses in these studies reveal that they perceive the most important caring behaviours to be expressive (i.e. feeling oriented)—for example, listening to the patient. The nurses' perceptions contrast with what the patients say is most important. The caring behaviours patients value most are instrumental behaviours (i.e. action oriented)—for example, giving medications on time, notifying medical staff when necessary and explaining what is physically wrong with the patient. That is, patients were more concerned than nurses with behaviours that indicated technical competence as a demonstration of caring, rather than emotional care. The results of the most recent study of this nature (Chang et al 2005) revealed an agreement between nurses and cancer patients that 'being accessible' was the most important nurse caring behaviour, although there was still discrepancy in their views.

One explanation for the discrepancy in nurses' and patients' perceptions of caring may relate to the use of the Care-Q instrument (Larson 1986) that was used in the studies. The instrument includes items describing both expressive and instrumental behaviours. Nurses who placed the expressive items in priority (the Q-sort methodology) may have assumed technical competence was present (McKenna 1993). Another possible reason is that behaviours (not meanings) were investigated, and that patients were challenged by technical aspects of care, while nurses were challenged by personalising their care through expressive behaviours (Swanson 1999). Chang et al (2005) speculate that the agreement on the most important behaviour may have resulted from nurses and patients being paired in their study and therefore more likely to know each other's preferences.

While patients in the studies cited did not report expressive (interpersonal) behaviours as the most important caring action, the absence of respect and regard for the patient as a person (e.g. being treated like an object) was viewed by patients as non-caring (Wiman & Wikblad 2004, Rieman 1986). Studies that have explored patients' perceptions of nursing care (McCabe 2004, Williams & Iruita 2004, Hegedus 1999, Webb & Hope 1995, Fosbinder 1994, Appleton 1993) demonstrate that patients *do* value nurses' interpersonal skills. More importantly, there is evidence of a positive correlation between nurse caring and patient satisfaction (Wolf et al 2003).

Overall, the evidence indicates that patients do want to interact with nurses who are genuine, not hurried, and are available and willing to talk (Shattell 2004)—that is, patients want nurses who are accessible and approachable.

Consider the following story:

At 20 years of age, I was shocked when I received a diagnosis of cancer. Cancer was something that happened to old people, not young uni students like myself. The diagnosis did provide an explanation for my fatigue and lack of usual enthusiasm for life, but was one that I was not at all prepared to hear. The good news was that the medical staff thought that the diagnosis had been made early enough in the progress of the disease for there to be a good likelihood of remission. But getting to remission required a series of chemotherapy treatments that not only made me feel incredibly sick and very tired, but that also resulted in my loss of hair.

My family and friends were incredibly supportive throughout the whole ordeal. So were the majority of the nursing staff. It was one nurse who really upset me by her lack of caring concern for my welfare.

Donna worked in the chemo clinic and I had only met her fleetingly on previous visits to the clinic. Having chemo required daily visits during each course of treatment. When Donna approached me that morning in order to prepare the intravenous line that would deliver the medication, I noticed that she looked very tired and not 100% well. I overheard her talking to one of her colleagues about her big night the previous evening, as she relayed having too much to drink with her friends in the pub. She was complaining of feeling hung-over, but came to work nevertheless. She did not say much to me personally, although she kept talking to her colleagues as she prepared the equipment for me.

It was when she attempted to insert the needle that I began to get distressed. Her hands were not that steady as she went about her work. She was fumbling with the equipment. She did not seem to know what she was doing, although we had every reason to believe that she was usually a competent nurse. Each attempt to insert the needle was creating more pain and anxiety in me. Side effects of the medications were bad enough. Why did I have to suffer because of this nurse's lack of skill? After three attempts to insert the needle, she called for assistance. My Mum and I just looked on in fear. Another nurse came over to the bedside and assisted. Donna laughed about her inability to insert the needle. I did not see the humour in the situation.

Donna's actions that morning indicated to me that she did not care. How could she when she did not arrive for work prepared to focus her energy on the patients? I thought to myself that she should have called in sick, rather than expose vulnerable patients to herself that morning. I received my chemo okay that morning, but am still angry about Donna's actions. Her behaviour seemed like a lack of caring and I was not impressed. It is not that I am a prude; my friends and I enjoy our evenings in the pub. It was that Donna should have realised that she had responsibilities to her patients that morning and she failed to meet them to the best of her capability.

The story demonstrates that caring involves technical competence; the patient's distress was created by a lack of demonstration of the same. But the real reason for the patient's distress in this story was that Donna's technical capacity was compromised that morning by her own state of health and behaviour. In effect, she was not really 'available' to patients that day. To this patient, that meant that she did not care.

The previously mentioned studies exploring the nature of caring in nursing demonstrate that both instrumental and expressive nursing behaviours are needed for patients to feel cared for. As Dunlop (1986) points out, caring cannot be understood as compassion and concern while ignoring physical aspects of nursing. In fact, technical competence has been identified as a precedent to a caring relationship (Coffey 2006), and for some patients (such as those in an emergency department) competence is synonymous with caring (Baldursdottir & Jonsdottir 2002). The combined results of the reviewed studies suggest that caring involves psychosocial and technical skills. This sentiment is expressed well by Roach (1985) who states:

> While competence without compassion can be brutal and inhumane, compassion without competence may be no more than meaningless, if not harmful, intrusion into the life of a person or persons needing help (p 172).

Patient–nurse relationships in nursing practice

There are also claims that centralising the interpersonal relationship between patient and nurse is a new situation (see, for example, Barthow 1997, Porter 1994, May 1992b, Ramos 1992, Salvage 1990). Previously, nursing work was organised according to tasks in order to protect nurses from emotional involvement (Menzies 1961). Under such a system, nurses were discouraged from relating to individual patients because doing so has the potential to distract them from completing their allocated tasks (May 1993). For the most part this system was impersonal, with nurses focusing on their functional role in healthcare (i.e. a job), not on their professional responsibility to relate to patients and personalise their care.

Nevertheless, the basis for relating to patients is not really new or revolutionary in nursing. It may come as no surprise that Nightingale's *Notes on Nursing*

(1859) contains numerous references to the need to understand idiosyncrasies of individual patients. Nightingale iterates and reiterates both how to relieve the anxieties of sick people and also how 'not to' exacerbate their worries or concerns. She is even prescriptive about how to talk to sick people. For example, she stresses the need for eye contact through her recommendation to be seated while talking. She warns of the problems of false reassurance, referred to as 'chattering hopes', stating that there is 'scarcely a greater worry which invalids have to endure' (p 54). She admonishes friends, visitors and attendants from attempting to cheer the sick by 'making light of their danger and by exaggerating their probability of recovery' (p 54). The language of today's nursing may have changed from the time of Nightingale, but the underlying message remains the same. The patient is a unique individual with idiosyncratic concerns and worries, and nurses need to understand the patient's point of view.

It was in the early 1950s that Peplau wrote what was to become the seminal work that specifically addressed patient–nurse relationships. *Interpersonal Relations in Nursing* (Peplau 1952/1988) outlined a theoretical framework and structure for therapeutic patient–nurse relationships. Peplau articulated how the nursing relationship could be a vehicle for a 'corrective human experience' for patients. In keeping with Peplau, Travelbee (1971) expanded the interpersonal aspects of relating to patients, referring to such activities as 'therapeutic use of self as an art'.

Peplau's philosophy of relating continues to have relevance for contemporary scholars (McNaughton 2005, Stockman 2005). Carroll (2004) used Peplau's framework in a metasynthesis of qualitative research of patients feeling understood when unable to speak due to mechanical ventilation. The results revealed the importance of individualising care and knowing the patient. Findings from a multinational study by Arthur et al (1999) revealed that nurses value the development of a trusting relationship that enables patients to express their concerns and feelings. Furthermore, in contemporary times, there is evidence that the philosophy of *primary nursing*, which centralises the patient–nurse relationship, is an organisational factor associated with improved patient outcomes (Aiken et al 2002). (Aiken's investigations are reviewed further in Ch 11.) The system operates on the notion that relationships between nurses and their patients will develop, and that such relationships enable individualised care and promote continuity of care. That is, the nurse comes to 'know the patient'.

The 'move to relate' has not been without its critics. There are suggestions that requiring nurses to relate to patients as subjective beings is a questionable form of control and surveillance (May 1992b, Armstrong 1983). In support of this contention, May (1992a) cautions nurses that transforming patients from objects (of physical care) to subjects (with psychosocial needs) carries with it the risk of 'inventing' living and coping problems for patients when such 'problems' are matters of daily living. Solving problems such as these through the development of therapeutic relationships becomes a vehicle for nurses to legitimate their interpersonal work.

Additional criticism of the move to relate involves the 'burden' of the emotional work involved in relating to patients (Mackintosh 2000). This burden has the potential to drain nurses of their energy, especially because this type of work is often unacknowledged in an efficiency-driven healthcare system. Healthcare organisations need to acknowledge the importance of nurses' endeavours to relate to patients, and provide support systems to cope with the potential stress and burden (see Ch 11).

The extent to which a nurse becomes 'burdened' throughout the relationship is dependent both on clinical context and the level of interpersonal involvement that is negotiated between them. Patients will reveal themselves to nurses selectively and some relationships will progress to deeply moving levels, while others remain therapeutically superficial. Some patients will require direct aid and assistance with managing their lives, while others will need information and advice in order to cope with and problem-solve challenges related to their health. Still others may simply need the supportive and comforting understanding of another human being. Each has a different level of involvement and commitment that is negotiated. The negotiation process is fully described in the next chapter.

What makes the relationship therapeutic in nursing spans a range of possibilities and this is why context-free rules cannot be applied. There are many ways that nurses help through their interactions with patients. According the Benner (1984 p 48), 'helping [in the nursing context] encompasses transformative changes in meanings, and sometimes simply the courage to be with the patient, offering whatever comfort the situation allows'. This description provides useful guidance in understanding the range of form and purpose patient–nurse relationships can encompass. It reinforces the notion that 'being with' a patient, fully present and involved, is helpful in itself.

Consider the following story, told by a nurse:

Tony, aged 5, was hospitalised as a result of serious injuries he sustained in a car accident. He was a passenger in the car driven by his mother, who also sustained injuries and required hospitalisation in a different facility to Tony. Although Tony's mother was in hospital, her injuries were minor. Because Tony's injuries were to his head and spine, he was initially admitted to the intensive care unit of the hospital, but eventually was transferred to a general medical ward. This is when we first met.

Tony's father remained by his son's side day and night throughout the entire hospitalisation. He did not say much and most of our interactions were either non-verbal or limited to brief and factual information about Tony's condition. I noticed that Tony's father looked increasingly tired and drained as the days went by. The dark circles under his eyes were noticeable. He walked with a slumped posture.

After 5 days on the ward, Tony's condition deteriorated, necessitating a transfer back to the intensive care unit. This setback was overwhelming for Tony's father. I could see it in his face. Initially, I concerned myself with the details of getting the transfer underway. After the transfer was complete, Tony's father returned to the ward area to collect his son's belongings. He didn't look at me and seemed quite distant. I wanted to say something to him in an effort to offer some degree of comfort, but knew better than to deliver a trite cliché such as 'It will be all right'. After all, how was I to know it would be? Instead, I approached him in the hallway as he was about to leave the ward area and told him how sorry I was that his son had to be transferred back to intensive care. I expressed my genuine sympathy for the turn of events that led to the transfer. He didn't respond, but rather looked at me with a vacant stare, as if he was looking through and past me. I wanted to say more. I could not leave it at just that. So I said: 'I can only imagine one-hundredth of what you must be feeling. It seems like Tony has taken two steps forward and three steps back.'

Tears welled in his eyes and he said, 'I keep hoping … but something always happens.' He began to cry and talk about how much he loved his son and how helpless he felt in this situation. I placed my hand on his shoulder and guided him to a private area of the ward. He expressed his thoughts and feelings about what was happening to his son, describing his condition in detail and expressing feelings of despair. Although I too felt extremely sad for Tony and his father, I maintained control over my emotions at the moment because I wanted to focus on him, not me (although I did cry later). I said nothing but simply placed my hand on his hand and squeezed it. It seemed enough. After a few minutes he composed himself, told me how much he appreciated my concern, thanked me and left the ward. I recall how helpless I felt about Tony's situation. It was likely that he would not walk again.

Although I felt helpless, I focused my energy on making contact with Tony's father. I *had* to make contact and was glad I found the courage to do so. In some small way I knew my concern for him and his son helped Tony's father. I could not change the situation, but I was there for him. I demonstrated that I cared and that I wanted to understand how he felt, no matter how helpless this made me feel.

The situations that nurses encounter often create feelings of helplessness within them when the patient's circumstances cannot be changed. Nurses may fear that because they cannot change the situation, there is nothing else that can be done. When this happens, nurses may avoid interaction and interpersonal contact, or limit contact with patients to those times when physical aspects of care require attention.

This story illustrates how conveying concern and understanding enables nurses to connect with patients and their families. It also demonstrates that the helpless feelings nurses sometimes experience, as a result of clinical realities that are devastating and sad, do not mean that *they* are helpless. Such feelings do not mean that nothing more can be done. The clinical reality of Tony's injuries was not altered, but the emotional pain that Tony's father was experiencing was shared by this nurse. The fact that nurses do encounter situations of human suffering means that they cannot avoid it. Not only must nurses face such realities, but also, on a personal and professional level, they need to learn how to make contact with people who are experiencing human pain and suffering. Being with patients in a manner that is wholly human and caring is more than just something that can be done. It may be everything.

The connection between Tony's father and this nurse came easily. There are other times in nursing where more direct intervention would be required and make a connection much more challenging. Understanding the patient's point of view is difficult when anger and frustration are being experienced. The challenge of even establishing helpful contact can be especially daunting when trying to help.

Consider the following story, told by a nurse:

As I came on duty to begin my night shift in the paediatric ward, I noticed two distraught women in the nursery. They were engaged in what appeared to be a heated discussion. One of the women was Eve, the nurse who was finishing her evening shift. The other woman was Tracey, the mother of one of the babies in the nursery. Tracey's child was hospitalised for respiratory problems. I caught only the tail end of their conversation and although I could not understand the content, I sensed hostility and anger in both of them. Tracey was walking away from Eve as

I entered the nursery. I sat down to receive the handover report from Eve and she began to tell me of her frustration with Tracey. 'It seems that I cannot do anything to make her happy,' Eve said. She then went on to tell of the numerous complaints made by Tracey. I listened to Eve, knowing in the back of my mind that I would have to listen to Tracey as well. I told Eve I would try to sort out the situation and would see her the next day. She seemed relieved.

After the report I went to find Tracey. She was packing her baby's belongings and informed me that she was taking her baby home. I knew from the report that Tracey's baby had not taken any fluids by mouth during the previous shift and was at risk of dehydration. I was quite concerned about Tracey's plan to leave. Slowly I said, 'I know you are upset …', but was cut off mid-sentence by Tracey.

'That nurse is typical of everything here, just typical. You bet I'm upset.' She continued to pack her belongings. 'And I don't want to discuss it. I'm going home with my baby.'

At this point I felt at a loss, but also knew I had to try and make contact with Tracey, even though she was shutting me out.

'Look,' I said in an almost pleading manner, 'I want to help but I don't know what is going on. I don't know what is wrong.'

Tracey picked up her belongings and her baby and said, 'Well, it's too late to start worrying now.'

I protested, 'I *am* worried, even if it is too late. I am concerned for you and your baby.'

'Don't give me that, nobody cares around here, not you nor any of the other nurses,' she said.

I blurted out, 'Oh, is that what's wrong?'

She looked straight at me for the first time, 'Yes, that's exactly what's wrong.'

I knew I had to think fast. The contact that I had made with her seemed tenuous and I wanted to strengthen it. I did not want this mother to leave. 'Please, let's talk,' I said. 'I was just about to have a cup of coffee. Come with me and I'll get you one too.' To my relief she agreed. I added, 'And I'll get a bottle for your baby.'

We went together into the kitchen area where I prepared coffee for us and a bottle for Tracey's baby, who had been crying the entire time we had been talking. I didn't want to take over but thought it essential to get the baby settled. Her distressed baby could have been half of Tracey's problem. When the bottle was ready I asked Tracey if she would like to feed her baby.

She replied, 'Look, that's what I've been trying to do all evening. He just won't take anything. I can't do it, and he'll end up needing a drip.'

I sensed her anger and frustration, which was now starting to escalate again. 'Okay,' I said, 'I'll feed the baby and you drink your coffee.' I noticed how directive I'd become, but decided that Tracey needed some concrete assistance in settling her baby. Besides, it was becoming increasingly difficult to carry on a conversation in the presence of the crying baby.

'Nobody has been able to feed him today and they said he may need a drip. They expect me to feed him but what can I do when he keeps fussing and refusing to suck,' she explained. She felt useless and helpless, while at the same time responsible. She was trapped by the circumstances. I decided to take over a bit more. In proceeding to feed her baby, I explained how his respiratory problems were interfering with his ability to suck. Thankfully, Tracey's baby began to feed and settle. At this point I turned to Tracey and said, 'You must be so frustrated and angry. I know I would be if I were you.' I held my breath, hoping that this statement would connect with Tracey. She nodded and looked at me; some of her anger was dissipating. I continued, 'Sometimes it's hard for us to know exactly when to take over and when to let mothers care for their own babies.'

I really didn't expect her to have much sympathy for the plight of the nurses, but fortunately I had struck a chord with Tracey. She responded by saying, 'Right now, I do need for you to take over and care for my baby. I can't bear the thought that he would get a drip because I am unable to feed him.' With this statement I began to understand what this mother was going through.

Eventually, Tracey's baby settled and I managed to put him to bed and get him off to sleep. Tracey also prepared to settle for the night. She was lying down in the bed next to her baby's cot as I prepared to leave the nursery. As I began to exit, she called me over and whispered, 'Thank you.' Even though I now had what seemed like a hundred other chores to complete, I knew I had spent my time wisely. I looked at my watch. Twenty minutes was all that it had taken to turn these events around. I had taken the time to become involved in what might have been a most unfortunate situation. I had taken the time to understand. I felt satisfied.

Situations like this are demanding of nurses. They must contain their natural instincts to defend themselves, their colleagues and their nursing care. Tracey was distressed because she felt unable to care for her baby. She felt responsible for her baby's deteriorating condition and blamed the nurses for not assuming what she perceived to be *their* responsibility.

When this nurse arrived on the scene, the situation was almost out of control. By involving herself in a non-defensive, concerned manner she was able to make contact with Tracey and begin to see the situation through her eyes. This took effort, energy and time, all of which she knew were well spent in the end. She offered both practical assistance and an understanding ear. Often nurses believe that no time exists to listen to and understand what patients are experiencing. While this is sometimes the case, lack of time can become an easy excuse for not becoming involved in difficult and emotionally draining interactions. The work involved in managing own emotions in this way is referred to as 'emotional labour', and is discussed in Chapter 3.

Practical know-how in relating to patients

The skills that are described throughout this book are designed to enable nurses to develop practical know-how in relating to patients. While it is important for nurses to *know that* it is important to communicate with patients, they also must *know how* to do so. The theory of how to relate serves little purpose in the absence of interpersonal skills that promote therapeutic relationships. The skills are techniques that will enable the development of the type of relationships that have been described in this chapter as helpful and caring.

The techniques are presented in a 'micro-skills' manner, meaning they are broken down into component parts. Learning the techniques is supported by experiential activities interspersed throughout the text. This style of presentation has been influenced by writers in the counselling field, such as Egan (2007) and Ivey and Ivey (2003). Describing skills in this way runs the risk of it appearing that they can be applied mechanistically. However, the skills cannot be used in such a prescriptive manner.

There are no context-free rules about interacting with patients. Nurses must consider a host of variables when they make contact with patients. Sometimes, a discussion about feelings is suitable to the context, while at other times such discussions are inappropriate. Throughout this book, guidelines and theory about how to establish interpersonal contact with patients are presented. However, each interaction, like each patient and each nurse, will be unique and dynamic in its own right.

CHAPTER SUMMARY

Taking the time and expending the effort to understand the world as the patient experiences it results in nursing care that integrates the patient's experiences. The most effective way to review the material that has been presented in this chapter is through the following story, which illustrates the art and science of nursing relationships. It is told by an experienced nurse:

I was in my second undergraduate year at university when I met Margaret. We met during my clinical placement at a large public healthcare facility that was established to provide rehabilitation services for people who were disabled and/or chronically ill. There were over a thousand patients in this facility and the sheer mass of this humanity hit me like a tonne of bricks on the first day. We were taken on a grand tour of the entire facility on that day and told that the average age of the residents was 72. It was 'so young', we were told, because there were a few patients in their thirties and forties who were suffering from progressive conditions such as multiple sclerosis. To me the place looked like an enormous nursing home.

Although I had an overview of all patients who lived in this facility, I only came to recognise the 50 who resided in the ward to which I was assigned, and one of these patients became well known to me. Margaret caught my attention on that first day I was on the ward. She was a frail looking lady who sat in a wheelchair the entire day, being transported from bed to dining table and back to bed at various times during the day. Margaret captured my attention because she kept repeating the same phrase over and over again. 'Why am I being chastised?' she kept saying. The word 'chastise' struck me as quaint and curious, as if it was a relic from a bygone era. I had to look in a dictionary to find its meaning. Once I discovered the meaning of the word, I became intrigued by Margaret's thought that she was being punished. 'Punished for what?' I thought. What is making Margaret feel she is being punished? I thought to myself that being a permanent resident of this facility could be perceived as punishment, but there was more than this in Margaret's experience.

I set out to learn more about Margaret. It did not take long for me to get to know her. The fact that I was willing to sit with her and listen to her was sufficient to establish a rapport. During the 2 days a week that I spent on the ward, I sat next to her and listened, mostly to her thoughts about being punished. For what, I still did not know. I accepted her feelings, although in the back of my mind there were nagging thoughts about the reason for them.

Whenever we talked, I could not get past her expression of the feeling that she was being chastised, so I went to the records to learn more about Margaret. There I saw the words 'legally blind' and 'nearly deaf'. I began to wonder how much sensory input Margaret was receiving and how much this was contributing to her feelings. I located material in my textbooks that described the possible effects of reduced sensory input (in Margaret's case, near blindness and near deafness). I learnt that one of these effects is suspicious feelings.

I also discussed Margaret with the regular staff working in this ward. They told me that Margaret was a 'bit crazy' and definitely 'paranoid'. Because I thought there was more to Margaret than her suspicion, labelling her as paranoid did not satisfy me. Although the label of 'paranoid' seemed insufficient to me, I could see how easily such a label could dismiss Margaret's reality. I still wanted to learn more about Margaret and only she could help me to do so. Week after week I came to Margaret, sat next to her, expressed my interest in her and then just listened.

Eventually, Margaret began to share with me more than just her feelings of being punished. We talked about her family and discussed other things. I learnt more about Margaret, beyond her paranoia. I think me just being there, showing interest in her and listening to her was enough to enable her to open up and share her thoughts. As I listened to Margaret's story, I began to piece together bits of what she said.

She mentioned that when she entered this facility her handbag had been taken away and put into a room somewhere. She often spoke of the handbag and the room where it was held. I began to realise that the handbag was significant. I asked, 'What's in the handbag?' She told me it contained a card that had her nephew's address written on it. Her nephew, who lived in the next state, was her only living relative. Margaret's husband had died and so had all of her brothers and sisters. She had no children. Her nephew was her only link with her family and she didn't have his address! Margaret wanted desperately to write to this nephew but could not.

Through my perseverance and with the aid of my clinical instructor, I located the room that held Margaret's possessions. They had been taken from her when she was admitted and placed for 'safe keeping' in this room. Fortunately, I was able to retrieve the handbag and, sure enough, inside was a card from her nephew that was sent to her shortly before Margaret entered this facility. Margaret was ecstatic about the find. With it came the possibility of re-establishing contact with her family. I penned Margaret's words to her nephew and made sure the letter was posted to him. Margaret seemed to settle after this, although she continued to complain about being punished and I continued to wonder why this feeling persisted.

While the contact with her nephew had helped to calm Margaret, she remained quite anxious about being in this facility. So I kept listening. One day she mentioned that sitting near the window hurt her eyes. Her diminishing eyesight was the result of cataracts and the bright summer sun through the window created discomfort for her. Each day after lunch she was wheeled to the window to 'enjoy the sunshine'. But instead of enjoying this afternoon ritual, Margaret found the experience quite uncomfortable. Could this be perceived by Margaret as punishment? I explored my hunch with Margaret, directing my questions towards the subject of her daily seating near the window. She confirmed my hunch. In Margaret's mind, the afternoon ritual of being placed in the sun was equivalent to a daily punishment. For what reason, she was not certain. But in her mind she thought it was because she had done something wrong and this was punishment for the transgression. With this revelation came my understanding of Margaret's reality. Her feelings of being punished made more sense to me.

My next plan of action was to try to get the other staff on the ward to appreciate Margaret's experience. I spoke with the nursing staff and they realised what was happening to Margaret. They agreed that placing her in direct contact with the sunshine was counterproductive to what was intended by the move. Even placing her near the sun but not in its direct flow would help her. No longer would Margaret be placed in the direct sunlight.

When it came close to the time that I would be leaving this placement, I could hardly contain my feelings of sadness. Saying goodbye to Margaret was going to be difficult for me. When the time finally came to do so, Margaret reached into her 'newly found' handbag, pulled out an embroidered handkerchief and placed it in my hand. 'Here,' she said, 'this is for you.' In the back of my mind I recalled the warnings I had heard about accepting gifts from patients. I ignored the warnings, placed the handkerchief in the pocket of my uniform and thanked Margaret. We had shared a special understanding and the handkerchief became a symbol of this understanding. I cherished this gift because it served as a reminder of the importance of being interested in patients, listening to and accepting their reality and, most importantly, understanding their experiences.

The nurse in this story demonstrated concern and compassion for Margaret. In addition, she came to know Margaret as a case, a patient and a person. She used understanding that generated from case knowledge when she connected Margaret's feelings with her sensory deprivation through loss of vision. She had learned in her studies that derogatory labels such as 'paranoid' could lead to nurses rejecting and ignoring patients. This is an example of patient knowledge because Margaret's behaviour is viewed in the social context of healthcare organisations. She came also to know the person who was Margaret. Through understanding that contact with her family mattered to Margaret, this nurse came to know something of Margaret's life value system.

Her relationship with Margaret enabled this nurse to feel the sadness that Margaret was experiencing in relation to the loss of contact with her family. She also felt empathic understanding of Margaret's feeling of being punished. She then went one step further and functioned, with the aid of her clinical supervisor, as a useful resource for Margaret in locating her family contact details.

In this final sense they both functioned as advocates for Margaret by working through an organisational system that disabled Margaret from contacting her relatives. Although still a student, this nurse functioned with professional autonomy and responsibility because she had come to know the person who is the patient. And she made a difference as a result.

REFERENCES

Aiken LH, Clarke SP, Sloane DM, Sochalski J 2002 Hospital nurse staffing and patient mortality, nurse burnout, and job dissatisfaction. Journal of the American Medical Association 288(16):1987–1993

Appleton C 1993 The art of nursing: the experience of patients and nurses. Journal of Advanced Nursing 18:892–899

Armstrong D 1983 The fabrication of the nurse–patient relationship. Social Science and Medicine 17:457–460

Arthur D, Pang S, Wong T, Alexander MF, Drury J, Eastwood I et al 1999 Caring attributes, professional self concept and technological influences in a sample of registered nurses in eleven countries. International Journal of Nursing Studies 36:387–396

Australian Nursing and Midwifery Council (ANMC) 2002 Code of Ethics for Nurses in Australia, ANMC, Canberra

Australian Nursing and Midwifery Council (ANMC) 2003 Code of Professional Conduct for Nurses in Australia, ANMC, Canberra

Australian Nursing and Midwifery Council (ANMC) 2005 National Competency Standards for the Registered Nurse, ANMC, Canberra

Baldursdottir G, Jonsdottir H 2002 The importance of nurse caring behaviors as perceived by patients receiving care at an emergency department. Heart and Lung 31:67–75

Barthow C 1997 Negotiating realistic and mutually sustaining nurse–patient relationships in palliative care. International Journal of Nursing Practice 3:206–210

Benner P 1984 From novice to expert: excellence and power in clinical nursing practice. Addison-Wesley, Menlo Park, CA

Benner P, Tanner C, Chesla C 1992 From beginner to expert: gaining a differentiated clinical world in critical care nursing. Advances in Nursing Science 14(3):13–28

Benner P, Wrubel J 1989 The primacy of caring: stress and coping in health and illness. Addison-Wesley, Menlo Park, CA

Bidmead C, Cowley S 2005 A concept analysis of partnerships with clients. Community Practitioner 78(6):203–208

Bishop AH, Scudder JR 1999 A philosophical interpretation of nursing. Scholarly Inquiry for Nursing Practice: An International Journal 13(1):17–27

Brilowski GA, Wendler MC 2005 An evolutionary concept analysis of caring. Journal of Advanced Nursing 50:641–650

Carper BA 1978 Fundamental patterns of knowing in nursing. Advances in Nursing Science 1(1):13–23

Carroll SM 2004 Nonvocal ventilated patients' perceptions of being understood. Western Journal of Nursing Research 26(1):85–103

Chang T, Lin Y-P, Change H-J, Lin C-C 2005 Cancer patient and staff ratings of caring behaviors. Cancer Nursing 28(5):331–339

Cheung J 1998 Caring as the ontological and epistemological foundations of nursing: a view of caring from the perspectives of Australian nurses. International Journal of Nursing Practice 4:225–233

Coffey S 2006 The nurse–patient relationship in cancer care as a shared covenant: a concept analysis. Advances in Nursing Science 29(4):308–323

Duffy JR, Hoskins L, Seiferty RF 2007 Dimensions of caring: psychometric evaluation of the Caring Assessment Tool. Advances in Nursing Science 30(3):235–245

Dunlop M 1986 Is a science of caring possible? Journal of Advanced Nursing 11:661–670

Egan G 2007 The skilled helper, 8th edn. Brooks/Cole/Thomas Learning, Boston, MA

Eriksson K 2002 Caring science in a new key. Nursing Science Quarterly 15(1):61–65

Florin J, Ehrenberg A, Ehnfors M 2006 Patient participation in clinical decision-making in nursing: a comparative study of nurses' and patients' perceptions. Journal of Clinical Nursing 15:1498–1508

Fosbinder D 1994 Patient perceptions of nursing care: an emerging theory of interpersonal competence. Journal of Advanced Nursing 20:1085–1093

Gadow S 1980 Existential advocacy: philosophical foundation of nursing. In: Spiker SF, Gadow S (eds), Nursing: images and ideals, pp. 79–101. Springer, New York

Gallant MH, Beaulieu MC, Carnevale FA 2002 Partnership: an analysis of the concept within the nurse–client relationship. Journal of Advanced Nursing 40:149–157

Hanson MD 2004 Using data from critical care nurses to validate Swanson's phenomenological derived middle range caring theory. Journal of Theory Construction and Testing 8(1):21–25

Hegedus KS 1999 Providers' and consumers' perspectives of nurses' caring behaviours. Journal of Advanced Nursing 30:1090–1096

Henderson S 1997 Knowing the patient and the impact on patient participation: a grounded theory study. International Journal of Nursing Practice 3:111–118

Ivey A, Ivey M 2003 Intentional interviewing and counselling, 5th edn. Brooks/Cole, Pacific Grove, CA

Jenks JM 1993 The pattern of personal knowing in nurses' clinical decision-making. Journal of Nursing Education 32(9):399–415

Jenny J, Logan J 1992 Knowing the patient: one aspect of clinical knowledge. Image: Journal of Nursing Scholarship 24(4):254–258

Jonsdottir H, Litchfield M, Dexheimer M 2004 The relational course of nursing practice as partnership. Journal of Advanced Nursing 47:241–250

Kyle TV 1995 The concept of caring: a review of the literature. Journal of Advanced Nursing 21:506–514

Larson PJ 1986 Cancer nurses' perceptions of caring. Cancer Nursing 9(2):86–91

Leininger M (ed.) 1984 Care: the essence of nursing and health. Charles B Slack, Thorofare, NJ

Liaschenko J 1997 Knowing the patient? In Thorne SE, Hayes VE (eds) Nursing praxis: knowledge and action, pp. 23–38. Sage, Thousand Oaks, CA

Liaschenko J, Fisher A 1999 Theorizing the knowledge that nurses use in the conduct of their work. Scholarly Inquiry for Nursing Practice: An International Journal 13(1):29–41

Luker KA, Austin L, Caress A, Hallett CE 2000 The importance of 'knowing the patient': community nurses' constructions of quality in providing palliative care. Journal of Advanced Nursing 31:775–782

McCabe C 2004 Nurse–patient communication: an exploration of patients' experiences. Journal of Clinical Nursing 13:41–49

Mackintosh C 2000 Is there a place for 'care' in nursing? International Journal of Nursing Studies 37:321–327

May C 1992a Individual care? Power and subjectivity in therapeutic relationships. Sociology 26(4):589–602

May C 1992b Nursing work, nurses' knowledge, and the subjectification of the patient. Sociology of Health and Illness 14(4):472–487

May C 1993 Subjectivity and culpability in the constitution of nurse–patient relationships. International Journal of Nursing Studies 30(2):181–192

McKenna G 1993 Caring is the essence of nursing practice. British Journal of Nursing 2(1):72–76

McNaughton DB 2005 A naturalistic test of Peplau's theory in home visiting. Public Health Nursing 22(5):429–438

Menzies I 1961 A case study of the functioning of social systems as a defence against anxiety. Human Relations 13(2):95–123

Mok E, Chui PC 2004 Nurse–patient relationships in palliative care. Journal of Advanced Nursing 48:475–483

Morse JM, Solberg SM, Neaner WL, Bottoroff JL, Johnson JL 1990 Concepts of caring and caring as a concept. Advances in Nursing Science 13:1–14

Newman M 2002 The pattern that connects. Advances in Nursing Science 24(3):1–7

Nightingale F 1859 Notes on nursing: what it is and what it is not. Reprinted 1992, Lippincott, Philadelphia, PA, originally published by Harrison & Son, London

Parsons T 1951/1987 Illness and the role of the physicians: a sociological perspective. In: Stoeckle JD (ed.), Encounters between patients and doctors: an anthology, pp 147–56. MIT Press, Cambridge, MA

Peplau H 1952/1988 Interpersonal relations in nursing. Macmillan, London, originally published by GP Putnam and Sons

Porter S 1994 New nursing: the road to freedom? Journal of Advanced Nursing 20:269–274

Radwin LE 1995 'Knowing the patient': a review of research on an emerging concept. Journal of Advanced Nursing 23:1142–1146

Ramos MC 1992 The nurse–patient relationship: theme and variations. Journal of Advanced Nursing 17:496–506

Reynolds WJ, Scott B 1999 Empathy: a crucial component of the helping relationship. Journal of Psychiatric and Mental Health Nursing 6:363–370

Rieman DJ 1986 Noncaring and caring in the clinical setting: patients' descriptions. Topics in Clinical Nursing 8(2):30–36

Roach SM 1985 A foundation for nursing ethics. In Carmi A, Schneider S (eds) Nursing law and ethics, pp 170–7. Springer-Verlag, Berlin

Sahlsten MJM, Larsson IE, Sjöström B, Lindencrona CSC, Plos KAE 2007 Patient participation in nursing care: towards a concept clarification from a nurse perspective. Journal of Clinical Nursing 16:630–637

Salvage J 1990 The theory and practice of the 'new nursing'. Nursing Times 86(4):42–45

Shattell M 2004 Nurse–patient interaction: a review of the literature. Journal of Clinical Nursing 13:714–722

Smith M 2004 Review of research related to Watson's theory of caring. Nursing Science Quarterly 17(1):13–25

Sourial S 1997 An analysis of caring. Journal of Advanced Nursing 26:1189–1192

Speed S, Luker KA 2004 Changes in patterns of knowing the patient: the case of British district nurses. International Journal of Nursing Studies 41:921–931

Stockman C 2005 A literature review of the progress of the psychiatric nurse patient relationship as described by Peplau. Issues in Mental Health Nursing 26:911–919

Swanson K 1993 Nursing as informed caring for the well-being of others. Image: Journal of Nursing Scholarship 25:352–357

Swanson K 1999 What is known about caring in nursing science: a literary analysis. In: Hinshaw AS, Feetham SL, Shaver JL Handbook of clinical nursing research, pp 31–60. Sage, Thousand Oaks, CA

Tanner C, Benner P, Chesla C, Gordon DR 1993 The phenomenology of knowing the patient. Image: Journal of Nursing Scholarship 25(4):273–280

Tarlier DS 2004 Beyond caring: the moral and ethical basis of responsive nurse–patient relationship. Nursing Philosophy 5:230–241

Travelbee J 1971 Interpersonal aspects of nursing, 2nd edn. FA Davis, Philadelphia, PA

Watson J 1985 Nursing, human science and human care: a theory of nursing. Appleton-Century-Crofts, East Norwark, CT

Watson J 1999 Postmodern nursing and beyond. Churchill Livingstone, Edinburgh

Webb C, Hope K 1995 What kind of nurses do patients want? Journal of Clinical Nursing 4:101–108

Wilkin K, Slevin E 2004 The meaning of caring to nurses: an investigation into the nature of caring work in an intensive care unit. Journal of Clinical Nursing 13:50–59

Williams AM, Iruita VF 2004 Therapeutic and non-therapeutic interpersonal interactions: the patient's perspective. Journal of Clinical Nursing 13:806–815

Wiman E, Wikblad K 2004 Caring and uncaring encounters in nursing in an emergency department. Journal of Clinical Nursing 13(4):422–429

Wolf ZR, Miller P, Devine M 2003 Relationship between nurse caring and patient satisfaction in patients undergoing invasive cardiac procedures. Medsurg Nursing 12(6):391–396

CHAPTER 2

The patient–nurse relationship

INTRODUCTION

The skills described in the following chapters offer nurses a range of alternatives when interacting with patients. The skills of listening, understanding and exploring are not ends in themselves, but useful ways to establish and build relationships between patients and nurses. Using such skills effectively increases the possibility that patients and nurses will connect and relate in meaningful ways. These skills enable nurses to understand patients' experiences. Operating from within patients' experiences enhances the possibility that nursing interventions will be individualised and context-specific, as opposed to mechanical, procedural or task-oriented.

Technical proficiency in skill use holds no guarantee that skills will be used in ways that are beneficial to patients. A view that skills can be used merely as techniques applied in a rational, objective manner loses an essential element—that the skills only make sense when viewed within the subjective reality of a relationship between two human beings: nurse and patient. When viewed as techniques, devoid of the subjective experience of the relationship, interpersonal skills lose their most crucial quality—that they are relational and interactional.

General guidelines for the appropriate utilisation of each skill are presented in the following chapters, but these guidelines may not provide enough direction for nurses as they try to determine which skill is most fitting under a given set of circumstances. This is because the 'best' approach can be determined only within the context of the relationship between patient and nurse. No single response is ever correct in itself; no magical formula can be applied out of this context.

Nurses' personal styles; personality factors of both patient and nurse; the patient's immediate situation and their perception of it; how patients are responding to nurses; and how nurses are responding to patients—these are but a few of the contextual variables that need to be considered when determining

25

the 'best' way to respond helpfully to patients. It is through direct involvement in the relationship, 'being there', that nurses can develop appropriate responses. There is no available blueprint for skill use.

Chapter overview

This chapter addresses the whole of the relationship between patient and nurse so that skills can be placed within this context. It begins with a discussion of the distinction between helping, counselling and psychotherapy, as all are relevant to nursing practice, depending on clinical context. Next are the characteristics of the helpful relationship between nurse and patient, focusing on mutual understanding and collaboration as essential features. Then specific aspects of the relationship are reviewed, including social versus professional relationships, interpersonal distance versus involvement, therapeutic superficiality versus intimacy, and mutuality and reciprocity. The various types of relationships that may develop are reviewed and the focus of skill use in each type of relationship is explored. The final section of this chapter traces how relationships progress from beginning to end by highlighting critical issues at each stage of relationship development.

HELPING RELATIONSHIPS IN NURSING CONTEXTS

The therapeutic nature of the relationship between nurse and patient was presented in Chapter 1 as being useful to the patient. In this regard, the process of patient–nurse relationship can be considered to be that of *helping*. In nursing contexts, helping means that nurses come to know patients in order to provide knowledgeable assistance and direct aid, as well as interpersonal support and comfort (see Ch 8).

Helping is something that people do everyday for other people. In everyday life, friends sometimes do not have the knowledge and skill to help: nurses are expected to be knowledgeable and skilful in helping.

Helping is a term that is used interchangeably with counselling and psychotherapy. As a result, the distinction between these three processes— *helping, counselling* and *therapy*—is often blurred. The nursing literature uses all three terms, referring to the helping relationship and process, the counselling role of the nurse and the therapeutic patient–nurse relationship. No one description clearly captures the essence of the purpose of patient–nurse relationships because nurses relate to people in a variety of life situations—from people facing life crises, to those in need of standard and routine healthcare, to those whose behaviour is deemed to be abnormal. Thus, the processes of helping, counselling and therapy all fit the nursing context, with no singular process providing clear direction for patient–nurse relationships in general.

Helping is the term preferred by Benner (1984), who states that the term *therapeutic* has inherited meaning from the psychoanalytic therapy perspective (a theory of psychotherapy) in which the therapist purposefully distances self. In addition, the term therapeutic implies that something must be fixed and this is not always the case, as sometimes just connecting interpersonally with a patient is all that is required to be helpful. Because of its association with therapy, the term therapeutic is often replaced in the nursing literature with the terms helping and counselling. However, in the clinical specialty of mental health nursing, the term therapeutic is the most fitting, because processes based on psychotherapy clearly fit this clinical context.

Regardless of whether a nurse is helping, counselling or conducting psychotherapy, there are characteristics of the relationship that are common. These characteristics are referred to as helpful, but could as easily be called therapeutic.

CHARACTERISTICS OF HELPFUL PATIENT–NURSE RELATIONSHIPS

No single definition could possibly capture the rich and complex nature of the relationships between patients and nurses. Each relationship is distinct, because both patient and nurse are distinctive and the way they interact and relate is unique. Each participant brings particular experiences to the relationship.

Rather than imposing artificial limits by specifying a definition of the relationship, various facets of the patient–nurse relationship are described here. The facets include the characteristics of social versus professional relationships, interpersonal distance versus involvement, therapeutic superficiality versus intimacy, and mutuality and reciprocity.

Social versus professional relationships

When the suggestion is made to beginning nurses that they are 'to be professional' in their relationships with patients, they sometimes state a preference 'to be friends' with patients. In saying this, these nurses could be revealing a desire to remain in the comfortable and familiar arena of social relationships, where the rules for relating are predictable. It may also be that an emphasis on problem solving and goal setting (two processes often considered to be 'professional') contributes to the preference for 'being friends'. A common distinction made between the social relationships of friendship and professional relationships is that the professional relationship is goal-directed. Fears of 'not knowing what to do' and anxieties about 'how can I help to solve patients' problems?', especially when such problems seem overwhelming, are logical responses to being asked to form professional relationships with patients.

The most likely reason for the expressed desire 'to be friends' with patients, as contrasted to being professional, probably emanates from a preconceived notion that 'to be professional' is to be distant, detached, aloof and cool. This aura of the professional stance, that of the detached observer who also has the answers, involves expectations that these nurses may be unwilling to accept. Being professional is sometimes equated with denying or abandoning the personal, human side of the nurse. These beginning nurses could be saying, 'How can I leave myself behind when I interact with patients?'

Nurses do not, and cannot, leave themselves behind when they enter the healthcare setting, but neither are they there to be friends with patients, in the strictest sense of the word. This is not to say that nurses cannot be friendly, sociable and personable with patients, or that professional relationships do not have similarities with social relationships. Nevertheless, professional relationships are different from other types of personal relationships, such as friendship.

Some of the ways that social relationships differ from professional relationships include the following: the nurse usually initiates the professional relationship with patients; there are time and space limits to professional relationships, in that they do not go on for life; and interactions are confined to a particular setting, be it a hospital setting or a patient's home. The final, and perhaps the most significant, difference is that patient–nurse relationships are formed with a focus on the needs of one of the participants only—the patient. Nurses are expected to meet their own needs for social contact, inclusion and affection outside of their relationships with patients. This is not to say that these needs might not be met through relationships with patients, but more to emphasise that the relationships are not used as the primary source of nurses' social-need fulfilment.

Differences in focus, intensity and perspective

Gadow (1980) offers a useful analysis in differentiating personal and professional relationships by describing these differences in terms of focus, intensity and perspective.

In professional relationships, the nurse's focus of concern is away from self and towards the other—the patient. Emotions are expressed and genuine feelings of distress for the patient's situation are felt (as in social relationships), but these emotions are not expressed by nurses for the purpose of obtaining relief or attention from patients. Nurses' concern and interest remain for the patient. There is no expectation that the patient is mutually concerned about the nurse, as would be the case if nurse and patient were friends involved in a personal relationship. In friendships, there is equal concern; for the professional, concern is one-sided (Gadow 1980).

In addition, the intensity of the situation is experienced differently in personal and professional relationships. In professional relationships, nurses may become emotionally aroused, and feel the patient's concern, distress, or sense of urgency. Therefore, nurses may experience emotional intensity along with the patient in a given situation, but in a reflective manner rather than the immediate way that patients experience the intensity of their situations (Gadow 1980). The reflective nature of nurses' experience of the intensity of a situation means that nurses use their experience of patients' distress as a way of considering what would be of help to patients. Nurses integrate this experience with their knowledge of how to be of help. Helping to alleviate patients' distress is *why* nurses share and experience patients' distress. In personal relationships, more value is placed on sharing experiences than helping (Gadow 1980). Professional relationships are experienced by nurses as more purposeful than friendships (Ramos 1992).

The final difference in Gadow's analysis is that of perspective. The professional maintains an objectivity that is impossible for friends to sustain. While objectivity does not equate with distance and lack of connection with the patient, it does relate to the one-sided nature or focus of these relationships. That is, in professional relationships, nurses remain focused on patients rather than on their own subjective experiences. This is not to say that nurses should disregard their own subjective experiences, but rather the significance of these experiences is placed in the context of how it affects the patient and the relationship.

Gadow's emphasis of shifting motivation from the self (i.e. the nurse) to the other (i.e. the patient) is consistent with the findings of a study into clinicians of various professional groups who are known to be capable of forming compassionate relationships with patients (Graber & Mitcham 2004). These clinicians described levels of interpersonal involvement, from superficial to intimate, on the basis of the degree to which they shifted focus and concern from themselves to the patient. Increasing focus of concern for the other, with decreasing concern for the self, was associated with greater levels of involvement and intimacy. This capacity to shift focus from the self, putting the interest of the other ahead of one's own, is considered a central aspect in caring relationships (Tarlier 2004, Noddings 1984).

It is not the level of personal involvement that differentiates friendship from professional relationships, but the form and direction of the involvement. The amount of personal involvement in the two types of relationship may be equal. Both types of relationship rely on active demonstration of personal qualities, so the notion that nurses' professional relationships are devoid of their personal selves is rejected. In fact, nurses rely on their personal qualities and style of relating.

This idea challenges the notion that to be professional is to maintain a distanced stance in which nurses share little of their personal selves. By sharing themselves, nurses share their humanity with patients. Experienced clinicians (Graber & Mitcham 2004, Benner 1984) do judge the 'correct' level of engagement with each patient, because not all relationships will reach the same degree of personal involvement. This brings forward the next facet of patient–nurse relationships: interpersonal distance versus involvement.

Interpersonal distance versus involvement

The very fact that a relationship exists between patient and nurse implies a degree of interpersonal involvement, which includes the process of 'knowing the patient' (Mok & Chui 2004). Yet nurses are often warned of the dangers of becoming emotionally 'involved' with patients. The warning is based on the notion that a 'professional' demeanour requires emotional detachment in order to maintain objectivity in decision making.

The reasons usually given for warnings about involvement are brought into question by Benner's (1984) research into expert clinical nursing practice. The experts in this study involved themselves with patients by identifying with them and imagining that they or someone they loved was in a similar predicament (Benner 1984 p 209). Identification invokes involvement in the situation, not as a passive observer but as an active participant. Through identifying with patients, nurses involve themselves in a personal way in patients' experiences. This involvement, of being close to the heart of the situation, enables nurses to notice what is significant and to notice subtle changes in patients. Rather than hampering nurses' clinical judgment, involvement enhances it.

In addition to the need for objective decision making, nurses are also advised of the dangers of involvement with patients because it is perceived that such involvement will result in an emotional draining, leaving nurses unable to cope with the sometimes harsh reality of nursing. Nurses may believe that they can protect themselves from hurt, from the emotional aspects of illness, from depletion of their own internal resources, through distancing strategies that remove them from the situation emotionally and numb them from the reality of pain and suffering. Interpersonal distancing and lack of involvement has been shown to be a defensive strategy used by nurses in an effort to cope with the distress of nursing (Jourard 1964, Menzies 1961).

When the defensive strategy is removed and efforts to relate are made, nurses do need to be capable of managing their emotional responses to patients' vulnerability and suffering. In remaining focused on the patient, they cannot allow their own emotional responses to dominate a clinical situation. Such management, termed 'emotional' labour, is starting to be recognised as an aspect of nursing work (Smith 1992), and is reviewed in Chapter 3, 'Nurse as therapeutic agent'.

Interestingly, the expert nurses in Benner's study did *not* become drained or depleted by their involvement with patients, but they also had the experience of feeling affirmed and stronger for it (Benner 1984). This is consistent with the clinicians in Graber and Mitcham's (2004) investigation in that interpersonal involvement with patients sustained and supported these clinicians, and also helped with treatment efforts. Committed and involved patient–nurse relationships enabled nurses in Coffey's study (2006) to feel professional satisfaction, while patients reported feeling confident and secure as a consequence. Both nurses and patients agreed that the relationship had a positive effect on their physical treatment.

The expert nurses in these studies (Coffey 2006, Benner 1984) did know how to retain a sense of their 'otherness' that kept their focus on patient needs, but not at the expense of their own welfare. Likewise, nurses in Henderson's study (2001) were able to describe the need for determining the right level of emotional engagement and detachment in their relationships with patients. These nurses have come to terms with what has been referred to as the 'paradox of helping' (Brammer 1988 p 47). They were able to be involved enough to participate— emotionally, spiritually and intellectually—in their relationships with patients, yet remained distanced enough to maintain control and use their involvement to assist patients. In doing so, they set appropriate boundaries in their professional relationships with patients.

Professional boundaries

There are various types of boundaries in nursing practice that provide a safe space in which nurses can function. First, there are legal boundaries, which specify the scope of nursing practice. For example, unless authorised to do so as a nurse practitioner, prescribing medications is outside the scope of most nursing practice. In addition, there are ethical boundaries of nursing practice that are specified in codes of practice (ANMC 2003). The boundaries that pertain to interpersonal relationships between nurses and patients are not as easily codified as these other types of boundaries. Nonetheless, they are important to understand and consider when forming relationships with patients.

The boundaries that surround the patient–nurse relationship cannot be rule-governed at all times, as their negotiation requires professional judgment. For example, a nurse may choose to disclose a personal experience in the interest of offering the patient hope or reassurance. The judgments are made on the basis of the guiding principle for the establishment of the relationship—to be of benefit to the patient. Therefore, the standard by which actions should be judged is whether they are in the 'best interest of the patient' (Peternelj-Taylor & Younge 2003). Actions that are obviously harmful to the patient, such as having sexual relationships with nurses while in their care, are clear boundary violations. Actions such as this are considered exploitative because the nurse is satisfying personal needs through the relationship. Boundary violations can carry professional repercussions such as loss of nursing registration.

Boundary crossings, unlike boundary violations, are more difficult to judge (Peternelj-Taylor & Younge 2003, Sheets 2000). There are subtle ways in which nurses may not act in the best interest of the patient. For example, nurses may disclose their own personal problems to patients in an effort to unburden their own anxieties. Complaining about work conditions to patients can be a boundary crossing if done for the purpose of sparking patient sympathy for nurses' overwork. That is, the motivation is not on the patient but rather on meeting the nurse's need; when this happens there is a risk of overinvolvement.

Overinvolvement

When nurses are overinvolved, they can no longer retain a sense of 'otherness' that enables them to maintain a sense of control. Overinvolved relationships become close personal friendships in which the nurse relinquishes the professional role and the patient relinquishes the patient role (Morse 1991). The nurse functions as omnipotent rescuer and leaps in and takes over, assuming the patient's burdens and problems, and failing to perceive the resourcefulness of the patient (Benner & Wrubel 1989). In overinvolved relationships, nurses overextend themselves—often to their own personal and professional detriment (Morse 1991). When nurses sacrifice some professional control for the bonds of friendship, they feel less satisfied and less helpful to the patient (Ramos 1992).

It is important for nurses to recognise when they are at risk of overinvolving themselves with patients. Nurses are at risk of overinvolvement when they believe they are the only ones who can help a patient, when they try to rescue patients, when they cannot imagine a relationship with a patient ending, and when they feel overextended or overwhelmed by a relationship with a patient.

If overinvolvement does occur, it is equally important to reflect on the situation and learn from the experience, as do most nurses (Morse 1991). Talking it over with a trusted colleague (see Ch 11) not only provides support, but also enhances and accelerates learning from the experience.

It does happen that patients and nurses develop into lifelong friends even though their initial meeting was not purely social in nature. However, if this becomes an everyday occurrence in a nurse's life, it does signal a need for self-reflection (see Ch 3). It could indicate that the nurse is unable to focus energy on patients. Nurses who 'make friends' with the majority of patients they meet may be treating their own needs as more important than their patients' needs.

There is an art to knowing what can be offered without an overextension of personal resources. Through reflective practice, nurses learn how to offer what they can without dictating results and with a clear recognition that they are not the only ones who contribute to patients' wellbeing (Benner & Wrubel 1989 p 376). The key to avoiding overinvolved relationships is not to avoid involvement altogether, but rather to find the right kind of involvement (Benner & Wrubel 1989). The degree of involvement varies with the type of relationship that is formed between nurses and patients, and these types of relationship are covered later in this chapter.

Issues of social versus professional relationships and distance versus involvement help in bringing forward the next facet of patient–nurse relationships: therapeutic superficiality versus intimacy.

Therapeutic superficiality versus intimacy

All relationships between patient and nurse begin at a level of superficiality. Relationships at this level are characterised by minimal self-disclosure and focus primarily on 'safe' (non-personal) content areas because there is minimal knowledge and understanding of each other, and trust has yet to be established (Coad-Chapman 1986). Social exchanges and chit-chat are common at this level.

It is important for nurses to recognise the value of such interactions, believing that they are not really benefiting patients during these interchanges (remember the focus on task-oriented 'doing'). Because deep and meaningful interaction is not occurring, they fail to perceive the relevance of these superficial exchanges. Social interactions are valuable because they are a way for nurses and patients to get to know each other. In fact, patients use social conversation as a way of connecting with nurses and building a relationship (Shattell 2005, Williams & Irurita 2004). Being friendly and informal helps to break down authoritarian barriers sometimes associated with professional roles (Hunt 1991). In addition, patients feel affirmed and uplifted by nurses who are friendly and light-hearted, thus aiding their recovery (Gaenellos 2005).

Therapeutically intimate relationships (Graber & Mitcham 2004, Williams 2001, Kadner 1994, Savage 1992, Coad-Chapman 1986) are characterised by a high degree of mutual involvement, trust and self-disclosure of a personal nature. Patients and nurses feel free to share their thoughts, feelings and perceptions when involved in such a relationship. Topics are of a personal nature, feelings are expressed openly and freely, and both nurse and patient are committed to the relationship.

Some relationships remain at a superficial level, with nurses providing technical care and patients being satisfied with that care (Morse 1991). Ramos (1992) described this level as instrumental, while Graber and Mitcham (2004) term it practical. Whatever term is used, this level of involvement is characterised by the nurse focusing on the task at hand. For example, a patient visiting an outpatient clinic for a routine pap smear would not expect, nor probably desire, any more than a nurse who listened, explained the procedure in understandable language, and provided privacy and comfort during the procedure. Therapeutic intimacy is not warranted.

Other relationships develop beyond this level and become profoundly moving experiences for both patient and nurse. For example, a situation in which a nurse connects with and enables a patient to face dying with dignity, meaning, peace and comfort involves a deeply meaningful, often intimate, relationship between them.

The main differentiation between the two types of relationships is the content of the interactions, and the level of trust and self-disclosure. At a superficial level, very little is known beyond the formal roles of patient and nurse. At the intimate level of involvement, the formalised roles fade into the background and patient and nurse become known to each other as unique beings. There is a feeling of unity with the patient (Graber & Mitcham 2004).

Therapeutic intimacy in the nursing context is characterised by a high degree of openness and self-disclosure, accompanied by an expectation of acceptance and understanding (Williams 2001, Kadner 1994). The extent of self-disclosure is greater for the patient than the nurse (Kadner 1994, Savage 1992). This is in keeping with the notion that the relationship is formed not for its own purpose but for the aid of the patient. The focus of a therapeutic relationship remains on the patient.

Closely related to the concept of therapeutic intimacy is the concept of trust (Williams 2001). Trust implies a willingness to place oneself in a relationship that may increase vulnerability (Peter & Morgan 2001)—that is, the trusting person takes a risk in self-disclosure on the understanding that the other person will behave in certain ways (Hupcey et al 2001). In the nursing context, patients expect that they can rely on nurses—that is, they have confidence that nurses will be there to help them. Patients expect that nurses will not only care for them with technical competence, but will also care about them as demonstrated by concern and commitment (de Raeve 2002).

An awareness that different levels of interpersonal involvement exist between themselves and patients enables nurses to feel confident in maintaining a relationship at a superficial level and, at times, in choosing to engage in a relationship that progresses to a more intimate level. Descriptions such as 'therapeutic intimacy' imply an expectation that all relationships between nurse and patient should reach this level of involvement, or that nurses should at least attempt to have their relationships with patients reach this level. Not only is such an expectation unrealistic, and often inappropriate, it also fails to acknowledge the central characteristics of mutuality and reciprocity in the relationship.

Mutuality and reciprocity

The level of interpersonal involvement between nurse and patient cannot be mandated. It needs to be mutually agreed upon by both nurse and patient (the negotiation process in which this happens is discussed later in this chapter). There must be freedom to determine how they will relate; their involvement cannot be preordained and outcomes cannot be predetermined because these remain unpredictable at the outset of the relationship. While nurses aim to understand patients' experiences, they also need to appreciate patients' desire for the relationship and felt need to connect with the nurse.

Establishing the right level of involvement is not simply a matter for nurses because relationships are mutual endeavours between patients and nurses. Mutuality is the sharing of commonalities, including mutual goal setting. Each participant, nurse and patient, influences the level of involvement. This is referred to as *mutuality*. Mutuality is the midpoint between nursing care that is determined by the nurse without reference to the patient, and care that is determined by the patient independent of the nurse. The former is paternalistic, while the latter is autonomous (Henson 1997).

Although it is more common for nurses to initiate the relationship, either participant, nurse or patient, may make the initial overtures. The other participant must respond in some way to this initiative. For example, the nurse solicits the patient's participation in the relationship by exploring the patient's experience, and the patient responds by disclosing information. Or, the patient solicits the nurse's help and the nurse responds by providing assistance. This call-and-response exchange is referred to as *reciprocity*.

Reciprocity and mutuality are essential to establishing the human connection needed for a therapeutic patient–nurse relationship (McGilton & Boscart 2007, Mok & Chui 2004, Tarlier 2004, Hagerty & Patusky 2003). Therapeutic reciprocity, the mutual exchange of meaningful thoughts and feelings, involves nurse self-disclosure in an effort to assist the patient (Marck 1990). At times, the mutuality needed to sustain the relationship is not present; in these situations, there is a unilateral relationship.

Mutual versus unilateral relationships

A unilateral relationship is one in which one participant is unwilling or unable to develop the relationship to the level desired by the other participant (Morse 1991 p 456). When patients' conditions warrant a quick response, nurses engage in unilateral decision making without taking time to take patient understanding into account (Ramos 1992 p 502). Nurses may continue their efforts to relate at a deeper level, despite the patients' unwillingness or inability to be engaged in the relationship. Likewise, patients may try to engage a nurse in a relationship even when the nurse is unwilling or unable to make an investment in the relationship (Morse 1991).

When relationships between patients and nurses are mutual, there is a shared sense of responsibility and commitment to maintain the relationship. Mutual relationships between patients and nurses vary in their degree of intensity and involvement, and this raises questions about how and why some relationships remain on a superficial level while others progress to the level of therapeutic intimacy. The process used in determining the level of involvement is one of negotiation between patient and nurse (Ramos 1992, Morse 1991).

The negotiation of mutual relationships

Through negotiation, both nurse and patient make a choice to move the relationship to deeper levels of involvement and commitment. The negotiation is based on patients' and nurses' perceptions of the situation and of each other.

From patients' perspectives, it is the seriousness of the situation (as they perceive it), their feelings of vulnerability (perceived absence of personal resources), and their degree of dependence that affect whether they seek interpersonal connection and involvement with nurses. When patients perceive their situation as serious, rendering them dependent on nurses for care, they are likely to make overtures and efforts to find a nurse whom they feel they can trust, and on whom they can rely. In addition, when patients interpret that the demands of the situation outweigh their perceived capabilities for meeting these demands (i.e. they are vulnerable), they are likely to seek involved relationships with nurses. When patients perceive their situation as minor or routine, that it does not require them to become dependent on the nurses and they feel they can cope, they expect no more than routine, technical nursing care (Morse 1991).

Nurses base their decision about entering into a more than superficial relationship on their evaluation of the patient's needs and available support systems (i.e. their evaluation of the patient's situation). Because this evaluation may be different from the patient's interpretation, the importance of understanding (see Ch 6) is reinforced.

In addition to their evaluation of the patient's situation, nurses also base their choice about becoming involved with a particular patient on whether or not they sense a personality 'click', as well as their estimation of the patient as a person (Fosbinder 1994, Ramos 1992). Nurses choose to become involved with patients who touch or appeal to them on a personal or emotional level (Morse 1991).

As such, there is often a 'perceived fit' between nurses and patients who develop relationships beyond a superficial level (Hagerty & Patusky 2003).

The process of negotiation

Patients seek active connections with nurses by being friendly, likeable, cooperative and an easy patient who does 'not rock the boat' (Shattell 2005, McCabe 2004, Iruita & Williams 2001). Unfortunately, they also express reluctance to do so when nurses seem too busy and patients do not want to bother them (Chang et al 2005, Shattell 2005, McCabe 2004). Nonetheless, patients do want nurses who are friendly and genuinely interested in them as a person, and who are available and willing to interact with them (Shatell 2004).

Patients make connections with nurses by engaging in everyday chit-chat that helps them to get to know each other (Shatell 2005, Williams & Iruita 2004, Hagerty & Patusky 2003). They may ask the nurse personal questions, which are aimed at having the nurse self-disclose. Self-disclosure is associated with trust and patients look for nurses whom they like and on whom they feel they can depend. Likewise, patients determine if the nurse is a 'good person' by looking for indications of kindness, empathy, enjoyment of nursing and nursing competence. They test the nurse's ability to keep a confidence by sharing a minor secret. If a nurse passes the test of dependability and trustworthiness, the patient makes friendly overtures to build the relationship (Morse 1991).

It can be seen from this description of the negotiation process that, although patients may not be able to choose which nurses are assigned to their care, they do have a choice about nurses with whom they become involved. Depending on the healthcare setting, nurses may or may not be able to influence which patients are assigned to their care, but the preceding description of the negotiation process indicates that nurses choose those patients with whom they become involved.

The depth of the relationship is determined by many factors, and nurses who realise which factors are operating in a relationship are in a position to establish appropriate relationships. The goal is not to form as deep a relationship as possible, but rather to create conditions that keep possibilities open. Unaware nurses may inadvertently hinder the development of a relationship or try to deepen relationships under circumstances where this is not warranted.

Dislike between patient and nurse

Just as it is unrealistic for nurses to expect that each relationship with a patient will be deeply meaningful, it is equally unrealistic to expect that they will like every patient with whom they come into contact. The reverse side of the coin of mutually satisfying relationships is revealed whenever nurses and patients are unable to form *any* level of relationship because they dislike each other. This feeling may be unilateral or mutual.

When it is the nurse who feels antipathy towards a patient, there is often a sense of accompanying guilt. Nurses may feel they are remiss in their professional responsibility when they dislike patients. This feeling can be offset by a realisation that nurses' responsibility is to provide adequate care for patients, irrespective of whether they actually like an individual patient. If nurses allow their dislike of a particular patient to interfere with actually caring for that patient, they are failing in their 'duty of care'. More often, however, it is the relationship between the nurse and patient that falters, and not the nursing care that is provided.

It is more than likely that a nurse who senses disaffection towards a patient will either try to ignore it or, worse, blame the patient for the difficulty. Either response has the potential to have a negative effect on the relationship between this patient and this nurse.

Nurses who sense dislike for a particular patient first need to admit the feeling to themselves and learn to accept it as a natural part of being a person. Through self-exploration (see Ch 3), nurses may be able to unravel their reasons for feeling negative about a patient. Even if they are unable to discover why they are reacting this way, nurses who engage in self-reflection are able to separate what may be 'their' problem from what is an aspect of the patient.

Talking to colleagues is another useful way to learn more about these reactions to patients. Most experienced nurses probably have encountered unpleasant feelings towards patients, and those who have may be able to offer valuable insights into how to manage the situation effectively. In seeking such insights, nurses are demonstrating self-awareness and willingness to learn and grow (see Ch 3). In time, it may happen that a nurse develops ways of coping with situations that engender dislike of patients. Unless there is recognition and acknowledgment of the difficulty, such growth is unlikely to occur.

Admitting negative feelings about particular patients to colleagues serves another potentially useful purpose. Usually, there are other nurses working in the same area, with the same patients, who do not react negatively to that particular patient. What rubs against one nurse's grain may roll easily off another nurse. Often an agreement can be reached so that those nurses who do not feel disdain towards a particular patient can care for that patient.

Sometimes, however, all nurses working in a particular locality dislike the *same* patient, often referred as a 'difficult patient' (see Ch 10 for a full discussion). When this happens, it is useful for all nurses caring for this particular patient to discuss the situation with each other in an effort to develop a workable way of relating to that patient. Neither nurses nor patients should be blamed when they do not get along, because of what may be a 'personality clash'. Reflecting on the situation, talking it over with colleagues and developing ways of working with and around the potential problem are the best approaches.

TYPES OF RELATIONSHIPS

Through the process of negotiation, different types of patient–nurse relationships are developed and are characterised by their level of involvement and commitment (Ramos 1992, Morse 1991). Ramos (1992) identifies three types of relationship: instrumental, protective and reciprocal. Graber and Mitcham (2004) refer to levels of interactive involvement as practical, social, personal and transcendent. These descriptors bear remarkable resemblance to three types of helpful patient–nurse relationships referred to by Morse (1991): the clinical relationship, the therapeutic relationship, and the connected relationship.

Each type is characterised by the level of involvement and the extent to which patient *and* nurse become known to each other. In this respect, each type of relationship is associated with the different sources of knowledge that nurses use in clinical practice. These sources, identified by Liaschenko and Fisher (1999) as case knowledge, patient knowledge and person knowledge, are described in Chapter 1. The level of involvement determines the degree to which the patient is known as a person. The types of relationship outlined by Morse (1991), Ramos

(1992) and Graber and Mitcham (2004) are discussed here in terms of the type of knowledge that is used. In addition, the types of relationship are described in relation to the skills that are the subject of subsequent chapters (listening, understanding, exploring and intervening).

Relevance of skill focus and type of relationship

Each set of skills—listening, understanding, exploring and intervening—is used in each type of relationship. It is not simply a matter of the type of skill used, but rather the focus of its use. In specifying a focus for skill use, there is a danger that these specifications will be used as prescriptions (i.e. hard and fast rules that require rigid adherence), but they should be used as guidelines that are fluid and open to change. These guidelines are presented in an effort to fit the skills into the particular context of the type of relationship negotiated between patient and nurse. The focus of skill use in each type of relationship is summarised in Table 2.1.

TABLE 2.1 Types of knowledge and focus of skill use in various levels of involvement			
	Level of involvement		
Morse (1991) Graber and Mitcham (2004) Ramos (1992)	**Clinical Practical** **Instrumental**	**Therapeutic Social** **Protective**	**Connected Personal transcendent** **Reciprocal**
Type of knowledge (Liaschenko & Fisher 1999)	Case knowledge	Case knowledge and patient knowledge	Case knowledge, patient knowledge and person knowledge
Listening	Content	Content and obvious feelings	Content and underlying feelings
Understanding	External view of the clinical situation	External and some internal patient response	Primarily internal, from patient experience
Exploring	Factual data, not feelings	Factual data and patient perceptions of the immediate situation	Personal meanings of both the situation and the effects on patient life
Intervening: comforting, supporting and enabling	Explanations and factual information Reassuring presence and manner	Sharing information Mobilising resources	Sharing own interpretations Providing support Concrete and specific feedback

The clinical relationship

In clinical relationships, nurses and patients interact in a routine or standard manner. Nurses perform technical care that is usual or standard for the circumstances. These relationships are characteristically short in duration, and involve a health situation that is perceived by nurse and patient to be minor and routine. The patient's vulnerability and dependence is almost non-existent, and the nurse follows clinical protocols in a technically competent manner.

There is little negotiation involved in this relationship, although there is implicit agreement to keep the relationship at this level (Ramos 1992, Morse 1991).

Focus of skill use in clinical relationships

A clinical relationship is not cold and distant, as the words technical, routine and standard might imply. Because the care is routine, that does not mean that the patient is treated as a 'number' or a 'case', reduced to an object. The nurse is concerned and interested, conveying this by being friendly and cordial. Social exchanges and chit-chat are often part of the interactions in these types of relationships.

During interactions in a clinical relationship, attending and listening skills are present, but the focus of listening remains primarily on content (see Ch 5). Unless directly stated by patients, feelings usually are not discussed or explored. Understanding is external (see Ch 6), based on the nurse's clinical knowledge, rather than internal, subjectively based understanding. Exploration (see Ch 7) is focused on factual data, although strict adherence to a prescribed form or format is potentially alienating to the patient. Intervening skills are of the stabilising type (see Ch 8), reassurance is provided through the nurse's manner and presence, and explanations and factual information are shared. The nurse's self-awareness (see Ch 3) during clinical relationships is focused primarily on clinical knowledge of the patient's situation, although personal biases and values may impinge on the relationship. For example, nurses may believe that patients should not complain about minor, routine procedures; they may become judgmental of patients as a result.

The therapeutic relationship

Therapeutic relationships between patients and nurses are formed in the majority of situations (Ramos 1992, Morse 1991). Morse (1991) considers this level as mutual, while Ramos (1992) refers to it as unilateral because the nurse maintains most of the control. This type of relationship is usually of short or average duration, with the patient facing a situation that is perceived by the patient as neither life-threatening nor serious. The patient's internal and external resources for meeting the demands of the situation are adequate. Although the nurse's perspective is primarily that the patient *is* a patient, there is also recognition and understanding of the patient as a person.

Focus of skill use in therapeutic relationships

In attending, listening and exploring, the nurse focuses on both content and feelings, when these emotions relate directly to the patient's health situation. For example, when patients are anxious prior to surgery, the nurse perceives the anxiety and explores further in order to determine the patient's need for information and/or reassurance. Understanding skills (see Ch 6) enable nurses to focus on the patient's subjective experience of the health event, and exploration (see Ch 7) is therefore focused on both factual data and the patient's perception of the situation. Interventions are aimed primarily at maintaining and stabilising the patient's resources; nevertheless, there is the possibility that information shared by the nurse will alter the patient's perception of the situation (see types of interventions in Ch 8). Because the therapeutic relationship is more involved than the clinical relationship, nurses' self-awareness is focused on how they are affecting the patient.

Connected relationships

A connected relationship is one in which the nurse and patient become involved to the degree that they perceive each other as people first, and their roles as patient and nurse become secondary. At this level of involvement, nurses understand the meaning of the clinical situation for the patient as a person (Ramos 1992). Usually, these types of relationships take time to develop, but a degree of connection may happen in a short time when patients' situations are extreme, in terms of seriousness, vulnerability and/or dependence (the factors affecting negotiation). Both nurse and patient choose to enter connected relationships, and trust and commitment are deep and complete. In a connected relationship, nurses often choose to 'go the extra mile' for patients, and act 'above and beyond' the call of duty (Ramos 1992, Morse 1991). Patients describe these types of relationships as 'friendships' (Fosbinder 1994).

A major difference between therapeutic and connected relationships is that the nurse functions as a source of support in the connected relationship, whereas in the therapeutic relationship nurses are support mobilisers and enhancers. This is because, in the therapeutic relationship, patients' supportive resources are present, even if not immediately available. In a connected relationship, the nurse is involved and committed, although the relationship does not necessarily extend beyond the patient's contact with the healthcare setting. These relationships are memorable for both patient and nurse, and nurses in connected relationships feel that they have made a significant difference to the patient (Morse 1991). Although they require a great deal of energy, nurses leave these relationships feeling energised by the strong bond (Ramos 1992).

The following scenario is an example of a connected relationship, told in the first person by the nurse:

When I heard Pat's story of how she received a gunshot wound to her spine at close range, from her husband during a domestic argument, I felt anger towards her husband and a deep sense of sympathy for Pat. There was virtually no hope that she would ever walk again, as the bullet had severed her spine. She was out of intensive care, out of immediate life-threatening danger, when we met. I was working as a consultation-liaison mental health nurse and the nurses had referred Pat to me for supportive counselling. I liked her the moment I met her and felt an affinity towards her. She was a physically beautiful woman of 35, who sustained a charm and graciousness that would be difficult for most people under the circumstances. We instantly 'hit it off', and over the next 3 months of her hospitalisation became quite close.

The fact that I often thought about her when I was off duty did not seem remarkable to me; I often thought about patients when I was at home. But there was something different about our relationship. We came to know each other on a deeply personal basis, and I no longer thought of her as a patient. I also got to know her family very well and was treated like part of their network. Her parents, three sisters, brother-in-law and three nieces were an extremely close-knit family. They maintained a continual presence at Pat's side, supporting and caring for her in every possible way. They sensed my deep commitment to Pat, and expressed appreciation for it.

Neither Pat nor her family ever spoke of Pat's husband, the person I held responsible for putting her in a wheelchair. Not surprisingly, he had not been in to see her. My anger towards him grew as I became closer to Pat. 'How could anyone have done this to her?' My sense of injustice and my firm belief in the senselessness of firearms in the home kept my anger strong. But Pat never demonstrated any anger; in fact, she never talked about 'what happened'. She accepted her situation, the complex physical problems that accompany a spinal injury, her life in a wheelchair and her altered future with equanimity and remarkable resilience. I admired her strength and supported it, for it was keeping her going against enormous odds.

When her nightmares began, and the events of the shooting were vividly replayed in them, her fear and anguish started to seep through. She shared her nightmares and her feelings with me. I encouraged her to talk about what happened only to the extent that she could make meaning and begin to build her life again. Although she expressed anger and sadness, she never dwelled on these emotions. Perhaps she knew I felt the same way; perhaps it was that I always listened—quietly encouraging her to 'get it out' while containing my own emotions. She told no one else of the emotional pain, because she knew the others who were closest to her, her family, were bearing their own anguish. She never wanted to be a burden, and this internal resource saw her through the long rehabilitation process.

When Pat was discharged from hospital to the rehabilitation centre, I stayed in touch with her and her entire family, as there were ongoing health issues with a number of them. Her sister in particular would always stop by to see me when she was at the health centre. When my own personal circumstances necessitated a relocation from the area, I drove to the rehabilitation centre to say goodbye in person to Pat and her sister. She told me of the plans that were underway to have her home converted for a wheelchair. Divorce proceedings were underway and she was making plans to return to work.

We sat in the garden of the centre and relived our relationship. She thanked me for all that I had done to help her to adjust to her new life. I thanked her for sharing so much of herself with me. I told her that my own life was enriched by seeing her strength and resilience. We knew we had touched each other in a 'special' way. I knew that Pat would continue to live a full, although dramatically altered, life. That I may have had something to contribute to this outcome filled me with great professional satisfaction.

This story illustrates the reciprocity that can exist in therapeutically intimate relationships. Not all relationships reach this level of involvement. In fact, most do not. This story also illustrates the essence of this book: the significance and value of taking the time to understand patients as people, of taking the time to notice, of being concerned enough to explore and understand their world as they experience it. Interpersonal skills enable nurses to make contact with the private, subjective experiences of patients.

Focus of skill use in connected relationships

In connected relationships, nurses attend and listen to the entirety of the patient's story, and are able to perceive themes by relating content to underlying feelings (see Ch 5). Understanding is primarily internal (see Ch 6), with the nurse developing awareness of the deeply personal, subjective experience of the patient. Exploration is focused on meanings, and exploration that is based on cue recognition and perception (see Ch 7) is frequent. Interventions are aimed at the nurse as being the source of support (see Ch 8), and the nurse's interpretation of the situation is shared with the patient, in order to assist the patient in making sense of what is happening in the situation. Self-disclosure is high, characteristic of therapeutic intimacy, and the nurse is free to share concrete and specific feedback (see Ch 8) about the relationship. There is 'you–me' talk as nurse and patient feel safe in sharing their immediate reactions about how they are experiencing each other. Self-awareness skills (see Ch 3) focus on the nurse as participant in the relationship, and both nurse and patient experience change as a result of their relationship.

Summary of skill use in various types of relationships

Each type of patient–nurse relationship is qualitatively different from the other. In each, nurses use the same skills, but the focus of skill use alters as relationships become more involved and intense. A high degree of self-disclosure on the nurse's part is inappropriate in a clinical relationship, yet significantly helpful in the connected relationship. The focus of listening extends from content only in clinical relationships to themes and meanings in connected/reciprocal relationships. Understanding is primarily external in clinical relationships and primarily internal in connected/reciprocal relationships. Exploration moves from the safe areas of content in clinical relationships to the intimate area of feelings and meanings in connected relationships. Interventions in clinical relationships are of the stabilising type, while mobilising interventions characterise connected relationships.

THE PROGRESS OF THE RELATIONSHIP

It is important that nurses understand not only the various types of relationships that are formed with patients, but also how these relationships develop and progress. An ability to track the progress of development of relationships enables nurses to time their responses accordingly. For example, without trust—the major issue in beginning relationships—challenging (see Ch 8) may alienate patients and reflecting feelings (see Ch 6) could be perceived by patients as intrusive. Tracking the progress of relationships means paying careful attention to the major issues of relationship development and to how patients are responding to the efforts of the nurses.

The progress of relationships is described in terms of phases of development: prior to interacting; establishing the relationship; building the relationship; and ending the relationship. The major themes and issues that are characteristic of each phase serve as signals and signposts in the progress of relationships. These are indicators for nurses to notice, to be concerned about, and to respond to with an awareness of their significance to the development of relationships.

Not all relationships pass through each phase, and not all issues will be relevant. The phases and their central themes and issues are presented as a guide to tracking the progress of the relationship. They are not definitive, but rather present a probable scenario. For this reason they should be treated with caution. Using the concept of phases of development runs the risk that they will be perceived as rigid, adhered to as dogma or, worse, applied in a procedural, step-by-step manner. Relationships between patients and nurses are fluid, flexible and dynamic. No one picture could ever capture the complexity and variety of these relationships. The phases presented here should be viewed with these qualifications in mind.

Prior to interacting

The primary issue prior to interacting with patients is nurses' awareness of their own current thoughts, feelings and attitudes that may affect how they approach patients. Hearing about patients in a handover report or reading about them in their healthcare records sets up certain expectations, thoughts and feelings.

When there is knowledge of a particular patient, the nurse examines what, if any, thoughts, feelings and attitudes are engendered by such knowledge. For example, there may be fear and anxiety associated with caring for a patient with a known history of mental illness. These preliminary thoughts and feelings need not be negative (e.g. a nurse may enjoy caring for patients of a particular age group, gender or clinical condition).

Self-awareness skills (see Ch 3) are especially critical during this phase of relationship development. Any or all of a nurse's thoughts, feelings and attitudes prior to interacting with a patient may affect the relationship, for better or worse. For this reason self-awareness is where the relationship begins.

Establishing the relationship

In the initial phase of interacting, the major issue between patient and nurse revolves around trust. Both patient and nurse evaluate each other at this time, with questions such as:

- Can I be myself with this person?
- Will I be accepted?
- How trustworthy is this person?
- Will they like me?

The initial phase of the relationship is thus characterised by uncertainty and mutual exploration to decrease this uncertainty, as both patient and nurse assess each other. Nurses assess patients in terms of their current health status and their needs for nursing care (most often accomplished by a formal nursing assessment), *and* in terms of whether or not they feel they can work with the patient (Morse 1991). Similarly, patients assess nurses in terms of deciding if they can trust the nurses and whether they can work with them. This mutual assessment provides the avenue for negotiating the relationship.

Trust

The formation of trust is essential if the relationship is to progress beyond a superficial level because trust enables patient and nurse to place confidence in each other. Interpersonal trust means that one person in the relationship believes that the other person can be relied and depended upon. In the nursing context, trust can be specific to the patient's health problem and not encompass all areas of their lives as would be more likely with friendships (Hagerty & Patusky 2003). Unlike trust in friendships, trust in healthcare relationships is strongly connected to confidence in the healthcare provider's competence and knowledge, in addition to expressive caring behaviours such as listening and being sincerely interested in the patient as a person (Hupcey & Miller 2006).

Building trust is not simply a matter of the patient trusting the nurse; nurses must also be able to trust patients. It is a mutual process; it must be reciprocated. Trust is fostered when nurses believe in patients' competence and skill in knowing what is best for them in their management of their health (Bova et al 2006). Nurses demonstrate their trust in patients by treating them with respect and regard (see Ch 3), and accepting and supporting them as capable human beings.

From the patients' perspective, nurses must be perceived as trustworthy. Nurses are fortunate because their professional role is viewed as trustworthy by most patients. Patients expect that nurses will care for them, meet their physical needs and provide comfort. In fact, when nurses 'don't seem to care', patients will often express shock and dismay, feeling betrayed by an apparent failure of the nurses to fulfil their role.

In this respect, trust is associated with meeting the patients' expectations that they will be respected, listened to, and treated as an individual (Hupcey & Miller 2006, Hupcey et al 2004). Nurses can rely on patients' inherent trust in their role only to a limited extent. They must live up to patients' expectations that they are trustworthy through consistent actions, behaviours and attitudes.

Another important aspect in developing trust is for nurses to share their thoughts and reactions to patients' self-disclosure. Without feedback from nurses, patients who are sharing information about themselves may feel naked and vulnerable. Have you ever shared something of yourself, your thoughts, feelings or reactions with another person only to be met with a silent, stone-faced response? Under such circumstances, it is unlikely that you felt trust in this person. Likewise, patients rely on responses from nurses, and understanding responses (see Ch 6) are the most trust-enhancing. Moralising, evaluative and judgmental responses, early in the relationship, lead to patients feeling rejected.

Mutual assessment

In this initial phase of the relationship, nurses and patients assess each other in an effort to determine if they will get along—if there is any commonality or shared interest between them (e.g. whether they are both lovers of opera)—and if they feel they can work together. Patients may question the nurse's motivation to nurse, ask how much nursing experience the nurse has and generally observe the nurse to determine what kind of person they are.

Patients test nurses as to their dependability and their ability to keep a confidence (Morse 1991). All of these are strategies used to determine how far the involvement between patient and nurse will proceed. The patient bases the decision about whether to trust the nurse on what is determined during this phase. Nurses also assess patients during this initial phase in order to choose consciously whether to make an emotional investment in the patient (Morse 1991). This personal assessment is not the same as a formal clinical assessment, which is designed to elicit information that has a direct bearing on patients' nursing care.

The initial interview

Most frequently, the relationship between patient and nurse begins with an interview, during which the nurse collects pertinent data about the patient. Depending on the setting, the data that is to be collected is often specified on a formal nursing history/assessment form. Patients are usually the source of information, although if they are unable to interact (e.g. if they are unconscious), family and friends are used as the source of information. The initial information received by the nurse forms the basis for nursing-care planning.

Because this interview is also the time during which patient and nurse begin to get to know each other, the process of how the interview is conducted is as significant as the content. The climate established during this initial contact is crucial to the subsequent formation of the relationship. This interview sets the tone and establishes some of the ground rules on which the relationship will operate.

A rapid series of questions, asked in succession, may leave patients feeling intruded upon and bombarded by the nurse. Patients may form the impression that their role is to be obedient in providing answers. Lack of an explanation by a nurse about why the information is being collected may create confusion and uncertainty about the nurse's intentions. An initial interview conducted in an automatic, routine manner may create the impression that a nurse does not care about patients as people.

While this section cannot describe all the aspects of an initial nursing assessment (e.g. observation of physical signs), it does describe ways of conducting the initial interview with the recognition that it serves to establish the relationship between nurses and patients, as much as it serves to establish an adequate nursing database. These general guidelines for conducting the initial interview relate to its process and how it is conducted rather than to its content.

Exploration skills (see Ch 7) will predominate during this interview; however, the skills of attending and listening (Ch 5), as well as responding with understanding (Ch 6), will also feature in the interview.

Process aspects of the initial interview

It is essential that nurses establish the interview within the context. This is done by proper introductions and explanations of the meaning of the interview. Nurses who introduce themselves and clearly describe their role in the particular healthcare setting help to establish this context. While this may appear obvious, it is striking how often this is overlooked or brushed aside too quickly.

A clear description of the nurse's role in the setting includes more than a simple statement of name and title. It includes a description of how often the patient is likely to interact with and see this particular nurse. Is the interview being conducted by a student of nursing who is present in the setting for that day only? In this case, the patient will not see this nurse again, and should be informed of this fact, without having to wonder or ask. Is the interview being conducted by a permanent member of the hospital nursing staff who is about to go on days off? Again, this should be explained clearly. It is disconcerting for the patient to share information with a relative stranger, who is then not seen again, without an explanation of why this occurred.

An explanation of why the information is being sought, provided in a manner that the patient is likely to understand, also helps to set the interview within a particular context. Saying 'I need some information about you so that the nurses can care for you while you are here' is hardly adequate for a patient who is unfamiliar with the particular setting. A better way would be to explain to the patient that nurses need to know 'how a particular health situation concerns you personally, how it is affecting your day-to-day functioning and how it is likely to affect you in the future', followed by an explanation that the information is used to make nursing care specific to the particular patient.

If nurses are unsure or unclear about why they are collecting the information, other than to meet a requirement of the particular healthcare agency, it is not likely that the explanation will be adequate. For this reason, nurses are encouraged to think through what they need to know about patients and why they need to know this in order to provide nursing care.

Lastly, in establishing a context for the interview, it is important to explain to patients what will be done with the information they share. The information that relates directly to the patient's nursing care will be recorded and shared with other nurses and other healthcare professionals, and this practice of sharing information should be explained to patients. Not every detail of patients' stories needs to be shared, and it is best if patients are reassured that information that will be shared will be reviewed with them at the completion of the interview.

This raises an interesting point about confidentiality in the patient–nurse relationship. How can patients come to trust nurses if they believe there is little information that will be kept in confidence? In fact, one of the ways that patients test nurses' trustworthiness is by sharing a minor secret to see if it will be held in confidence (Morse 1991). For this reason, nurses are encouraged to question the sometimes established norm of 'telling all' to other nurses.

Confidentiality is not merely keeping patient information inside the confines of a particular setting, but also considering what should be shared, through reporting and recording, with other nurses and other healthcare professionals. Information that has no direct bearing on the nursing or other healthcare of the patient should be considered confidential and treated as such.

Each of these aspects—introducing self, explaining the purpose of the interview and informing patients how the information will be handled—helps to set the context and climate of the interview. Once the 'stage is set' in this manner, the specific data collection, the exploration phase, can begin.

In beginning the exploration phase of the initial interview, it is best to start with 'safe' topics that allow some rapport to be established, before moving into more sensitive areas. Delving into deeply subjective experiences is inappropriate as a beginning focus when the relationship is new and possibly fragile. It is unlikely that patients will share highly personal information before trust has been established—the sharing of such information is a sign that the patient is beginning to trust the nurse, or at least wants to know if the nurse is trustworthy.

During the interview, it is important that nurses bear in mind that patients are the experts on how their health situation is affecting their lives, although the nurse may have a clinical understanding of what is most pertinent. For example, patients may not perceive the significance of a question relating to how many stairs must be negotiated in their living quarters, but for some health situations this factor is very important. Nurses rely on their clinical knowledge in directing the interview, but need to mix nurse-led with patient-led exploration (see Ch 7).

The initial interview provides an opportunity for nurses to share information with patients. This is done by asking patients what questions are on their minds, as well as correcting any misinformation or misunderstandings they may have about their current health situation. Sharing information at this time also balances the interview, establishing a climate of reciprocity.

Building the relationship

Once the relationship is established, both nurse and patient know where the other stands and have an idea of what to expect from the relationship. The uncertainty that characterises the beginning of the relationship is reduced. It is at this point that nurses often experience a different type of uncertainty—an uneasiness and sense of pressure about 'doing something' for the patient. Because they have encouraged patients to disclose and share their experiences, nurses may feel that they now must take action and do something about what the patient has shared. When nurses experience their sense of responsibility in this manner, this may lead to taking on and assuming patients' burdens. Under such circumstances, nurses run the risk of feeling helpless, powerless and out of control. Taking on patients' burdens is also one of the warning signals of overinvolvement. These highlight the two central issues in building the relationship: control and power.

Control

An attitude that it is the nurses' responsibility to solve patients' problems for them reflects issues of control. Indicators that nurses may be too controlling in their interactions include:

- talking more than listening
- evaluating more than understanding
- leading more than following, and
- advising more than informing.

In order to manage effectively the issue of control, nurses must remind themselves that their role in the relationship is not that of rescuer, but rather that of facilitator—one who eases burdens by enabling patients to increase their access to their own resources. Through facilitating, nurses focus less on having the answers and more on enabling patients to maintain control and develop their own answers. Helping patients to feel in control has been shown to increase their comfort (Williams & Iruita 2004). In believing their role is a facilitating one, nurses do not relinquish their responsibility to patients, but assume their responsibility in a collaborative manner. In doing so, nurses operate from a position of partner in care, as distinct from the position of a provider of care.

This is not to say that every patient will want or need to be in control, or will be able to develop their own resources. Some patients prefer nurses to provide answers and offer solutions. In some clinical situations, it is appropriate for nurses to assume control because of the patient's clinical condition, desire and orientation, or a combination of these factors.

In building the relationship, the major focus is to develop a congruence between what the patient wants in the way of help and assistance and what the nurse offers. There could be difficulties experienced in the relationship if nurse and patient are operating from incongruent perspectives. For this reason, nurses are encouraged to reflect on how the patient is approaching the relationship compared to how they are approaching it. It is pointless to force patients into collaboration if they believe that nurses are experts with the solutions to their problems. Likewise, to take over and exclude patients from decision making when they want this level of influence is equally pointless.

Power

Another issue in building the relationship is power, which refers to the power that is developed through meaningful connection with patients. Simply put, power is the ability to do or act to secure desired outcomes (Oudshoorn 2005). Nurses who are trusted and regarded favourably by patients have power to influence these patients, and its appropriate use will enable rather than control patients. This type of enabling is often referred to as patient empowerment and is discussed in Chapter 8 in relation to providing information and support.

Nurses should remain conscious of the fact that they have legitimate authority, by virtue of their position. It is important that they recognise the power differential between themselves and patients (Oudshoorn 2005, Peter & Morgan 2001). This it true not only because of position power, but also because patients are often dependent and vulnerable, thus decreasing their own sense of power. Unfortunately, research evidence demonstrates that nurses exert power over patients in ways that further disempower patients, such as acting as if they know best, not consulting patients with changes to care delivery, and controlling and dominating interactions (Barrere 2007, Oudshoorn et al 2007, Shattell 2004, Henderson 2003, Hewison 1995).

Appropriate use of nurses' influencing power in their relationships with patients is an empowering process. Empowerment means relating to patients in such a way that they feel capable and competent, thus facilitating them to exert influence and control. Benner (1984) refers to the concept of caring power, which is used to empower patients, rather than dominate, control or coerce them. Nurses have the potential power to:

- transform patients' views of their situations
- reintegrate patients with their social world
- remove obstacles or stand alongside and support and enable patients
- solicit patients' resources
- bring hope, confidence and trust, and
- affirm the human capacity to cope.

All of these processes are powerful in their own right. Nurses engaged in these processes are not operating from a traditional view of 'power over', but rather the empowerment that comes from belief in, regard for and strengthening of patients. In this sense, empowerment is similar to the characteristic of respect (see Ch 3).

Ending the relationship

One of the major factors differentiating social relationships from professional ones is that professional relationships between patients and nurses are usually time-limited. Most patients and nurses are aware that, at some point in time, each will disengage from the relationship. Relationships between patients and nurses end for a variety of reasons: patients recover and are discharged from the healthcare setting; they are referred to another setting for follow-up care; nurses may depart from the clinical setting; and sometimes relationships end with the death of the patient. Whatever the reason for ending the relationship, there is a need to disengage and bring a sense of closure to it. The central issues involved in ending the relationship are emotionality and review.

Emotionality

Frequently, emotions are aroused during the disengagement process, and it is at this stage that both patients and nurses are most likely to express emotions about each other and the relationship. Emotions may range from sadness and frustration to satisfaction and happiness. Most often, there is a mixture of emotions. Nurses experience satisfaction when patients recover, especially if they have played a role in that recovery. While there may be a degree of sadness in saying goodbye, this is frequently offset by the feeling of satisfaction and happiness for the patient.

Depending on the type of relationship that has developed and the degree of connection and commitment between patient and nurse, the emotionality that often accompanies saying goodbye may or may not be present. In clinical relationships, there may be no emotions involved, except perhaps feelings of gratitude expressed by the patient. In connected relationships, emotions may run high as both patient and nurse have come to know each other intimately.

Handling these emotions is a matter of bringing them into awareness (see Ch 3) and expressing them openly. Nurses who are able to express their feelings about the relationship that has developed are behaving in an authentic, congruent manner (see Ch 3). In an effort to encourage the patient to reciprocate in expressing emotions, nurses may choose to reflect feelings (see Ch 6).

Review

Regardless of whether there is any emotionality in saying goodbye, the ending of the relationship is most satisfying when there is a review of what happened during the relationship. Various scenes may be relived and shared, or it may be a simple matter of reassuring the patient that all is now well. Reviewing what happened during their relationship does not mean that nurses and patients should relive every interaction, but rather briefly recount significant events. Such a review brings a sense of closure to the relationship.

At times, there is no opportunity to say goodbye to patients. If nurses feel unsettled when this happens, it is often helpful to share this experience with a colleague who also knew the patient (see Ch 11). Vicariously reliving the relationship with colleagues may help to bring a sense of closure to the relationship.

CHAPTER SUMMARY

The essential nature of relationships between patients and nurses is that of mutual understanding. In developing relationships with patients, nurses not only focus on understanding patients' experiences, but also on understanding the level of involvement desired by patients. Relationships that develop between patients and nurses differ in their level of involvement, and nurses are encouraged to establish a level of involvement that is appropriate to the circumstances.

Negotiating the 'right' level of involvement is based on the patient need, level of vulnerability and degree of dependency. Regardless of the level of involvement, all the skills presented in the following chapters are used in patient–nurse relationships, but the focus of their use alters depending on the type of relationship formed. With an appropriate focus, skills are employed within the context of the relationship between patient and nurse.

Critical issues emerge at various phases of development of relationships, and awareness of these issues enables nurses to address them. The issues of self-awareness, trust, mutual assessment, control, power, emotionality and review have been presented with an emphasis on the need for collaborative efforts between patient and nurse. All skills included in this book are presented from this point of view.

REFERENCES

Australian Nursing and Midwifery Council (ANMC) 2003 Code of Professional Conduct for Nurses in Australia. ANMC, Canberra

Barrere CC 2007 Discourse analysis of nurse–patient communication in a hospital setting: implications for staff development. Journal for Nurses in Staff Development 23(3):114–122

Benner P 1984 From novice to expert: excellence and power in clinical nursing practice. Addison-Wesley, Menlo Park, CA

Benner P, Wrubel J 1989 The primacy of caring: stress and coping in health and illness. Addison-Wesley, Menlo Park, CA

Bova C, Fennie KP, Watrous E, Dieckhause K, Williams AB 2006 The health care relationship (HCR) trust scale: development and psychometric evaluation. Research in Nursing and Health 29:477–488

Brammer LM 1988 The helping relationship: process and skills, 4th edn. Prentice-Hall, Englewood Cliffs, NJ

Chang T, Lin Y-P, Change H-J, Lin C-C 2005 Cancer patient and staff ratings of caring behaviors. Cancer Nursing 28(5):331–339

Coad-Chapman A 1986 Therapeutic superficiality and intimacy. In: Longo DC, Williams RA (eds), Clinical practice in psychosocial nursing: assessment and intervention. Appleton-Century Crofts, East Norwark, CT

Coffey S, 2006 The nurse–patient relationship in cancer care as a shared covenant: a concept analysis. Advances in Nursing Science 29(4):308–323

de Raeve L 2002 Trust and trustworthiness in the nurse–patient relationship. Nursing Philosophy 3(2):152–162

Fosbinder D 1994 Patient perceptions of nursing care: an emerging theory of interpersonal competence. Journal of Advanced Nursing 20:1085–1093

Gadow S 1980 Existential advocacy: philosophical foundation of nursing. In Spiker SF, Gadow S (eds) Nursing: images and ideals, pp 79–101. Springer, New York

Gaenellos R 2005 Sustaining well-being and enabling recovery: the therapeutic effect of nurse friendliness on clients and nursing environments. Contemporary Nurse 19(1–2):242–252

Graber DR, Mitcham MD 2004 Compassionate clinicians: taking patient care beyond the ordinary. Holistic Nursing Practice 18(2):87–94

Hagerty BM, Patusky KL 2003 Reconceptualizing the nurse–patient relationship. Journal of Nursing Scholarship 35(2):145–150

Henderson A 2001 Emotional labor and nursing: an under-appreciated aspect of caring work. Nursing Inquiry 8(2):130–138

Henderson S 2003 Power imbalance between nurses and patients: a potential inhibitor of partnership in care. Journal of Clinical Nursing 12:501–508

Henson RH 1997 Analysis of the concept of mutuality. Image: Journal of Nursing Scholarship 29:77–81

Hewison A 1995 Nurses' power in interactions with patients. Journal of Advanced Nursing 21:75–82

Hunt M 1991 Being friendly and informal: reflected in nurses' terminally ill patients' and relatives' conversations at home. Journal of Advanced Nursing 16:929–938

Hupcey JE, Clark MB, Hutchinson CR, Thompson VL 2004 Expectations for care: elders' satisfaction and trust in health care providers. Journal of Gerontological Nursing 30:37–45

Hupcey JE, Miller J 2006 Community dwelling adults' perception of interpersonal trust vs trust in health care providers. Journal of Clinial Nursing 15:1132–1139

Hupcey JE, Penrod J, Morse JM, Mitcham C 2001 An exploration and advancement of the concept of trust. Journal of Advanced Nursing 36:282–293

Iruita VF, Williams AM 2001 Balancing and compromising: nurses and patients preserving integrity of self and each other. International Journal of Nursing Studies 38:579–589

Jourard SM 1964 The transparent self. Van Nostrand, Princeton, NJ

Kadner K 1994 Therapeutic intimacy in nursing. Journal of Advanced Nursing 19:215–218

Liaschenko J, Fisher A 1999 Theorizing the knowledge that nurses use in the conduct of their work. Scholarly Inquiry for Nursing Practice: An International Journal 13(1):29–41

Marck P 1990 Therapeutic reciprocity: a caring phenomenon. Advances in Nursing Science 13(1):49–59

McCabe C 2004 Nurse–patient communication: an exploration of the patients' experiences. Journal of Clinical Nursing 13:41–49

McGilton KS, Boscart VM 2007 Close care provider–resident relationship in long-term care environments. Journal of Clinical Nursing 16:2149–2157

Menzies I 1961 A case study of the functioning of social systems as a defence against anxiety. Human Relations 13(2):95–123

Mok E, Chui PC 2004 Nurse–patient relationships in palliative care. Journal of Advanced Nursing 48:475–483

Morse JM 1991 Negotiating commitment and involvement in the nurse–patient relationship. Journal of Advanced Nursing 16:455–468

Noddings N 1984 Caring: a feminine approach to ethics and moral education. University of California Press, Berkeley, CA

Oudshoorn A 2005 Power and empowerment: critical concepts in the nurse–patient relationship. Contemporary Nurse 20:57–66

Oudshoorn A, Ward-Griffin C, McWilliam C 2007 Client–nurse relationships in home-based palliative care: a critical analysis of power relations. Journal of Clinical Nursing 16:1435–1443

Peter E, Morgan KP 2001 Explorations of a trust approach for nursing ethics. Nursing Inquiry 8(1):3–10

Peternelj-Taylor CA, Younge O 2003 Exploring boundaries in the nurse–client relationship: professional roles and responsibilities. Perspectives in Psychiatric Care 39(2):55–66

Ramos MC 1992 The nurse–patient relationship: theme and variations. Journal of Advanced Nursing 17:496–506

Savage J 1992 Nursing intimacy: an ethnographic approach to nurse patient interaction. Scutari Press, London

Shattell M 2004 Nurse–patient interaction: a review of the literature. Journal of Clinical Nursing 13:714–722

Shattell M 2005 Nurse bait: strategies hospitalized patients use to entice nurses within the context of the interpersonal relationship. Issues in Mental Health Nursing 26:205–223

Sheets VR 2000 Staying in the lines. Nursing Management 31(18): 28–30, 32–34

Smith P 1992 The emotional labour of nursing. Macmillan Press, London

Tarlier DS 2004 Beyond caring: the moral and ethical basis of responsive nurse–patient relationship. Nursing Philosophy 5:230–241

Williams A 2001 A literature review on the concept of intimacy in nursing. Journal of Advanced Nursing 33:660–667

Williams A, Irurita V 2004 Therapeutic and non-therapeutic interpersonal interactions: the patient's perspective. Journal of Clinical Nursing 13:806–815

CHAPTER 3

Nurse as therapeutic agent

INTRODUCTION

That nurses have a sense of agency is the basis on which they form relationships with patients. A sense of agency means that nurses understand and appreciate that they can make a difference to patients' lives, and that they know how to use their professional influence and knowledge to the benefit of patients. While such power could be used to harm the patient, a nurse's professional agency is employed in service to the patient (i.e. for therapeutic benefits).

In developing therapeutic agency, nurses need a wide and varied repertoire of interpersonal skills and an understanding of their use as well as practical know-how. In employing their agency, nurses need an awareness of how effectively they are using their skills because such awareness enables them to evaluate their own performance. Nurses who are able to reflect upon and evaluate their own performance are in a position to learn, grow and become more skilled and effective in their interactions with patients, thus increasing their potential for therapeutic agency.

The previous chapters have outlined a moral imperative for nurses to focus their attention on patients during their interactions. This may be interpreted to mean that nurses should disregard or forget themselves whenever they engage in nursing care. By focusing on patients, at the exclusion of themselves, nurses run the risk of failing to recognise the significance of how *they* are affecting patients and how patients are affecting *them*. In the process, nurses may fail to attend to their own reactions and responses, erroneously perceiving their subjectivity to be superfluous or irrelevant to patient care.

The skills presented in the following chapters of this book can be learnt, developed and refined. Nevertheless, the skills are only as effective as the person using them. Each nurse employs the skills in a unique way. Effectively relating to patients involves more than simply using the right skill, at the right time, with the right patient. *What matters and makes a difference are not the skills themselves, but the nurse who is using the skills.* Each nurse develops a style of relating to patients that is 'right' for that particular nurse. Nurses who focus solely on the skills without awareness of their own personality run the risk of contrived performance that lacks spontaneity and a personal touch. For these reasons, the initial focus of interpersonal skill development is placed on communication competence, emotional intelligence, self-awareness and reflective practice.

Chapter overview

This chapter begins with a discussion of the importance of communication competence in developing a sense of therapeutic agency. Nurses with such competence have the ability to be responsive to what others are thinking, feeling and perceiving, along with an ability to express what they are thinking, feeling and perceiving. Emotional intelligence and emotional labour are reviewed as they relate to communication competence. The importance of understanding in developing such competence, particularly in light of the concept of the 'use of self' in nursing, is then reviewed. The use of self as a therapeutic agent is discussed next. This is followed by a brief overview of reflection and reflective practice, as such processes are an effective means of increasing self-awareness and understanding. Reflective processes involved in developing self-understanding are then reviewed, with an emphasis on the interactive nature of these processes. The processes for developing greater self-understanding include introspection, feedback from others and self-sharing.

The following section provides an overview of the facets of the self that are of critical significance in patient–nurse relationships. The qualities and traits of effective helpers are also reviewed because self-understanding enhances the development of these. Challenges frequently encountered when learning interpersonal skills are then discussed. The final section, self-assessment of interpersonal skills, provides useful guidelines for evaluation of present skill level and suggested directions for further skill development.

THERAPEUTIC USE OF SELF

Therapeutic use of self is the direct expression of the art of nursing. Use of self requires creative thinking in response to the uniqueness of each individual patient. For example, nurses who are natural comedians can effectively use humour for those patients who are coping through finding a funny side to their circumstances. Other nurses will find that their strength lies in the area of providing explanations to patients who want more information. As such there is no one description or definition that captures the use of self as an art, as each nurses enactment of agency will be as unique as the nurse as a person.

The development of the art of using oneself will be a career-long process for nurses whose therapeutic agency is realised. Nonetheless, there are basic requisites for the development of therapeutic agency. These are: communication competence, emotional intelligence and skill in labouring the emotions, as much of what makes people unique is how they feel and respond emotionally. Because nursing care situations often involve strong emotions, nurses must be skilled in effectively managing their own feelings (emotional labour) if they are going to be of value to the patient.

Communication competence

Nurses must be competent communicators if they are going to develop their own personal sense of agency and use their interactions with patients to be of assistance and to provide help. Communication competence involves two types of skills: those of being responsive (i.e. able to listen to and understand what others are saying); and those of being assertive (i.e. able to state their point of view and express their needs). People who are competent communicators are able to express their own ideas, opinions and feelings, while also having the ability to understand the expressed ideas, opinions and feelings of other people. That is, they are skilled at balancing both assertive and responsive skills in their interpersonal interactions with others. Figure 3.1 depicts communication competence along two axes, assertiveness and responsiveness. The competent communicator will have a balance of both types of interpersonal skills and will lie in the upper outer quadrant of the matrix.

FIGURE 3.1   Communication competence

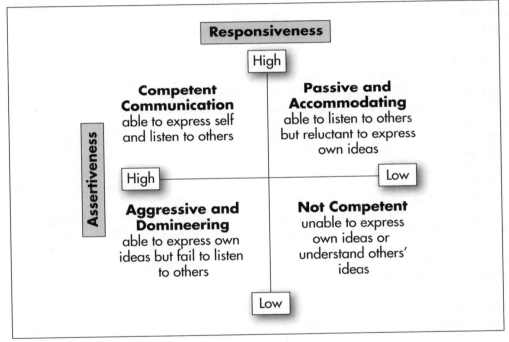

Overly assertive people who are not able to listen and understand others' opinions and ideas are usually considered aggressive or domineering in their communication, as they often do not listen to others as they continue to emphasise their viewpoint. As such, they are prone to override others' views. Highly responsive people, those people who are very adept at understanding others yet are unable to state their own ideas, often are considered passive or accommodating in their interpersonal interactions. As such, they often miss opportunities to be heard. Neither type of person is competent in communication, as they lack a balance between the skills of responding and the skills of asserting.

Nurses need to be competent communicators because they need to be both responsive and assertive as they enact their therapeutic agency. For example, they are often in a position to advocate on behalf of a patient, thus needing to use the skills of assertion. Likewise, empathic expression, developed through the use of responsive skills, is necessary to understanding the experience of patients. Responding skills are covered primarily in Chapters 5 and 6, and the skills of assertion are reviewed fully in Chapters 10 and 11.

Emotional intelligence

Competent communicators possess what is termed 'emotional intelligence'—the capacity to recognise their own emotions, as well as those of others, and to monitor those emotions and manage their feelings in themselves and in their relationships (Goleman 1996). People who are emotionally intelligent possess internal qualities of resilience, initiative, optimism and adaptability (Goleman 1998). In their interactions with others, they acknowledge the significance of human feelings and are able to use their hearts as well as their heads when deciding how to act. Emotional intelligence has been discussed as important in nursing because nursing work requires the capacity to understand the emotional realities of patients (McQueen 2004).

There are five dimensions of emotional intelligence—self-awareness, self-regulation, motivation, empathy and social skills—which are hierarchical and interdependent (Goleman 1998). That is, self-awareness is the basis on which all the other dimensions are developed. Self-awareness includes accurate assessment of self, along with self-confidence. Self-regulation involves control over one's emotions and being trustworthy. Motivation includes commitment, initiative and optimism. Empathy (see Ch 6), a central dimension in emotional intelligence, includes not only understanding other people but also maintaining a service orientation towards others. Finally, the social skills necessary for emotional intelligence include conflict management, cooperation and collaboration (see Ch 10).

Developing emotional intelligence is essential to becoming a competent helper (Ivey & Ivey 2003). Unlike IQ, emotional intelligence is largely learnt and increases with age and experience (Goleman 1998). The potential to become emotionally competent is largely determined by emotional intelligence, as such intelligence spurs motivation to keep improving in social interactions, especially in the workplace (Goleman 1998). This continual improvement results in ongoing professional development. In fact, emotional intelligence is associated with superior work performance (Goleman 1998).

Emotional intelligence is receiving attention in the nursing and healthcare literature (Akerjordet & Severinsson 2007, McCallin & Bamford 2007, Skinner & Spurgeon 2005, McQueen 2004, Henderson 2001). Emotional intelligence is evident in stories told by nurses that reveal how they use their knowledge (Kooker et al 2007). Other research findings reveal that emotional intelligence has a positive relationship with the level of clinical performance (Codier et al 2008), nurses seeking a deeper understanding of practice (Askerjordet & Severinsson 2004) and nurses choosing collaborative solutions in conflict situations (Jordan & Troth 2002).

Emotional labour

One aspect of being emotionally intelligent is the ability to self-regulate and manage emotional responses, especially in relation to the context in which they occur. The link between this dimension of emotional intelligence and the concept of 'emotional labour' has been made in the nursing literature (McQueen 2004). Emotional labour involves keeping natural emotional responses concealed in order to demonstrate an emotional response that is in keeping with the context of service provision (Hochschild 1983). Such labour involves regulating and displaying emotions that are considered professionally desirable (Larson & Yao 2005).

Nurses do learn to appropriately manage their emotional responses to patients, especially when there is a perceived gap between what they *do* feel and what they believe they should feel (Smith 1992). For example, if nurses respond to physical deformity of a patient with disgust, they hide these feelings from the patient as they serve little useful purpose in trying to be of help. In this sense, emotional labour is considered to be necessary to therapeutic relationships (McQueen 2004).

Emotional labour involves regulating one's emotions along with employing what is called 'surface acting' and 'deep acting' (Hochschild 1983). Surface acting is the overt expression of an emotion not felt by the person, yet thought to be needed in the situation. For example, if a nurse is feeling overtaxed by a heavy workload and a patient apologetically asks for help, stating 'So sorry to bother you …', a nurse may conceal their stress and say 'no bother at all' in a calm, pleasant manner. Deep acting involves a shift in emotional response within the nurse. For example, taking on a patient's perspective and trying to understand a situation from the patient's perspective may result in the nurse changing their views and feelings about the situation.

Like emotional intelligence, the concept of emotional labour is also receiving attention in the nursing and healthcare literature (Yang & Chang 2007, Mann & Cowburn 2005, Timmons & Tanner 2005, de Raeve 2002, Bolton 2000). The concept has been studied to reveal how this type of work may affect retention of nurses (Yang & Chang 2007) and work-related stress (Mikolajczak et al 2007, Mann & Cowburn 2005) in an effort to reveal the potential negative effects of this type of work. In contrast, a recent study of medical doctors revealed that emotional labour can have both positive and negative effects on wellbeing at work (Martinez-Inigo et al 2007).

While the link between the self-regulation of emotional intelligence and emotional labour has been made (McQueen 2004), Goleman (1998) asserts that emotional labour is not sufficient to explain the self-regulation of emotional intelligence and its effect on job performance. This may be because the workers in the original study on emotional labour (Hocshchild 1983) suppressed their emotions in service to their company, so money was not lost through poor customer service. In contrast, nurses are called to manage their emotions at work in service to the patient. The work satisfaction that is felt when enacting a professionally compassionate role, in keeping with the ideals of a caring profession, is the reward nurses often receive when they manage emotions in service to the patient.

Emotional labour has been criticised in the nursing literature as problematic because inauthentic behaviour, as occurs in surface acting or 'faking it', could disrupt the building of trust in the patient–nurse relationship (de Raeve 2002) (see Ch 2). One recent study demonstrated how nurses did manage a 'work persona' and a 'personal persona' to both the patients' and their own benefit (Macintosh 2007). The nurses in another study (Bolton 2000) not only engaged in emotional labour, but also emotional work through empathy (Ch 6) that was offered as a form of authentic caring behaviour. Emotional labour has been linked to the expression of empathy in other clinical situations as well (Larson & Yao 2005).

The complexities of emotion in nursing work are acknowledged and understood through concepts of emotional intelligence and emotional labour. Both concepts highlight the importance of self-awareness and self-understanding when nurses are interacting with patients.

THE IMPORTANCE OF SELF-UNDERSTANDING

An understanding of self in relation to patients, termed *personal knowing* (Carper 1978), is considered fundamental to the formation of therapeutic relationships in nursing. Personal knowing assists nurses in attending to the mutual relationship, not simply the patient in the relationship. A failure to take into account the effects nurses themselves have on patients, and their relationships with them, can lead to mistaken assumptions and judgments about what patients are experiencing.

Personal knowing, referred to here as self-understanding, is developed for the purpose of becoming authentic, congruent and open with patients. If nurses are authentic with patients, they are sincere and genuine, not only as people who care what happens to patients, but also as people who are unafraid to show that they are human. The more nurses are aware of themselves, the more likely it is that their interpersonal skills will be used in an authentic and natural manner. Self-understanding enables nurses to act in ways that are in harmony with who they are, and congruent with and true to their unique nature and style. Openness with patients is the ability to accept patients as they are, rather than how nurses may want them to be.

Consider the following story:

Sylvia is an experienced registered nurse who prides herself on her ability to care for seriously injured and impaired victims of brain damage. Peter had become one of those patients whom all the nurses on Sylvia's ward had come to dislike. He was labelled as uncooperative and difficult. Because some alleged his injuries had been self-inflicted, he engendered little sympathy from the nursing staff. They did not like caring for Peter and often complained bitterly to each other about their negative feelings towards him.

One day during change-of-shift report, Sylvia began to listen to her colleagues' complaints and negative judgments about Peter. She had been thinking about how some patients are labelled as difficult because of a journal article that she read. She came to realise that Peter had fallen into this unfortunate category. To her colleagues' relief and surprise, she asked to be assigned to care for Peter. Little did they realise that Sylvia was challenging herself to try and understand Peter as a person rather than a label.

That day when she entered his room she noticed, for the first time, the frightened and uncomfortable look on this young man's face. His primary manner of communication was through blinking his eyes as he had sustained an unstable neck injury. His hands were restrained because he was in the habit of pulling at tubes and equipment. Sylvia stood there for a moment, noticing and absorbing his situation.

Without even thinking, she suddenly realised the cool temperature of the room and noticed that Peter had nothing more than a light sheet draped over his naked body. She looked at him and said, 'I bet you are cold'. His eyes blinked furiously in the affirmative. She immediately went to get him a warm blanket. The look of relief on his face was incredible. Throughout the entire time, no one had noticed that Peter was cold. They did not notice because they had failed to perceive him as a person.

Sylvia no longer could say 'no' to the 'personhood' of Peter by thinking of him as a label. She began to question the dynamics that had led the nursing staff to label Peter and dismiss him as troublesome and difficult. Through reflection Sylvia had become more self-aware. Her awareness allowed her to put aside the labels used about Peter and to attend to his comfort needs.

This story highlights the importance of self-understanding—through active reflection and open acknowledgment Sylvia was able to take corrective action. Sometimes, nurses try to deny the existence of negative patient labels, claiming that such evaluations are unprofessional and therefore unacceptable. They do so in the erroneous belief that nurses, by virtue of being professional people, can rise above their natural human tendency to judge, or that at least nurses can put such judgments aside so that they do not interfere with their nursing care. Such denial is unfortunate because it diminishes self-understanding. Furthermore, there is empirical evidence that nurses' judgments about patients can and do influence patient care.

The results of numerous studies demonstrate how nurses' attitudes and interpersonal behaviour towards patients are affected by judgments made about patients. The judgments were based on patients' characteristics such as: the nature of their disease; their understanding of the situation and expressed interest; similarity of their values and nurses' values; social skills; ability to communicate; and gratitude for care (McAllister et al 2002, Woodward 1999, Olsen 1997, Carveth 1995, Grief & Elliott 1994, Forrest 1989, Baer & Lowery 1987, Armstrong-Esther & Browne 1986, Drew 1986, Sayler & Stuart 1985, Kelly & May 1982).

Johnson and Webb (1995a) found that nurses do judge the social worth of patients and that such judgment does have moral consequences. Nevertheless, their findings from a field study of nursing indicate that social evaluations of patients are not simply tied to personal characteristics of patients and their individual circumstances (e.g. bearing responsibility for their illness). Referring to the process as 'social judgement', Johnson and Webb (1995a, 1995b) describe a complex and dynamic system whereby evaluations of patients' social worth is negotiated and renegotiated throughout their interactions with nurses. That is, nurses' evaluations of patients can and do change over time.

More recent studies have shown how nurses make efforts to provide compassionate care even with patients for whom they feel little sympathy (McCann et al 2007, Camilli & Martin 2005). McCann et al (2007) found that nurses working in emergency departments held sympathetic views towards patients who have deliberately harmed themselves, and, more importantly, they did not discriminate against such people when providing care.

The evidence suggests that it is useful to encourage nurses to actively reflect on their evaluative perceptions of patients rather than deny or ignore that their judgments can and do affect patient care. Once negative evaluations are brought in to conscious awareness, nurses can explore their meaning and, like Sylvia in the story, take corrective action if necessary. Reflection will not prevent negative evaluations, but it will assist nurses in challenging or altering them.

The more nurses know about themselves, the more it is likely that they will come to accept themselves. The more nurses understand about themselves, the easier it becomes for them to understand patients. The more tolerant nurses are of themselves, the more tolerant they can be of patients. The more comfortable nurses are with themselves, the more comfortable they can be with patients. It is through coming to accept and understand their own perspective that nurses can come to accept and understand patients' perspectives. As nurses come to know their own experiences as human beings, they are better able to relate to the person who is the patient.

Self-understanding helps nurses to build emotional intelligence and a healthy self-concept. Self-understanding can lead to comfort with the self, and genuine liking of the self. This is no easy task to achieve. It often takes a long time and a person's relationship with the self is dynamic, not static.

Liking oneself is not the same as thinking one is all-good, without faults or failings. Liking oneself is about knowing one's strengths and areas for improvement, putting these together and concluding that what exists is acceptable, along with a continuous desire to grow and learn. When nurses know, understand and like themselves, they are less likely to hide behind their professional role, and more likely to make contact with patients on a genuinely human level.

Self-awareness versus self-consciousness

Completing Activity 3.1 often engenders feelings of self-consciousness and discomfort in people. This is because focusing on the self, especially the positive aspects, is usually a private affair and 'seeing yourself on paper', even when it is not shared with anyone else, brings the private into the open and often creates a sense of self-exposure and vulnerability.

Activity 3.1 WHAT DO I HAVE TO OFFER PATIENTS?   ➡301

PROCESS

1 Divide a blank piece of paper into two columns. In the first column, record a description of those aspects of yourself that you think are positive—ones you like about yourself. In the second column, describe those aspects of yourself that you would prefer to change—ones you do not always like about yourself. You do not need to share this list with anybody else. Be as honest as possible with yourself.

2 From your list of positive aspects, in the first column of your paper, reflect on how you could put these aspects to use in caring for and relating to patients.

3 From your list of negative aspects, in the second column of your paper, reflect on how these may affect your relationships with patients, for better or for worse.

4 Write a brief summary of how you could use your personal self in developing your professional self.

DISCUSSION

1 Which was easier: describing positive aspects of yourself or negative ones?

2 Which column contains more information?

- Frequently, when completing activities such as this, it is difficult to separate the 'you' that you want to be (ideal self) from the 'you' that exists (real self). How true was this for you in completing the activity?

- Ask someone who knows you well and whom you trust to describe what they see as positive and negative aspects about you. Compare what they say with your list and reflect on similarities and differences.

In bringing the self into awareness, even through an activity such as this, there is a danger of becoming preoccupied with self and uncomfortably self-conscious. Self-awareness can result in self-consciousness. There needs to be a balance between the self-consciousness that is experienced through focusing too much on self, and the lack of self-understanding that leads to alienation from the self. Achieving this balance is important for nurses because the risks of focusing too much on themselves are as great as the dangers of failing to take themselves into account at all.

Egan (2007) refers to the need to be 'productively self-conscious' when engaged in helping relationships. Productive self-consciousness has positive effects because it is the ability to be absorbed in an interaction, while simultaneously being aware of internal reactions and perceptions. It is the ability to raise self-understanding to a level that enhances reflection on the self, while not becoming so preoccupied with the self that there is a lack of ability to focus on the person being helped.

The relationship between self-understanding and professional growth

Nurses need to be able to evaluate how effectively they are relating to patients and self-understanding is essential in this assessment. Evaluation of performance in the use of the skills presented in the following chapters is best achieved through the process of self-assessment. In assessing their performance, nurses begin with an awareness of how they are interacting with patients. Through consideration of their *intentions*, *actions*, *responses* and *reactions*, nurses are able to evaluate their own performance in the interest of learning how to be more effective. Self-understanding is not simply a matter of perceiving the self as is; it is also a process of encouraging self-growth to become more effective in relating to patients. It would be irresponsible for nurses simply to accept themselves and not challenge themselves to change and grow through their nursing experiences. Through challenge comes change, and nurses willing to challenge themselves are open to personal and professional growth.

DEVELOPING THE SELF AS A THERAPEUTIC AGENT

When relating to patients therapeutically, nurses are deliberately using their interactions for the benefit of patients. This is the conscious 'use of self' as a therapeutic agent as nurses make choices and decisions in their interactions.

Benner et al (1996) define a nurse's clinical agency as an understanding of one's impact on what happens to the patient. A sense of agency is needed to influence and guide patients (Ch 8). Most importantly, this sense of agency develops through continual learning as a result of clinical experience.

In developing this sense of agency, nurses need to become aware of what they have to offer patients (e.g. they need to know their personal strengths and their personal areas for improvement). Self-understanding enables nurses to view themselves as human beings with failures, faults, successes and strengths—as people who have something to offer patients.

Self-understanding is an essential ingredient in the development of the nurse as a therapeutic agent. It is unlikely that nurses, or anyone else for that matter, will ever fully know and appreciate all facets of themselves. Nevertheless, nurses can develop their capabilities to engage in self-reflection, to perceive and accept input from others, and to openly disclose themselves to others to increase their self-understanding. In fact, engaging in these processes and being motivated to keep improving are essential to becoming emotionally intelligent (Goleman 1998).

When considering how to increase self-understanding, the process of introspection, or self-reflection, often comes to mind. This often begins with noticing what elicits a personal response. 'Why did I react negatively when that patient told me he wanted to die? Why did I want to leave the room? Was it that I felt helpless, or unsure about how to respond? Do I believe that self-destructive thoughts are unacceptable? Have I ever felt this way before? Why did I find it so hard to listen to what he was saying?' Often when something or somebody spurs a response, the tendency is to look to that person or thing, rather than to reflect on the self. Noticing and reflecting on thoughts about oneself involves introspection, which is one of the principal ways that self-understanding develops.

Paying attention to such thoughts and feelings (i.e. allowing them to enter into rather than forcing them out of awareness) encourages nurses to discover more about themselves. Introspection and listening to oneself mean trusting oneself, being honest with oneself, accepting oneself and sometimes challenging oneself. Nevertheless, introspection is only effective in increasing self-understanding when personal thoughts and feelings are used for the purpose of discovering more about oneself.

Many nurses interpret the need to maintain control over their emotions, as in the self-management of emotional labour, to mean that they should be void of emotions. Rather than deny their emotional responses, although they may be concealed from patients, it is better for nurses to be aware of and reflect on such reactions. Without awareness, it is likely that these emotions will be expressed inadvertently to patients. Nurses who keep in tune with their emotional responses have a greater chance of maintaining true control than those who try to control emotions by ignoring them.

More importantly, nurses' feelings and reactions to patients serve a purpose— they provide useful information in measuring how the relationship with a patient is progressing. For example, anger and frustration towards a patient, when left unexamined, may lead to labelling that patient. It could be that the feelings of anger and frustration are a result of the nurse's inability to understand what the patient is experiencing. Perhaps the patient is not conforming to the nurse's expectations of a 'good patient'. A host of other possibilities exist. Self-reflection enables nurses to discover what their emotional reactions might be revealing about *their* relationships with patients. Reflecting on personal thoughts and feelings triggered through interaction with patients provides useful sources of information about oneself.

REFLECTION AND REFLECTIVE PRACTICE

Reflection is an active exploration of personal experiences, consciously employed for the purpose of making sense of those experiences. Some people naturally engage in reflective processes, thinking deeply on life and their experiences of it. Other people may need guidance and assistance to be reflective. Professional nurses often are encouraged to engage in reflection because nursing knowledge is embedded in practical experience.

A spirit of inquiry sparks reflective nurses to think about their actions as they are engaged in clinical practice. In this sense, reflection is a way of functioning; it involves a here-and-now pursuit to make sense of the everyday world of nursing practice as it unfolds. This is reflection that 'looks on'. Reflection also involves thinking about experiences after they have occurred; this involves a there-and-then thinking process in order to use experience for the purpose of learning. This is reflection that 'looks back'. Reflection is also important prior to experience (Gustafson & Fagerberg 2004, Greenwood 1993), as nurses consider their intentions and plans for patient care. This is reflection that 'looks forward'.

Regardless of whether it occurs before, during or after clinical practice, reflection is a process for understanding and appreciating experiences (Clarke et al 1996). This is especially true when experiences are novel and/or formidable. Nurses do tend to reflect more when they consider care as troublesome (e.g. when there is an unexpected patient outcome) (Gustafson & Fagerberg 2004). More importantly, reflection is a way of challenging and changing perspectives (Peden-McAlpine et al 2005, Smith & Jack 2005, Taylor et al 2005, Gustafson & Fagerberg 2004, Atkins & Murphy 1993), the purpose of which is to improve practice. Such improvements are aided and enhanced by linking reflections to theory. In this sense, reflective processes accompany learning, encouraging nurses to develop theoretical understandings that will serve as guides for future action. They promote continuous professional development and the courage to try different approaches.

In addition to developing new insight and understanding, reflection has been shown to enhance nurses' capacity for empathy and appreciation of the uniqueness of the patient (Gustafson & Fagerberg 2004). In this sense, reflection is a process used both to protect the patient as a person (Maggs & Biley 2000) and to promote interpersonal competence in the nurse.

While the above studies do hold promise that reflection can result in learning and actual changes in practice, a study by Mantzoukas and Jasper (2004) demonstrated that nurses acknowledged the importance of reflection, yet they felt constrained in using reflection because ward culture invalidated reflective practice as a means of improving practice. Likewise, the participants in another study reported that while they engaged in reflective practice, they were unsure whether the process resulted in increasing their sense of clinical competence (Cirocco 2007). While there is evidence that reflection results in learning (e.g. Peden-McAlpine et al 2005, Taylor et al 2005), more empirical evidence is needed as to whether reflection actually results in changes to practice.

Nurses can reflect on various aspects of practice: the technical (e.g. treatment regimes); the practical (e.g. routines in care); the social and political (e.g. how healthcare resources are expended); and the personal (e.g. knowledge of the self) (Clarke et al 1996). 'The focus of reflection is *the self* within the context of the specific practice situation' (Johns 1999 p 242). In this respect, the processes of reflection are closely related to increasing self-understanding. Nevertheless, a certain amount of self-understanding is required for reflection to occur in the first place (Atkins & Murphy 1993).

Processes for reflection

Effective reflection requires active strategies to support the process (Maggs & Biley 2000, Wilkinson 1999, Johns 1995). This means that most successful reflection is accompanied by structured activities, such as keeping a professional diary or completing the activities in this book. Unless there is some means of tracking an individual nurse's reflections over a period of time, sustainable professional growth through reflection may be difficult to attain.

With increasing frequency, clinical supervision (Ch 11) is considered by many as an ideal method to encourage and support reflective practice (Kim 1999, Fowler 1998). Clinical supervision, whether conducted individually or in groups of nurses, is aimed at using reflective processes for the purpose of improving the quality of nursing care. It has been shown to be useful in the development of interpersonal skills (Tichen & Binnie 1995) and in increasing self-understanding (Begat et al 1997).

Pitfalls in reflection

Despite its obvious benefits, reflection does have its potential pitfalls. It is important to remember that effective reflection will inevitably lead to anxiety (Haddock & Bassett 1997) because the process of reflecting involves change and challenge. It requires nurses to show a willingness to be challenged to view experiences in different lights and to reconsider what may be long-held and cherished beliefs. The anxiety and discomfort that accompanies effective reflection points to the need for support systems to be in place (e.g. colleagues who serve as skilled facilitators and mentors) (Foster & Greenwood 1998, Carr 1996).

Another pitfall relates to the difficulty of reflecting after an event has taken place. This difficulty is called 'hindsight bias' (Jones 1995), a term that describes the way that people recall events that fit with the known outcome. For example, if a nurse were to interact with a patient who seemed distressed about a forthcoming procedure, only to discover that the distress involved another life event, then it would be difficult in retrospect for the nurse to recall that they initially associated the patient distress with the procedure. The nurse's recall of events would match what they now understand, not what was originally thought.

Taylor (1997) cautions nurses in the wholehearted embrace of reflection as a way of changing practice through empowerment and emancipation of nurses. The structural arrangements that are required for such emancipation may not be easy to attain, and reflection alone does not guarantee success in making such structural changes. In fact, reflective practices may result in nurses feeling less empowered by systems of healthcare delivery.

A final pitfall in the use of reflection is perhaps the most challenging of all in relation to beginning practitioners and students of nursing. It is that a nurse may need to be clinically experienced in order to benefit from reflection (Fowler 1998). This implies that the nurses who most need to learn in terms of clinical experience may be least able to benefit from the process of reflection. Nevertheless, structured reflection, especially under the guidance of a more experienced nurse, is a useful way for beginning nurses to assess their own interpersonal skills and to improve self-understanding through raised awareness of the impact of self on nursing practice.

Input from others/interactive reflection

There are limits to how far self-understanding can progress and develop through the use of introspection alone. Natural 'blind spots', the ease with which self-reflective thoughts can be ignored, dismissed and defended, along with the tendency to protect the self through self-deception, pose barriers in the use of the introspective process.

Other people provide useful information through the way they react and respond. For this reason, another effective way to complement, not replace, self-reflection occurs when nurses attend to feedback from others, be it solicited or unsolicited. Feedback from good friends is useful and can be solicited. Feedback from patients is another useful source of information, although nurses usually do not solicit it.

Input from patients

Patients are not only expressing information about themselves when they interact with nurses, they also are expressing information about how they perceive the nurse. Patients reveal how they feel and what they think about the nurses who are interacting with them by the manner in which they behave. What they choose to discuss, how freely they disclose information and how comfortable they seem during an interaction are examples of input that patients provide about how they see the nurse. The cues that indicate the effect nurses are having on them automatically surface throughout interactions. Nurses need to be receptive to such input from patients because this feedback informs them about themselves. In this regard, nurses need not actively solicit patient feedback.

Perceiving such input from patients begins with an awareness and understanding of its relevance. Next, nurses need to be open to receiving the information. Asking themselves questions such as, 'What is it about me that enables patients to openly express their feelings?', 'Why is this patient telling *me* this?' and 'Have *I* inadvertently communicated that I do not wish to hear what this patient is saying?' enables nurses to become open to input from patients.

It is natural for nurses to ignore or reject input and feedback about themselves when this information lacks congruence with personal images (what nurses believe they are or want to be). Nurses who are feeling inept may not notice when patients reveal that they *are* quite effective. For this reason, feedback and input from others, especially patients, may challenge nurses to reconsider their current perspectives.

Activity 3.2 FEEDBACK FROM PATIENTS

PROCESS

1 Reflect on a recent interaction with a patient. Record what happened between you and the patient.

2 Describe how this patient responded to you.

3 Through reflection about how this patient responded, try to determine what this patient was 'telling' you about how they perceived you.

4 Discuss the situation and your experience with another participant.

DISCUSSION

1 What are the various ways that participants interpreted how patients responded to them? What cues indicated these responses?

2 At the time of the interaction with the patient, how aware were participants that patients were actually revealing how they perceived the nurse?

3 How many participants described negative/ineffective interactions? How many described positive/effective ones? What does this say?

Self-sharing

Another process that is effective in increasing self-understanding arises out of a combination of self-reflection (introspection) and interactive reflection (input and feedback from others). It is the process of self-sharing—the disclosure of personal thoughts, feelings, perceptions and interpretations by openly expressing them to others.

How self-sharing increases self-understanding

Self-sharing enhances self-understanding because it triggers (and therefore solicits) feedback from others, and also because it intensifies self-reflection. When internal thoughts, feelings and attitudes are made external through open discussion, they are often internally clarified, expanded and accepted. Sometimes, self-sharing persuades nurses to internally challenge and alter their thoughts, feelings and attitudes. In this sense, self-sharing often transforms into a process of 'thinking aloud', and then having a dialogue with the self while using the other person as a sounding board.

At other times, self-sharing enables nurses to test the validity of their current thoughts, feelings and attitudes. In 'testing' their internal responses, nurses are asking others what they think or feel about these responses. This often leads nurses to reconsider their responses in light of what others think and feel.

The relationship between self-sharing and self-understanding is a circular one (see Fig 3.2). While a certain degree of self-understanding is helpful to begin self-sharing, it is not vital. Through self-sharing, further input is received, both from others and from the self, which is then useful in increasing self-understanding.

FIGURE 3.2 Relationship between self-sharing and self-understanding

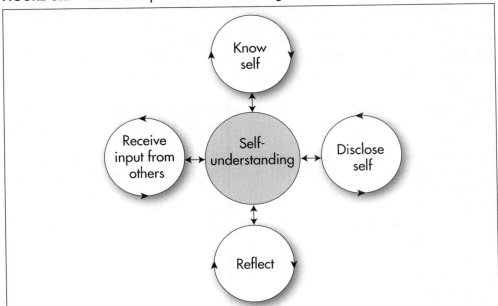

Risks of self-sharing

Despite its potential value for increasing self-understanding, disclosing oneself to others is not always easy to do. There are many reasons for keeping oneself to oneself, and choosing not to disclose. Activity 3.3 is designed to uncover some of the reasons why self-sharing may be difficult.

Activity 3.3 DIFFICULTIES IN SELF-SHARING

PROCESS

1 Working on your own, rank each of the following topics from 1 to 12, according to what is easiest for you to disclose about yourself (1) to what is hardest to disclose (12). Place these topics in the context of interacting with someone you do not know very well.
   a Talking about my fears
   b Sharing my hopes and dreams
   c Discussing my family life
   d Describing my previous health problems
   e Stating what I dislike about other people
   f Complaining about a mark on an assignment
   g Expressing my political views
   h Stating what I want or need
   i Expressing confusion or uncertainty

   j Describing how I like to be treated by others

   k Complaining about being treated unfairly

   l Telling others that I am not pleased about something they have done

2 Review your answers to step 1 and reflect on those items that you determined as easy to discuss (those ranked 1–5). Record your reasons for evaluating these items as easy to disclose.

3 Review your answers to step 1 and reflect on those items that you determined as difficult to disclose (those ranked 8–12). Record your reasons for evaluating these items as difficult to disclose.

4 Compare your responses with two other participants. Discuss your responses to steps 2 and 3. Summarise what is easy to disclose and what is hard to disclose, focusing on your reasons why this is so.

5 This step lists some of the reasons for lack of self-disclosure. Working individually, rate each of these reasons in terms of how often it is true for you. Use the following descriptions:

● Often

● Sometimes

● Rarely

If I tell others what I think and feel …

   a I may hurt them

   b They may take advantage of me

   c I may appear weak

   d I may become emotional

   e They may hurt me

   f They may talk to others about me

   g I may discover something about myself that I'd rather not know

   h They may use what I've said against me

   i I may discover problems I never knew I had

6 Working in the same groups of three as for step 4, discuss those items that you rated as 'Often' and 'Sometimes'. What similarities are there in your responses? What differences are there?

DISCUSSION

1 What are the major reasons for reluctance to self-disclose?

2 What are the major disadvantages in self-disclosure? What are the major advantages?

3 How does self-disclosure promote self-awareness?

The major difficulty in disclosing self is the exposure that it brings. Once people are exposed, they often feel vulnerable—especially if the disclosure has been about problem areas or negative thoughts, feelings and perceptions. There are risks of being rejected, being hurt and being challenged by others. This sense of vulnerability is not necessarily destructive to nurses because of its potential to increase feelings of empathy with patients, who often feel exposed and vulnerable when they disclose themselves to nurses. While there are obvious risks in exposing self, these are offset by its potential benefits.

The climate conducive to self-sharing

Because of the exposure and vulnerability that self-sharing can bring, it needs to take place in an atmosphere of trust and respect—trust in the sense that the disclosure will not be met with rejection and respect in the sense that disclosed information will be considered, and not dismissed or ridiculed.

As a general rule, there is ease and comfort with disclosure when it is likely that personal thoughts, feelings and attitudes will be understood and appreciated by the other person. This is more likely to happen when the other person shares similar experiences. For this reason, nurses often benefit by disclosing themselves to other nurses (see Ch 11). Through the process of self-sharing, nurses can be supported by other nurses. They also may be challenged at times to reconsider their perceptions, thoughts and feelings.

Self-disclosure with patients

Self-disclosure with patients (see Chs 5, 6 and 7) is different from self-sharing. Self-disclosure with patients is employed as a therapeutic skill and is therefore for the benefit of the patient, not the nurse. Although self-disclosure with patients may result in increased self-understanding for the nurse, this is not its primary focus. The intent of self-disclosing with patients is to promote interaction and increase interpersonal involvement with patients. The primary intent of self-sharing with people other than patients is increased self-understanding in the nurse.

AREAS OF SELF-EXPLORATION

It is important that nurses not only understand the processes for promoting greater self-understanding, but also that they recognise those areas of themselves that are most relevant to the nursing-care context. There are many facets of each nurse's personal self that are woven together to create the essence of the person who is the nurse. While many aspects of the self can be considered, those addressed in Activity 3.4 have a potential to affect the way that nurses approach helping patients.

Activity 3.4 BELIEFS ABOUT HELPING IN NURSING PRACTICE →301

PROCESS

For each of the following statements, record on a separate sheet of paper the response that most closely identifies your personal beliefs and attitudes. Use the following scale:

   3 For the most part, I *agree* with this statement

   2 I am *undecided* in my opinion about this statement

   1 For the most part, I *disagree* with this statement

   a Patients should be encouraged to accept that they have contributed to their own health problems.

   b What happens in patient–nurse relationships is more the nurse's responsibility than the patient's.

c   People are masters of their own destinies; solutions to whatever problems they have are in their own hands.

d   There are many social factors contributing to health problems that are beyond individual control.

e   Whether they realise it or not, people engage in behaviours that cause health problems.

f   Effective health education could prevent major health problems.

g   Patients should be encouraged to find solutions and take action on their own behalf when dealing with health problems.

h   It irritates me when I hear somebody say that patients caused their own health problems; most of the time people can't help it.

i   Providing advice to patients is an essential aspect of effective healthcare.

j   In my view of human nature, people are responsible for creating their problems.

k   People should be presented with options for healthcare so that they can choose what suits them best.

l   In recovering from an illness, it is essential that patients heed the advice of healthcare professionals.

m   Patients' health problems are most often of their own making.

n   Most people could change their problematic health habits if they really wanted to.

o   Patients cannot be held responsible for causing their own health problems.

p   Patients should determine their own goals when working with healthcare professionals.

q   Most health problems are the result of the personal choices people make in conducting their lives.

r   I don't have much time for patients who won't follow the advice of knowledgeable healthcare experts.

s   Diseases and illnesses are largely a result of biological and genetic factors, which are usually beyond individual control.

t   Patients should place themselves in the hands of qualified health professionals who know best what to do about health problems.

DISCUSSION

1   Reflect on your responses and consider whether you tend to hold people responsible for their health problems.

2   Consider your responses in light of whether you tend to think that people should take responsibility for their own healthcare.

3   In general, what do your responses reflect about your beliefs about health and healthcare?

Personal philosophy about health

Personal value systems, the 'shoulds' and 'ought tos' that direct individual behaviour, are part of all people's lives. These values and beliefs, which are personal and unique to the individual, assist a person in making choices and decisions about living. They provide direction about what is important, what matters, what is seen as significant and what is worthwhile. These values and beliefs are not static; they are altered, revised and adapted through life experiences. Nurses often find that their beliefs and values alter throughout their professional lives.

One aspect of personal value systems that is of particular relevance for nurses is their beliefs about health and helping. For example, nurses may feel less inclined to care for patients who they believe are responsible for their own health problems (Olsen 1997).

Activity 3.4 is designed to make participants think about how they would approach helping other people on the basis of two central issues: *blame* and *control* (Brickman et al 1982). Blame is the degree to which people are held responsible for causing their problems and control is the degree to which they are held responsible for solutions to their problems. Both involve questions of personal responsibility, and assumptions about personal responsibility have direct effects on the type of help offered.

Brickman et al (1982) developed four models of helping based on the issues of blame and control (see Fig 3.3). The view from within the 'medical model' is that people are neither responsible for creating their problems, nor are they responsible for solutions to their problems. The 'compensatory model' operates from beliefs that people cannot be blamed for their problems, but are held responsible for doing something about them. Beliefs within the 'enlightenment model' are that people are responsible for creating their problems, but need to rely on others in solving these problems. The 'moral model' holds people responsible for both creating their problems and developing their own solutions.

FIGURE 3.3 Models of helping

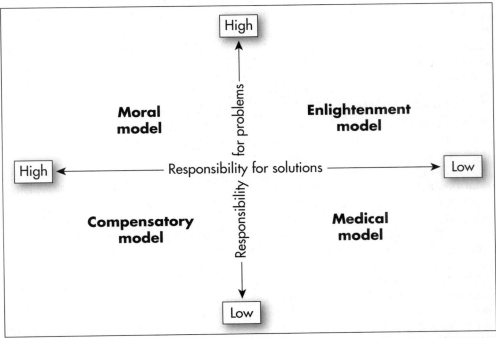

Source: Based on Brickman et al (1982).

Each stance results in an orientation to how to be of help to patients. The 'medical model' relies on expert advice and treats patients as passive recipients of assistance. Patients are expected to seek and heed such advice and assistance.

While people are not blamed for their problems, they may be blamed if they fail to cooperate with the solutions offered. Helping in the 'compensatory model' centres on the mobilisation of needed resources, and providing opportunities to compensate for what are seen as failures and weaknesses that are outside individual control. Acceptance of personal blame and a reliance on an external authority is the helping approach used in the 'enlightenment model'. The 'moral model' focuses helping on motivating people to change through persuasion, appeal, reprimand and reproach (Corey et al 1988, Cronenwett 1983, Brickman et al 1982).

In nursing practice, there is likely to be a mixed application of these models, as illustrated in the following examples. Nurses might hold active smokers responsible for problems such as lung cancer, while lung cancer acquired from passive smoking usually does not bring such blame. In both of these situations, people would not be held responsible for the possible solutions/treatment for the lung cancer. Nursing care would be provided to the active smokers ('enlightenment model'), although some nurses may question the use of healthcare resources on this population ('moral model'). The victims of passive smoking might be approached using the 'medical model', in which case they would not be held responsible for the cause or the solutions. A person with diabetes mellitus may not be held responsible for acquiring the disease, but will be expected to be actively involved in its control ('compensatory model'). An actively suicidal person may be blamed for the problem and expected to find solutions through effort and willpower ('moral model').

Help may not be effective if the person desiring help and the person offering help are operating from a different set of assumptions about personal responsibility (Brickman et al 1982). For this reason, it is important that nurses not only realise their own orientation to helping and its underlying assumptions, but also that they are aware of and understand patients' orientations to helping.

Personal values and beliefs

Nurses' personal values and beliefs directly affect their interactions with patients. They have the potential to restrict effective relationships with patients; however, they can also enhance these relationships.

One way that nurses' values and personal beliefs may hinder effective relationships with patients stems from the fact that these values and beliefs often function as perceptual filters. Perceptual filters allow some aspects of patients' stories to be accepted, while others are rejected. When values and personal beliefs function as filters, the skills of listening (see Ch 5) are most affected. Cultural stereotypes (see Ch 4), another possible hindrance in relating effectively with patients, often stem from values and personal beliefs.

Another way that personal values create interference occurs when nurses impose or project them onto patients, rather than keeping them in abeyance. When values and beliefs are imposed on patients, they are used as yardsticks for measuring patients. Whenever nurses make judgments about what patients 'should' or 'should not' be, there is a chance that they are evaluating patients in terms of their own value system. For this reason, nurses are encouraged to reflect on these types of judgments.

On the other hand, certain values and personal beliefs enhance and strengthen nurses' ability to relate to patients. For example, a personal belief that people are capable, worthwhile and dependable works in favour of establishing effective relationships with patients. Such beliefs help to create a climate of respect and regard for patients.

When relating to patients, nurses cannot be expected to abandon their values and personal beliefs; however, they need to be able to distinguish their own philosophical stance from that of a patient. The more aware nurses are of their own values and personal beliefs, the less likely it is that interference will occur, and the more likely it is that the values that enhance effective relationships will be strengthened.

Expectations of nursing

Most nurses enter nursing with some goal in mind. It might be to secure a job with the promise of sustained demand. It could be that part-time work is appealing. An advertisement in the local newspaper might have sparked interest in nursing in a 'Why not, I'm not doing anything else with my life?' fashion. Assuming there were options available, nursing is usually chosen because of an interest in people. In all likelihood this interest in people is directly related to a desire to be of help to them.

Activity 3.5 probably highlights a common myth about nursing: the belief that all benefits in nursing are for the patient, never the nurse. By focusing solely on their desire to help and to assist others, nurses fail to acknowledge the potential benefits of nursing for themselves.

Activity 3.5 EXPECTATIONS OF NURSING

PROCESS

1 Think of all the reasons why you chose nursing as a career. Record these on a sheet of paper. Do not place any identifying information about yourself on the paper.

2 Now complete the following sentences, recording your answers on the same sheet of paper:
   a If I could do anything as a nurse it would be to …
   b In my role as a nurse I see myself as …
   c Nurses help others because they …
   d My greatest disappointment as a nurse would be if I …

3 Collect all the sheets of paper and distribute them among all participants.

4 Record, on a sheet of paper visible to all participants, all the reasons identified by the participants for choosing nursing. If a reason is given by more than one participant, record how many times it is stated.

DISCUSSION

1 Discuss the responses to each of the items in step 2 of the process. Remember, you are not discussing your own responses, but rather the ones of the anonymous participant who authored the paper you received.

2 Do motivations to nurse and expectations of nursing focus exclusively on helping others or are there references to personal gains and benefits?

Activity 3.6 challenges the notion that nurses nurse solely because they are meeting the needs of patients. The 'ideal' nurse is often perceived as self-sacrificing, and so 'other-oriented' that there is a denial of self. Such an ideal does not exist in reality.

Activity 3.6 PERSONAL BENEFITS OF NURSING

PROCESS

1 On a sheet of paper that only you will see, answer the following questions:
   a What does nursing do for you?
   b What do you personally gain through nursing?
   c What benefits are there for you in nursing?
   d How does nursing satisfy you?

2 From your answers and personal reflection, list personal needs that are met through nursing.

DISCUSSION

1 How difficult was it for you to answer these questions?

2 What feelings did you experience while completing the activity?

3 Why is it important for nurses to realise that there are personal gains in nursing?

Personal needs

Forming meaningful relationships with patients and assisting them with health issues and problems often has benefits for nurses as well as patients. For example, nurses derive satisfaction in seeing patients recover from illnesses, especially when they know that they made a difference to the recovery. Does this mean that nurses meet their own needs through their nursing relationships? A recognition and acknowledgment of the personal benefits of nursing results in an affirmative answer to such a question.

Nevertheless, there are obvious risks involved because nurses' personal needs may interfere whenever relationships with patients are used as the *primary* source of meeting these needs. For example, relying on patients to satisfy the nurse's need for personal recognition, appreciation and validation is fraught with danger. For this reason, nurses need to develop awareness of potential trouble spots—those personal needs that may interfere in their relationships with patients.

Activity 3.7 NEEDS THAT MAY INTERFERE

PROCESS

1 Use one of the following descriptions to rate questions a–j:
   ● Hardly ever
   ● Sometimes
   ● Most of the time

How often do I …

    a Let people take advantage of me because I am afraid to say no to their requests?

    b Focus on problems and negative aspects of a situation, so I fail to take into account the positive side of people and their strengths?

    c Feel as if I must 'do something' to make other people feel better—to rescue them?

    d Think I need to have all the answers when other people discuss problems with me?

    e Worry about whether or not other people like me?

    f Feel the need to be needed?

    g Need to be in control of situations?

    h Want other people to take care of me?

    i Feel controlled by other people?

    j Act as openly with other people as I want them to act with me?

2 Review your answers. If the majority of your answers are 'Sometimes', go back and change them to either 'Hardly ever' or 'Most of the time'. All of the items will be true for most people *some* of the time!

3 Identify the items that are 'Hardly ever' and 'Most of the time'. Reflect on these in terms of how these aspects of yourself may affect your relationships with patients.

DISCUSSION

1 The items included in this self-assessment relate to three general areas of basic human needs: the need to feel attached to other people (included); the need to be in control; and the need for affection and affirmation from other people. Which one of these general areas of personal needs is predominant for you?

2 Discuss each of the three basic human needs and how, if they are predominant in a nurse, interactions and relationships with patients may be affected, for better or worse.

CHARACTERISTICS THAT HELP INTERPERSONAL CONNECTEDNESS

The focus of the preceding sections of this chapter has been on increasing self-awareness because such reflection leads to self-understanding, self-challenge and eventual acceptance of aspects that characterise each nurse. Other than considering how these aspects of the self potentially affect relationships with patients, no effort has been made to evaluate them (or the nurse they characterise) in terms of right/wrong, good/bad or desirable/undesirable. No evaluation has been attempted because nurses must first develop awareness of 'what is' before considering 'what should be'. Understanding 'what is' provides a starting point—a reference from which to work towards 'what should be'.

There are certain characteristics, personal beliefs, values and orientations towards helping that enhance nurses' abilities to relate effectively to patients. In this regard, they are the 'what should bes'. When they are present in the nurse, these characteristics help to facilitate interpersonal connections with patients because they help to create the necessary interpersonal climate for the development of patient–nurse relationships. The presence of this climate enables nurses to effectively use the skills and processes described in this book. If the facilitative climate is absent, the use of the skills may become hollow, mechanical and artificial.

From Activity 3.8, you may discover that people perceived to be helpful embody certain characteristics (what they are), demonstrate certain skills (what they do) and possess a degree of understanding about people (what they know). It is the personal characteristics associated with helpful people that are discussed here.

Activity 3.8 CHARACTERISTICS OF EFFECTIVE HELPERS

PROCESS

1 Think of someone in your life who you think is helpful to you (i.e. the person you go to for understanding, assistance and guidance).

2 Think about what this person is like. What personal characteristics do they possess? Focus on specific characteristics that are helpful to you. Describe these on a sheet of paper.

3 Now think about what this person does that you find helpful. What specific things does this person do? Describe these on your sheet of paper. Do not be concerned if there are similarities between answers to steps 2 and 3. In some instances, your answers may be exactly the same.

4 Review what you have written. Briefly summarise what, in your opinion, enables this person to be effective in helping you.

5 Compare your descriptions with those of all other participants by compiling an overall description of a person who is helpful. Record this in a place visible to all participants.

6 Select key words from the description and record them.

DISCUSSION

1 What are the similarities in participants' individual descriptions? What are the differences?

2 Focusing on the key words identified in step 6 of the process, describe personal characteristics that are essential for being a helpful person.

3 Is there anything you would add to this list of personal characteristics?

Characteristics that enhance the ability to be helpful include:
- authenticity and congruence
- respect and warmth, and
- confidence and assertiveness.

Self-understanding enables these characteristics to be fully realised and developed by nurses.

Authenticity and congruence

To be authentic means that nurses behave in ways that are reflective of their true selves. Authenticity means not hiding behind the role of nurse, but rather enacting the role in a manner that expresses the uniqueness of each nurse.

Frequently, when nurses try to use the skills described in this book, feelings of awkwardness and lack of authenticity accompany their first attempts. This is especially true if the skill being tried is unfamiliar and foreign to the nurse's current repertoire of skills. While a skill may be unfamiliar, the personal values from which it emerges may not be. For example, a nurse may be unaccustomed to reflecting feelings (see Ch 6) because of being raised in an environment where feelings were hardly ever expressed and never discussed openly. Unless this nurse believes that patients' feelings are important to understand and comes to realise that, for some patients, feelings are the most significant facet of their experience, the nurse may fail to try to use feeling reflections with patients. This nurse must tap into the authentic desire to help patients in order to overcome feelings of reluctance and awkwardness. That is, a genuine desire to be of help spurs the nurse to express concern and regard for patients through the use of (the skill of) reflecting feelings.

Congruence is related to authenticity because with congruence comes consistency between what nurses believe, how they feel and what they do. The skills described in this book are only effective if they are used in conjunction with an attitude that matches their intent. There is little point in pretending to listen through appropriate attending behaviour (see Ch 5) if a nurse is not currently interested in what a patient is expressing. A listening posture without an attitude of genuine interest lacks congruence. Attempting to understand (see Ch 6) without an open attitude to the uniqueness of each patient's experience also lacks congruence. A congruent manner is one in which the nurse's intent and related action are in harmony with each other.

The nurse's self-understanding is the key to demonstrating both authenticity and congruence. Without understanding and acceptance of who they are and how they are feeling at a given moment, and an examination of personal motives and intentions, nurses are at risk of losing touch with themselves. Authenticity and congruence cannot be demonstrated under such circumstances.

Respect and warmth

With respect comes a deep concern for patients' individual experiences—an acceptance of their perspective and feelings. Respect emerges from the value that each human being has inherent worth and dignity. Under conditions of respect, patients are more likely to feel free in expressing who they are and what they are experiencing. When they are respected, patients are free to be themselves; they need not fear that they will be placed against a standard of what they 'should' be experiencing.

Holding personal judgments in abeyance (see Ch 5) is one of the most striking ways nurses convey respect to patients. This highlights and reinforces the need for self-understanding. Unless nurses are cognisant of their personal values and beliefs, they may inadvertently judge patients against a personal value system.

Respect operates from an attitude of 'being for' patients. To be respectful is to assume the patient's goodwill (Egan 2007), and to believe that patients are doing their best to cope, to adapt and to change. Respect upholds an inherent belief in patients' capabilities and resources. An attitude that is suspicious of patients' motives and behaviours lacks respect if suspicion is the nurse's first reaction.

This is not to say that nurses cannot or should not challenge patients to transform their view of a situation (see Ch 8). Respect means not starting from the point of challenging, but rather developing an understanding of the situation (see Ch 6), then intervening to promote change if this is required.

Warmth is a feeling and is conveyed primarily through non-verbal behaviour that demonstrates an active interest in and regard for patients. It is designed to put patients at ease with nurses because, through the expression of warmth, nurses convey friendliness, approachability and interest. In this way, warmth is an active demonstration of respect because it conveys active concern. Warmth is not emotionally effusive or overly friendly behaviour. It cannot be feigned through insincere overconcern for patients; it requires authenticity and congruence in order to be effective.

Too much warmth creates a sense of false solicitude, lacking genuineness. Patients might become frightened at the prospect of a nurse whose concern seems extreme, especially if this occurs early in the course of the relationship. Too little warmth distances patients because this gives an impression of lack of concern and regard. Judging the 'right' degree of warmth, especially in the beginning of a relationship with a patient, can only be achieved by paying careful attention to how the patient responds to the nurse's demonstration of concern through warmth.

Confidence and assertiveness

Even when nurses are congruent and authentic, and able to convey respect and warmth, unless they also have an ability to express themselves confidently and assertively they may not be able to make interpersonal contact with patients. Knowing what to say and how to say it becomes inconsequential if nurses fail to use interpersonal skills because they are apprehensive and hesitant. Being confident and assertive is as important as being skilled and aware. High-level awareness and excellent technical ability are meaningless unless they are actually used when called for (Egan 2007). For example, nurses need to be assertive when they share perceptions and take the lead in exploring (see Ch 7), and challenge patients to reframe their perceptions (see Ch 8).

Assertiveness is most often presented as a means of resolving conflict (see Ch 10), defending individual rights if they have been violated. However, conflict is not the specific focus here. In the general context of patient–nurse relationships, being assertive means that nurses are able to take advantage of opportunities to make interpersonal contact with patients. While not always recognised, assertiveness and caring are compatible (McCartan & Hargie 2004).

While nurses often recognise the need to be assertive when advocating *for* patients (e.g. when another health professional is disregarding a patient's request), they often express concerns about being assertive *with* patients. Whenever nurses think 'I can't say *that* to a patient', they are experiencing concerns about what will happen. These concerns include a fear of upsetting patients, a discomfort with the expression of feelings, a perception that it is intrusive to ask personal questions and a reticence about delving into the subjective experiences of patients. Apprehensions such as these often inhibit nurses and may even restrict them from meeting their professional responsibilities to patients. For example, if a nurse is reluctant to explore a patient's apparent distress (out of fear of compounding that distress), vital information about the patient's experience may be missed or overlooked.

The concerns that inhibit nurses are often based on faulty assumptions such as 'patients will become *more* upset if asked to discuss their distress', 'nurses should be passive and obedient' and 'it is impolite to discuss sensitive and personal matters with a relative stranger'. In becoming assertive with patients, nurses need to overcome these concerns by challenging these assumptions.

Firstly, nurses do not have the 'power' to 'make' patients more upset simply on the basis of bringing patients' distress into the open (although this is different from abuse of power, which is discussed in Ch 10). When patients are distressed, they are often relieved to share their emotional pain with an interested and understanding nurse. Rather than compounding their tension, open discussion can actually provide comfort. Secondly, while it would be impolite to discuss highly personal matters with a stranger in a social situation, patient–nurse interactions are different from usual social interactions. In caring for patients, nurses need to discuss personal matters with them because this is part of their professional responsibility.

There is more to assertiveness than just being able to bring up sensitive and sometimes troubling subjects. At times, being assertive translates into making the decision 'not' to discuss something. For example, when a patient is coping by maintaining their emotions within manageable limits, a nurse can make an active decision *not* to explore or focus on feelings. Additionally, the discussion of feelings requires trust between patient and nurse (see Ch 6), and a nurse may choose to delay such discussion until trust is established. As long as the decision not to say something is based on an assessment of the situation, rather than the nurse's internal fear, assertiveness is present. Being assertive in relating to patients means that nurses have both the courage to say something and the wisdom to remain silent.

DEVELOPING A PERSONAL STYLE

Authenticity, congruence, respect, warmth and assertiveness are desirable characteristics that each nurse demonstrates in a unique manner. Although these characteristics help to create an interpersonal climate that enhances meaningful connections, they should not be construed as personality prescriptions for nurses. Each nurse develops personal capabilities for relating to patients.

Skills that are useful in establishing these relationships can be learnt and developed. There are certain conditions, such as respect and warmth, which enable nurses to use the skills most effectively. These conditions can be enhanced and developed. There are approaches to helping patients that can be employed (e.g. challenging patients to reframe their experiences) (see Ch 8). These approaches can be understood and developed.

Each nurse finds a way to use the skills, to express the necessary characteristics and to integrate a variety of approaches in a unique expression of that nurse's personality. Some nurses are good at challenging patients, and do so quite effectively and naturally, while other nurses find this approach difficult and are frustrated when they attempt to use it.

In developing a personal style, nurses must learn how to blend the skills and characteristics with their own personalities and to discover how their personal selves merge into their professional selves. A concerted effort to understand, practise and employ the skills results in this blending. Engaging in the processes of self-understanding accelerates the development of a personal style in relating to patients. Nevertheless, some unique challenges arise when nurses attempt to learn and develop the skills of interacting in a manner that is unique to them.

Developing a personal style of relating to patients poses certain learning challenges because beginning nurses have developed a characteristic style of communicating and relating to other people prior to entering nursing practice. Although these familiar patterns of interacting may be comfortable for the individual nurse as a person, they may not be suitable within the nursing context. In learning the skills and developing them for the nursing context, nurses are often challenged to alter or change their customary and usual patterns of interaction. In meeting this challenge, a total transformation of a nurse's particular manner is not necessary because such transformation may not reflect the nurse's personality. Nevertheless, alterations to existing patterns of interacting are often necessary in order to develop a personal style that is both authentic to an individual nurse and appropriate to the context of nursing care. While the person who is the nurse has not changed, the nursing-care context signals the need for a change in approach.

LEARNING THE SKILLS

The following chapters contain descriptions of a range of skills that enable nurses to interact effectively with patients. While theoretical understanding of the skills is a vital aspect of learning, understanding not accompanied by technical know-how in the use of the skills is insufficient. For this reason, learning the skills of interacting with patients is achieved most effectively through the performance of the skills.

Each nurse is encouraged to attempt each of the skills, see how they fit the particular nursing context and determine what alterations can be made to help them fit better. Some of the skills will be familiar and using them will come naturally because they already exist in the nurse's repertoire. Other skills will be foreign and nurses may feel awkward and unnatural when initially attempting to use these skills. Selecting some of the skills because they are comfortable to use and ignoring others because 'they don't feel right' limits practical learning opportunities and potential.

The need to 'unlearn'

More than likely, the skills presented in the following chapters will be recognisable as everyday activities. For example, listening (see Ch 5) is a process that people engage in daily, whether it be effective or ineffective. This familiarity with some skills, however, presents a specific dilemma to nurses as they approach learning how to fit skills into a nursing-care context as well as blending the skills with their personality.

Because nurses have been interacting with other people all of their lives they may believe that they already know how to talk to patients, and they may be disconcerted to find out there is more to learn. But these familiar patterns of interacting may not be effective within the nursing-care context. As a result, some nurses may fail to recognise and appreciate the alterations that may be needed to make their interactions with patients more effective.

Learning how to use interpersonal skills within the nursing-care context is often a matter of 'letting go' of habitual and automatic ways of interacting—ways that have become comfortable. For example, offering advice and giving solutions is a common response to someone who presents a problem. In Chapter 6, this way of responding is shown to be less effective than a response that demonstrates understanding. If offering advice and giving solutions is their customary way of responding to those in need, nurses are challenged to refrain from their usual way of responding. The necessity of letting go of familiar patterns and 'unlearning' ways that may have become entrenched presents a major hurdle in learning and developing effective interactive skills with patients.

Departing from the comfort zone of usual and customary patterns of interacting and attempting new and unfamiliar ways initially results in feelings of being untrue to oneself. Nurses may become confused by this apparent lack of authenticity, which has been discussed as a core condition for effective interactions. Nurses may feel inept, clumsy and overly self-conscious as they struggle to let go of the familiar and to meet the demands of learning new ways of interacting.

Such feelings are often unavoidable during initial attempts to use any new skill and this highlights the need for continuous self-assessment, which raises awareness and understanding of self. Through self-assessment, nurses come to appreciate what they are attempting in their interactions with patients, why they are attempting this and how it is affecting patients. Nurses are encouraged to promote their own growth as people and as nurses, and to challenge growth within themselves by trying various ways of interacting with patients, even when these ways initially feel awkward. With continuing practice, self-understanding and acceptance, as well as patience with the learning process, the skills will eventually become natural. At this point a personal style emerges.

Reactions to learning the skills

Some nurses fail to perceive and appreciate the significance of learning interpersonal skills simply because they *have* been interacting with other people all their lives. These nurses view the skills of interacting with patients as little more than commonsense and 'doing what comes naturally'. Because the skills used when interacting with patients are not exclusive to nursing, these nurses fail to perceive the importance of spending time learning them or recognising how the nursing-care context necessitates an alteration in interaction patterns.

Such reactions fail to take into account the fact that commonsense is not inborn, but learned behaviour. Toddlers do not have the commonsense to recognise the dangers of running onto a street full of moving vehicles. While the commonsense that nurses have developed throughout their lives could assist them in learning the skills, there is also a danger that this commonsense approach may inhibit learning. For example, commonsense may dictate that patients should not be worried or alarmed by what the nurse perceives to be a minor situation. Under such circumstances, the commonsense approach may be to try and talk patients out of their 'needless' worrying through the use of platitudes and clichés. While such an approach seems to have a rational, objective basis, it fails to acknowledge the reality of patients' experiences, and is therefore less effective than approaching patients by trying to understand their experiences.

In believing that interacting with patients is nothing more than commonsense, nurses may fail to develop the self-understanding necessary to recognise when their approach is not effective. They may fail to reconsider habitual and automatic responses and attitudes and to realise that the context indicates a need for a change in these usual approaches. In simply 'doing what comes naturally', nurses fail to learn how to develop skills specific to the nursing context.

At the opposite end of the spectrum are those nurses who accept the importance of learning how to interact with patients and immerse themselves in learning the skills. For these nurses, a different type of learning challenge may present itself. In attempting to learn the skills, these nurses may become reticent about saying anything to a patient out of fear of making a mistake and saying the wrong thing. If they do attempt to employ the skills, these nurses may have a stilted manner.

Most often this reaction is a result of a common misconception that talking to patients is somehow dramatically different from talking to people who are not patients. The nurses who become almost paralysed when trying to use the skills, or who use the skills in a stilted manner, often are stifled by a belief that 'being therapeutic' means being completely different from usual. The major consequence of this belief is that it retards development of a personal style.

The nurses who are resistant to learning new ways of interacting, because they believe that interacting with patients is nothing more than commonsense, assume that relationships with patients have no special features. The nurses who are reticent to interact with patients, out of fear of making a mistake, assume that relationships with patients are entirely different from other types of human interactions and that a common ground cannot be established. Both groups are misguided and are acting on false assumptions. The first response reflects a rejection of the professional self ('I'll just be myself'), while the second response fails to recognise the use of personal self ('I no longer *can* be myself').

While relationships with patients have characteristics that are different from social relationships such as friendship (see Ch 2), the person who is the nurse remains the same. Nurses must come to realise that their professional self emerges from their personal self (Leddy & Pepper 1998); neither is a separate entity.

These reactions to learning the skills of interacting within the nursing context highlight the need for continuous self-appraisal and self-challenge. By focusing their efforts on becoming more aware, nurses who react to learning the skills in the ways described in the preceding paragraphs are able to meet the challenges posed by these reactions. By reflecting on their responses, nurses not only become aware of their faulty perspectives (if any exist) on interactions with patients, but are challenged to review and revise these perspectives. The essential aim in developing such an awareness when interacting with patients is to be able to assess and evaluate how current perspectives and interpretations could be affecting the development of effective interpersonal skills.

SELF-ASSESSMENT OF INTERPERSONAL SKILLS

Active and ongoing self-assessment is an active strategy for reflection and is one of the most effective ways to increase interpersonal effectiveness as a nurse. Self-assessment draws on all of the processes for developing self-understanding that are described in this chapter. Nurses need to develop the ability to observe themselves as they participate in interactions with patients. This requires nurses to develop abilities to stand apart from themselves temporarily, and to tune their senses to recognise effective and ineffective interaction patterns. Observing feedback and input from patients, which indicates how patients are responding to the nurse's attempts to interact, adds to this self-evaluation. Discussion with other nurses about relationships with patients offers opportunities to be both reassured and challenged. Finally, the sharing of motives, intentions, thoughts and feelings, both with oneself and other nurses, offers further opportunities for growth in interpersonal effectiveness with patients.

Advantages of self-assessment

Self-assessment is a useful way to approach the development of skills for a variety of reasons. Firstly, focusing on self-assessing, especially when initially attempting to use the skills, helps to release nurses from the fear of saying the wrong thing. Through the process of self-assessment, 'mistakes', when made, are viewed as indicators for further growth and development rather than outright failures. Nurses who can recognise when they either miss the point or could be handling an interaction more effectively have an opportunity to recover and move the interaction back on track. When awareness is lacking, errors and omissions go unrecognised and future learning opportunities are missed.

Secondly, self-assessment has the advantage of using the nurse's firsthand experience in the interaction. Nurses who have participated in an interaction know best what happened. In this sense, 'being there' provides essential input. Nurses who 'were there' understand their own intentions during the interaction and can therefore evaluate an interaction in light of these intentions. In this regard, evaluation of performance is placed within the context of actual interactions, as opposed to employing rules that are context-free. This approach takes into account the specific factors relevant to a given interaction and places evaluation within the light of these factors.

Finally, and perhaps most importantly, developing the ability to self-assess enables nurses to engage in continual learning. Through awareness and self-assessment, nurses come to understand their personal strengths and areas for improvement, and performance is evaluated in terms of these personal aspects. When every interaction is viewed as an opportunity for learning, nurses engage in continuous professional growth. In this respect, self-assessment, the evaluation of one's own performance, is considered an essential ability, even a skill in its own right.

Self-assessment is useful in evaluating interpersonal effectiveness after an interaction has occurred, and this is the most common way in which it is initially developed. When developed to its fullest, self-assessment also enables nurses to determine how best to approach a given situation *during* an interaction.

During interactions with patients, nurses have a range of skill options to employ, assuming their repertoire of skills is extensive. For example, the choice to encourage a patient through attending and listening (see Ch 5), through the use of exploration (see Ch 7) or through the use of empathy expression (see Ch 6) depends on nurses' ability to evaluate their own performance in the immediate situation and to track the progress of the relationship (see Ch 2). Through maintaining an orientation towards self-assessment, the choices that are made have a sounder basis than those made by using either a trial-and-error approach or a standard textbook description.

Approaches to self-assessment

Beginning and experienced nurses are encouraged to begin their self-evaluation with an assessment of how they are currently functioning with their interpersonal skills. Activity 3.9 is designed to increase awareness of current interaction patterns. It relies on the process of introspection, discussed earlier in this chapter, and is therefore an activity that should be completed in solitude.

Activity 3.9 ASSESSMENT OF CURRENT SKILLS

PROCESS

1 Observe your interactions for approximately 10 days. Focus on situations in which you are aware of how you are interacting. These situations should contain interactions during which you felt you were effectively interacting with the other persons, and those that you felt were not as effective. These should be situations that illustrate how you typically communicate and interact with other people. Some examples of the type of situations you may observe include:
   - introducing yourself to a stranger
   - needing to clarify something that you have not understood
   - asking another person about themself
   - speaking in a group
   - asking someone for a favour
   - wanting to say 'no' to a request
   - giving or seeking information
   - receiving negative feedback about yourself
   - explaining why you did or said something
   - disagreeing with someone
   - seeking assistance from someone
   - expressing concern for someone else
   - wanting to help someone else, and
   - demonstrating to someone that you care about them.

2 Record these situations as soon as possible after they occur. Include a description of what happened, what you thought about what happened and how you felt about what happened.

3 After you have recorded these situations for about 10 days, review them in order to determine your major strengths when interacting with other people and those areas that you think you could improve.

DISCUSSION

1 Write a brief summary of your interactions, using the following as a guide:
   - what you observed about your interpersonal interactions (e.g. 'I notice that I don't always listen when I am worried about what I am going to say')
   - your strengths and areas for improvement (e.g. 'I am good at starting conversations with people I do not know'), and
   - your personal goals for improving your ability to interact and relate to others (e.g. 'I would like to be able to seek clarification so that I'm sure I understand').

In addition to reflecting on 'everyday' interactions, it is essential that nurses reflect on their interactions with patients. Interactions with patients are different from everyday interactions in the sense that nurses are often focused on being of help to patients. While helping others does occur during everyday interactions, this is not always the primary intent of such interactions.

In order to determine how best to approach situations with patients, nurses must be able to observe and reflect on the interaction, while simultaneously participating in the interaction. The complexity of self-assessment is often overwhelming as a result of these demands. Because the ability to become a participant–observer during interactions can be quite cumbersome to manage all at once, it is often useful to sort the process of self-assessment into manageable units. Although the ultimate aim is to combine all units, first mastering smaller units helps develop the art of self-assessment. The following approaches and activities focus on these smaller units: observing, perceiving, reflecting, evaluating and making alterations on the basis of the evaluation.

Reflection after interactions with patients

An effective approach to assessing performance, and one of the most commonly used approaches, is a reflective evaluation of an interaction after it has occurred. This approach to self-assessment is used after nurses have spontaneously participated in an interaction with a patient. Through reflection, nurses are able to identify skills that were used, assess the effects of these skills and, using patient responses and theoretical concepts as a guide, construct a probable explanation of why the skills were effective or ineffective.

Activity 3.10 is presented as a useful way for nurses to reflect personally on interactions with patients, be they positive or negative experiences.

Activity 3.10 GUIDE TO SELF-REFLECTION

PROCESS

1 Describe (either through speaking or writing) an interaction in terms of what happened. Do not think about why it happened. Just think about what happened between you and the patient.

2 Answer the following questions:
   a What did you say that was helpful to the patient?
   b What was your intent in saying this?
   c How did you know it was helpful?
   d What did you say/do that was not helpful to the patient?
   e What was your intent in saying this?
   f How did you know it was not helpful?
   g What could you have said that would have been more helpful?
   h What were you feeling during this interaction?
   i What do you think the patient was feeling during the interaction?
   j How would you have changed this interaction if you could do it again?

Nurses may fall into the trap of being overly critical of themselves whenever they reflect on their interactions with patients, because they place pressure on themselves to 'do it right'. Rather than viewing interactions as opportunities for growth, nurses who want to 'do it right' perceive interactions as tests of effective performance. This view often stifles personal and professional development.

Whenever nurses are asked to reflect on their interactions, there is a danger that they will recall only those interactions during which they felt ineffective. For this reason, it is important that nurses focus on positive, fulfilling and beneficial interactions, as well as on those interactions that could have been more effective. Satisfying and successful interactions are as informative as those that are not.

Focus on specific skills during an interaction

At times, nurses will want to develop a specific skill or related set of skills because they perceive these skills as difficult, uncomfortable to use or hard to understand. Under these circumstances, an effective way to self-assess is to focus on these skills during an interaction.

Activity 3.11 SELF-ASSESSMENT OF SPECIFIC SKILLS   ➡301

PROCESS

1 Identify which skill or set of skills is particularly difficult to understand or seems too uncomfortable to use.

2 Review the section of this book that covers this particular skill or set of skills.

3 During interactions with patients, look for opportunities when this skill or set of skills is appropriate to use or notice each time you use the skill or set of skills during an interaction with patients.

DISCUSSION

1 Each time you use the skill or set of skills:
 ● Evaluate its effects on interaction with the patient.
 ● Observe how the patient responds.
 ● Reflect on how you felt and responded.
 ● Make a note of the circumstances and immediate situation.

Maintaining an ongoing record

The previously described self-assessment methods are most effective whenever nurses keep track of a number of patient interactions. Such a record is sometimes referred to as a 'journal' or 'diary'. In maintaining such a record, nurses are able to develop their understanding and use of interpersonal skills by referring to a variety of situations and circumstances. When a variety of situations are evaluated, comparisons and contrasts can be made and patterns begin to emerge. Keeping track of various patient situations, and various ways of interacting in these situations, enables nurses to formulate a more complete understanding than simply focusing on isolated events or isolated skills.

Soliciting help from other nurses

In addition to the introspection that the previous approaches encourage, it is useful for nurses to solicit feedback from other nurses about how they are interacting with patients. The questions in Activity 3.10 can be used to prompt information from other nurses. The questions are exploratory. They refrain from passing judgment and encourage other nurses to reflect and determine how they are interacting.

This approach to helping other nurses is preferable to providing solutions and offering advice. When solutions and advice are given, nurses are not encouraged to generate their own solutions. Also, it is only the nurse who 'was there' during a given interaction who knows exactly what happened. Nurses who were not present, yet receive a reported account of what happened, are relying on the nurse giving the account and are processing the information through their own filters. It is preferable for the nurse who 'was there' to process the interaction through their own perceptual filters because this approach has the greatest possibility for promoting self-understanding. Other nurses may offer alternative perspectives, thus encouraging a reappraisal of the situation, but it is best to begin with attempting to understand.

PITFALLS IN SELF-ASSESSMENT

The tendency to judge or evaluate their performance is often automatic, even natural for nurses. Nevertheless, a negative evaluation can be quite troublesome when the perceived stakes are great. In evaluating their interactions with patients, the stakes are often high for nurses because of a need to maintain a positive professional image. Most nurses will want to be effective in their interactions with patients, and performance judged as ineffective may threaten a nurse's professional image and professional esteem. For example, when nurses recognise that they have blocked or inhibited an interaction with a patient, they may find this behaviour unacceptable in a professional sense. In order to preserve and maintain an image as effective professionals, they may overlook, diminish, justify or even reject flaws and mistakes in their performance.

Overcoming this potential pitfall is best achieved through recognition and continuous awareness that self-assessment is done for the purpose of professional growth and development. Continual reflection and evaluation of performance enables nurses to build on their experiences and learn from them. Through self-assessment, nurses determine what was right or wrong, effective or ineffective about their interaction skills and patterns. Nevertheless, this evaluation is not the end point of self-assessment. Self-assessment is employed primarily for the purpose of seeking ways to improve. Thus, it is not simply an evaluative process but a learning process. A commitment to continual learning is an essential aspect of professionalism.

Another potential pitfall in using self-assessment is a tendency to gloss over performance, perceiving it globally as either all good or all bad. Focusing exclusively on positive aspects is as much a pitfall as focusing exclusively on negative aspects of performance. Nurses who can focus only on mistakes or flaws in their interactions with patients are being too harsh in their self-evaluation. Nurses who can focus only on positive aspects of their performance are failing to recognise areas for improvement and learning which exist in the majority of situations.

The tendency to view performance globally as either all good or all bad is kept in check through the realisation that most interactions will contain a mixture of positive and negative aspects. Whenever nurses can perceive only one type or the other, their self-assessment lacks accuracy and completeness. If this happens, nurses are encouraged to reflect further in order to develop a balanced view of evaluation.

A final potential pitfall in using one's self as the assessor of performance emerges whenever nurses lack understanding of the criteria on which to base their evaluations. A lack of understanding of how and why interpersonal skills are used is addressed through further reading and discussion about the theory of effective interactions in nursing. Additionally, nurses may need to solicit assistance from an external authority (e.g. an experienced nurse or an educator), in developing appropriate criteria on which to base their self-assessment.

CHAPTER SUMMARY

Nurses need to become competent communicators who display emotional intelligence in their practice environment. In order to do so, they need to develop acute self-understanding whenever they engage in interactions and relationships with patients, because the primary tool they are using in these circumstances is themselves. Without self-understanding, nurses run the risk of imposing their values and views onto patients. *Values that serve the nurse may be detrimental or useless to patients.* There is a danger that without self-understanding nurses may confuse their own values with those of their patients. Although connected through the relationship, nurses need to maintain an identity that remains separate from the patients.

More than any other parts of nursing, interpersonal relationships with patients are likely to engender feelings within nurses. The processes of self-reflection provide assistance in handling such reactions to patients.

This chapter has reviewed three processes for developing self-understanding:

- introspection
- input from others, and
- self-sharing.

Nurses are encouraged to use these processes in their day-to-day encounters with patients. Reflection, both in solitude and through interaction with others as well as self-sharing, enables nurses to meet the challenges of self-growth.

Self-understanding is the primary means through which nurses are able to evaluate their effectiveness in relating to patients. Through self-understanding, nurses remain in touch with what they are doing, and how this is affecting patients for whom they care.

REFERENCES

Akerjordet K, Severinsson E 2004 Emotional intelligence in mental health nurses talking about practice. International Journal of Mental Health Nursing 13:164–170

Akerjordet K, Severinsson E 2007 Emotional intelligence: a review of the literature with specific focus on empirical and epistemological perspectives. Journal of Clinical Nursing 16:1405–1416

Armstrong-Esther CA, Browne KD 1986 The influence of elderly patients' mental impairment on nurse–patient interaction. Journal of Advanced Nursing 11:379–387

Atkins S, Murphy K 1993 Reflection: a review of the literature. Journal of Advanced Nursing 18:1188–1192

Baer E, Lowery BJ 1987 Patient and situational factors that affect nursing students' like or dislike of caring for patients. Nursing Research 36(5):298–302

Begat I, Severinsson E, Berggren I 1997 Implementation of clinical supervision in a medical department: nurses' views of the effects. Journal of Clinical Nursing 6(5):389–394

Benner P, Tanner C, Chelsea C 1996 Expertise in nursing practice caring, clinical judgment and ethics. Springer, New York

Bolton SC 2000 Who cares?: offering emotion work as a 'gift' in the nursing labour process. Journal of Advanced Nursing 32:580–586

Brickman P, Rabinowitz VC, Karuza J, Coates D, Cohn E, Kidder L 1982 Models of helping and coping. American Psychologist 37(4):368–384

Camilli V, Martin J 2005 Emergency department nurses' attitudes toward suspected intoxicated and psychiatric patients. Topics in Emergency Medicine 27(4):313–316

Carper BA 1978 Fundamental patterns of knowing in nursing. Advances in Nursing Science 1(1):13–23

Carr CJ 1996 Reflecting on clinical practice: hectoring talk or reality? Journal of Clinical Nursing 5:289–295

Carveth JA 1995 Perceived patient deviance and avoidance by nurses. Nursing Research 44(3):173–178

Cirocco M 2007 How reflective practice improves nurses' critical thinking ability. Gastroenterology Nursing 30(6):405–413

Clarke B, James C, Kelly J 1996 Reflective practice: reviewing the issues and refocusing the debate. International Journal of Nursing Studies 33(2):171–180

Codier E, Kooker BM, Shoultz J 2008 Measuring the emotional intelligence of clinical staff nurses. Nursing Administration Quarterly 32(1):8–14

Corey G, Coreu MS, Callahan P 1988 Issues and ethics in the helping professions, 3rd edn. Brooks/Cole, Belmont, CA

Crisp J, Taylor C (eds) 2009 Potter & Perry's fundamentals of nursing, 3rd edn. Elsevier, Sydney

Cronenwett LR 1983 When and how people help: theoretical issues and evidence. In Chinn PL (ed.) Advances in nursing theory development, pp. 251–270. Aspen, Rockville, MD

de Raeve L 2002 The modification of emotional responses: a problem for trust in nurse–patient relationships? Nursing Ethics 9(5):465–471

Drew N 1986 Exclusion and confirmation: phenomenology of patients' experiences with caregivers. Image: Journal of Nursing Scholarship 18:39–43

Egan G 2007 The skilled helper, 8th edn. Brooks/Cole/Thomas Learning, Boston, MA

Forrest D 1989 The experience of caring. Journal of Advanced Nursing 14:815–823

Foster J, Greenwood J 1998 Reflection: a challenging innovation for nurses. Contemporary Nurse 7:165–172

Fowler J 1998 Evaluating the efficacy of reflective practice within the context of clinical supervision. Journal of Advanced Nursing 27:379–382

Goleman D 1996 Emotional intelligence: why it can matter more than IQ. Bloomsbury, London

Goleman D 1998 Working with emotional intelligence. Bloomsbury, London

Greenwood J 1993 Reflective practice: a critique of the work of Argyris and Schon. Journal of Advanced Nursing 18:1183–1187

Greenwood J 1998 The role of reflection in single and double loop learning. Journal of Advanced Nursing 27:1048–1053

Grief CL, Elliot R 1994 Emergency nurses' moral evaluation of patients. Journal of Emergency Nursing 20(4):275–279

Gustafson C, Fagerberg I 2004 Reflection: the way to professional development? Journal of Clinical Nursing 13:271–280

Haddock J, Bassett C 1997 Nurses' perceptions of reflective practice. Nursing Standard 11(32):39–41

Henderson A 2001 Emotional labor and nursing: an under-appreciated aspect of caring work. Nursing Inquiry 8:130–138

Hochschild AR 1983 The managed heart: commercialisation of human feeling. University of California Press, Berkeley, CA

Ivey AE, Ivey MB 2003 Intentional interviewing and counseling: facilitating client development in a multicultural society. Brooks/Cole–Thompson, Pacific Grove, CA

Johns C 1995 The value of reflective practice for nursing. Journal of Clinical Nursing 4(1):23–30

Johns C 1999 Reflection as empowerment? Nursing Inquiry 6:241–249

Johnson M, Webb C 1995a Rediscovering unpopular patients: the concept of social judgement. Journal of Advanced Nursing 21:455–466

Johnson M, Webb C 1995b The power of social judgement: struggle and negotiation in the nursing process. Nurse Education Today 15:83–89

Jones PR 1995 Hindsight bias in reflective practice: an empirical investigation. Journal of Advanced Nursing 21:783–788

Jordan PJ, Troth AC 2002 Emotional intelligence and conflict resolution in nursing. Contemporary Nurse 13:94–100

Kelly MP, May D 1982 Good and bad patients: a review of the literature and a theoretical critique. Journal of Advanced Nursing 7:147–156

Kim HS 1999 Critical reflective inquiry for knowledge development in nursing practice. Journal of Advanced Nursing 29:1205–1212

Kooker BM, Schoultz J, Codier EE 2007 Identifying emotional intelligence in professional nursing practice. Journal of Professional Nursing 23(1):30–36

Larson EB, Yao X 2005 Clinical empathy as emotional labor in the patient–physician relationship. Journal of the American Medical Association 293:1100–1106

Leddy S, Pepper JM 1998 Conceptual bases of professional nursing, 4th edn. JB Lippincott, Philadelphia, PA

Macintosh C 2007 Protecting the self: a descriptive qualitative exploration of how registered nurses cope with working in surgical areas. International Journal of Nursing Studies 44: 982–990

Maggs C, Biley A 2000 Reflections on the role of the nursing development facilitator in clinical supervision and reflective practice. International Journal of Nursing Practice 6:192–195

Mann S, Cowburn J 2005 Emotional labour and stress within mental health nursing. Journal of Psychiatric and Mental Health Nursing 12:154–162

Mantzoukas S, Jasper MA 2004 Reflective practice and daily ward reality: a covert power game. Journal of Clinical Nursing 13:925–933

Martinez-Inigo D, Totterdell P, Alcover CM, Holman D 2007 Emotional labour and emotional exhaustion: interpersonal and intrapersonal mechanisms. Work and Stress 21(1):30–47

McAllister M, Creedy D, Moyle W, Farrugia C 2002 Nurses' attitudes towards clients who self harm. Journal of Advanced Nursing 40:578–586

McCallin A, Bamford A 2007 Interdisciplinary teamwork: is the influence of emotional intelligence fully appreciated? Journal of Nursing Management 15:386–391

McCann T, Clark E, McConnachie S, Harvey I 2007 Deliberate self-harm: emergency department nurses' attitudes, triage, and care intentions. Journal of Clinical Nursing 16:1704–1711

McCartan PJ, Hargie ODW 2004 Assertiveness and caring: are they compatible? Journal of Advanced Nursing 13:707–713

McQueen A 2004 Emotional intelligence in nursing work. Journal of Advanced Nursing 47:101–108

Mikolajczak M, Menil C, Luminet O 2007 Explaining the protective effect of trait emotional intelligence regarding occupational stress: exploration of emotional labour processes. Journal of Research in Personality 41:1107–1117

Olsen D 1997 When the patient causes the problem: the effect of patient responsibility on the nurse–patient relationship. Journal of Advanced Nursing 26:515–522

Peden-McAlpine C, Tomlinson PS, Forneris SG, Genck G, Meier SJ 2005 Evaluation of a reflective practice intervention to enhance family care. Journal of Advanced Nursing 49:494–501

Savage J 2004 Researching emotion: the need for coherence between focus theory and methodology. Nursing Inquiry 11:25–34

Sayler J, Stuart BJ 1985 Nurse–patient interaction in the intensive care unit. Heart and Lung 14:20–24

Skinner C, Spurgeon P 2005 Valuing empathy and emotional intelligence in health leadership: a study of empathy, leadership behaviour and outcome effectiveness. Health Services Management Research 18:1–12

Smith A, Jack K 2005 Reflective practice: a meaningful task for students. Nursing Standard 19(26):33–37

Smith P 1992 The emotional labour of nursing. Macmillan, London

Taylor B 1997 Big battles for small gains: a cautionary note for teaching reflective processes in nursing and midwifery practice. Nursing Inquiry 4:19–26

Taylor B, Holroyd B, Edwards P, Unwin A, Rowley J 2005 Assertiveness in nursing practice: an action research and reflection project. Contemporary Nurse 20:234–247

Tichen A, Binnie A 1995 The art of clinical supervision. Journal of Clinical Nursing 4(5):327–334

Timmons S, Tanner J 2005 Operating theatre nurses: emotional labour and the hostess role. International Journal of Nursing Practice 11:85–91

Wilkinson J 1999 Implementing reflective practice. Nursing Standard 13(21):36–40

Woodward V 1999 Achieving moral health care: the challenge of patient partiality. Nursing Ethics 6(5):390–398

Yang G, Chang C 2007 Emotional labour, job satisfaction and organization commitment amongst clinical nurses: a questionnaire survey. International Journal of Nursing Studies, doi:10.1016/ijnurstu.2007.02.001

CHAPTER 4

Considering culture

INTRODUCTION

The material throughout this book continuously emphasises the importance of understanding the patient as a person with a unique perspective of the world. Nurses who come to understand an individual patient are able to work through the patient's own unique perspective in order to 'see through the patient's eyes'. These perspectives of the world, be they those of nurse or patient, are based on cultural beliefs and values. Therefore, a central aspect of understanding another person is an appreciation of differences in cultural meaning. Differences in cultural understanding commonly lie outside conscious awareness. That is, cultural understandings are often taken for granted. It is for this reason that nurses need to develop conscious awareness and appreciation of cultural diversity when interacting with patients. Doing so forms the basis of culturally congruent nursing care. The development of cultural competence is an ongoing process for cultural congruence, as is the promotion of cultural safety in nursing practice.

Chapter overview

This chapter begins with a general discussion of culture and its specific relationship to healthcare. Concepts such as cultural safety and cultural competence are highlighted as vital processes in the development of culturally congruent care for patients. Challenges faced when there are language differences between nurse and patient are discussed, as are guidelines when using the services of interpreters when interacting with patients. The use of non-verbal communication, especially through touch, is considered in relation to language barriers.

WHAT IS CULTURE?

When considering the influence of culture, there is a tendency to think that culture is something that pertains to *others* and not the self. Likewise, it is often viewed as something that is 'exotic' or 'foreign', such as rituals pertaining to death and burial. Of utmost importance is the recognition that culture is something that pertains to every human being. Everybody has culture.

Culture encompasses a view of the world that is shared by a group of people and learnt through social interactions within the group. Culture includes a wide range of behaviours, values, beliefs, attitudes and customs, and is reflected in the language, dress, food materials and social institutions of a group. These values and beliefs are often taken for granted and are therefore not always in conscious awareness (Schim et al 2007, Rosenjack Burchum 2002).

Culture provides the framework for a particular society's way of life; it influences the way social life is regulated and guides interactions between members of a social group. Cultural understandings affect the way that members of the group make sense of the world. Culture has a vast influence on behaviour. A particular social group's culture is reflected in all aspects of everyday life, including customs, greetings, methods of communication, attitudes to the family, beliefs about marriage, attitudes to illness and approaches to healthcare. For example, a group of friends often develop ways of greeting each other and interacting that are unique to the group. Such behaviours form part of the group culture.

Healthcare organisations will also have particular cultures, with a shared language and customs that influence how care is delivered. The care practices within an organisation will reflect cultural values and beliefs. Those new to that culture must learn the cultural ways in order to become part of that group. The importance of organisational culture is recognised as influencing patient care, satisfaction and outcomes, as well as nurse satisfaction (see Ch 11).

Culture and ethnicity

Culture is often confused with ethnicity. They are not the same. Although members of an ethnic group usually share cultural customs and beliefs, ethnicity alone does not make a culture. Ethnicity refers to belonging to a certain race or group of people. It is usually biologically determined (e.g. a member of the Semite race of people). Ethnicity, which may shape a person's identity, is determined by birth. Culture, on the other hand, can be shared by members who choose to embrace a particular way of life. For example, the Australian culture is shared by many people of diverse ethnic backgrounds.

Activity 4.1 illustrates the difficulty in describing the 'typical Australian' and the futility of attempts to deny the diversity that exists within a particular group. There is always diversity within a cultural group and this is one of the problems with stereotyping; it denies individual and subgroup variation.

Activity 4.1 IS THERE AN AUSTRALIAN CULTURE?

PROCESS

1 Imagine that you have a friend from another country who is interested in migrating to Australia and wants to know more about the culture and way of life. What would you tell your friend about Australian attitudes to:
   a alcohol use
   b celebrations
   c sport and leisure

> d family life
> e work
> f parties (what people wear and do at parties)
> g relationships between males and females
> h friendship, and
> i dating?
>
> 2 Form groups of four to eight participants and compare answers. For each of the items considered, discuss with the group the following:
>   a Do all Australians everywhere have similar attitudes?
>   b Do my parents have similar attitudes to me?
>   c Would a poor Australian depict a similar picture to a wealthy Australian?
>
>
>
> DISCUSSION
>
> 1 Is there a typical Australian? In what way is this typicality a stereotype (i.e. an exaggerated caricature of Australia)?
>
> 2 Do you think that stereotypes apply to other cultures? Is there a stereotype of a 'typical English person', a 'typical Vietnamese person', or 'a typical American'?
>
> 3 Ask participants whose culture of origin is different from Australian to describe how they believe their cultures have been stereotyped.
>
> 4 What differences might there be in perceptions of what it means to 'be Australian' between people living in metropolitan, rural and remote areas of the country?
>
> *Source: Adapted from the cultural game, Who are we?, Multicultural Centre, Sydney Teachers College, now University of Sydney, Faculty of Education, Sydney, 1981.*

Cultural stereotyping

Stereotyping is categorising individuals into groups based on an oversimplified set of characteristics. For example, a stereotypic Australian male wears thongs and stubbies and has a beer in hand. Stereotypes are potentially useful because they can provide a sort of mental shorthand that allows processing and organisation of the enormous amounts of diverse information encountered in everyday life. The ultimate danger, however, involves generalisation of these stereotypes in their extreme forms, and an associated reluctance to recognise the extent to which individual differences do exist within all groups.

When nurses rely on stereotypes and act on them, they miss an opportunity to get to know the person on any more than a superficial level. The cost of not getting close enough to patients to gain insight into their respective individualities may result in a failure to identify and meet their specific needs, thus compromising quality nursing care.

The menace inherent in stereotypes is that they are intransigent, pervasive, self-fulfilling and self-perpetuating. Stereotypes also provide convenient shortcuts when there is a perceived lack of the time and energy necessary to gain an accurate view of the needs and problems of individual patients. If a patient is viewed by nurses as 'a typical hysterical Mediterranean patient', all interactions will be coloured by that perception. When nurses apply the stereotype of a 'druggie' (i.e. irresponsible, immature, needy and worthless), they avoid taking the risk of coming to know and value the patient. Nurses need to challenge continually their own use of stereotypes in order to minimise the influence they exert on patient–nurse interactions and nursing practice.

The tendency to stereotype can be lessened by recognising the influence that values have on behaviour (see Ch 3) and by appreciating the range of values that lie behind the behaviour of specific groups. To be truly culturally aware, it is important to recognise that while there are differences *between* different cultural groups, there are also as many or even greater differences *within* them. Nevertheless, cultural stereotypes do exist and they tend to be remarkably resistant to change.

More importantly, stereotypes can stigmatise people and affect their access to healthcare. Consider the following example:

Brenda has strong links to and relationships with Indigenous Australians as this is her heritage and identity. People sometimes find her background confusing as she has pale skin and blonde hair. When people seem genuinely interested, she always takes the time to explain the meaning of being an Aboriginal Australian. On the afternoon that she arrived at a hospital emergency department (ED) with her seriously ill 2-year-old son, she had no time to explain anything, although she ticked the box on the admission form to identify her son as an Indigenous Australian.

She came to the ED of a busy metropolitan hospital because her son was having an extreme allergic reaction to peanuts. That day her family and friends had come together for a children's birthday party for her 5-year-old daughter. The party was a large gathering of toddlers and preschoolers who enjoyed an afternoon's festivities. Near the end of the party, following the cutting and eating of the cake, she noticed her 2-year-old was showing signs of a severe allergic reaction. She had seen it before and knew exactly what to do.

Not knowing for sure what had caused the reaction, as she is extremely careful about her son's allergy, she administered adrenaline and set out for the local hospital, a 2-minute car trip from home. On the way, she remembered that she had decorated the cake with 'hundreds and thousands' that had been stored in a jar that previously contained peanuts. Her 2-year-old reacted immediately after eating the cake.

On arrival she quickly explained what was happening to the triage nurse in the ED. She told him of her son's history and the events of the day, stating that she and her son needed to be seen immediately as her son has severe allergic reactions to peanuts. The nurse's response was not in keeping with the seriousness of the circumstances and he asked her to be seated. She became quite distressed, stating in a loud voice that she and her son must be seen immediately. He replied, 'have a seat and wait like everybody else'.

Knowing she had no time and knowing of another hospital 2 minutes away she picked up her son, who by now was unable to walk, and went to the second hospital. There, her son was stabilised in the ED and admitted to the intensive care unit. Although he recovered physically, Brenda could not recover emotionally from her treatment in the ED of the first hospital.

She retained the services of a lawyer and obtained the ED record of her son's admission under the right to freedom of information. On the record she read: 'Aboriginal woman, dishevelled, wearing dirty clothes, with two-year-old child in her arms, loudly demanding to be seen immediately. Child appears dirty, unkempt and possibly neglected, not in keeping with developmental milestones as he is crawling. Strong smell of alcohol on mother's breath. Mother seems hysterical and believes child is having a reaction to peanuts. Not able to confirm allergy. Plan is to contact the children's services department and have the child seen by a social worker. Mother told to wait. Triaged to category 3.'

Brenda filed a formal complaint against both the hospital and nurse. She was pleased to hear that this resulted in action being taken against the nurse, who was removed from further triage duty. Brenda was satisfied knowing that this nurse would not have further opportunity to make decisions that could have dire consequences purely on the basis of a racial stereotype.

Brenda's story is extreme, but true. It illustrates what can happen when people make decisions on the basis of stereotyping. Had the nurse asked a few pertinent questions, he would have found logical explanations for the circumstances. First, attendees at a preschool children's birthday party will often have soiled clothing at the conclusion. Second, Brenda did have one glass of champagne at the commencement of the party, well over an hour before she arrived in the ED, so was unlikely to be inebriated as the nurse suggested. Third, her son was unable to walk because he was critically ill by the time he arrived at hospital. Unfortunately, the nurse made decisions not on these facts, but rather on his image of 'an Aboriginal' (i.e. a stereotype).

CULTURE AND HEALTHCARE

To interact effectively with members of different cultural groups, it is necessary for nurses to become more culturally aware and less ethnocentric. Ethnocentrism is a tendency to see the world as having one standard—that of one's own cultural group—and to judge other cultural groups in relation to it. An ethnocentric individual is unlikely to perceive or acknowledge differences in the ways that people view the world, and to fail to appreciate the advantages of living in a culturally diverse society.

Culturally aware nurses realise that much of their world is socially constructed and that the way it is constructed largely depends on cultural beliefs. In becoming culturally aware, nurses develop an understanding and acceptance of the differences that exist between different groups of people and are more willing to investigate the practices and rituals that are associated with different cultural groups. Some of the more fundamental of these practices include the care of the body after death, religious rituals, beliefs associated with food and childbirth customs.

The initial step in developing cultural awareness is to increase understanding of one's own culture. This is best done through the process of reflection about the origin and nature of a personal value and belief system. For example, nurses might reflect on how illness was perceived and managed in their family of origin. Of central importance is a reflection on how members of the cultural group 'expect' people to behave when ill. For example, in some cultures people do not complain when in pain, while in others a dramatic outward expression of pain is accepted as 'normal'.

In addition to becoming familiar with their own culturally influenced values, nurses can increase their understanding of culture through conscious recognition and appreciation of the diversity that exists across cultures. In order to gain this understanding, nurses need to gain experience (e.g. through reading material on different cultures, travelling, and social or professional interaction). Listening with an accepting, open mind to patients' cultural viewpoints is perhaps the best way to develop awareness and understanding.

Perceptions of health and illness

The influence of culture is particularly evident when considering the meaning of illness, because beliefs and explanations about health and illness are often culturally determined (see illness representation, Ch 9). For example, some groups of people believe that illness is a punishment for past wrongdoings, with suffering being a means of atonement. Other groups of people may share a belief that illness is nothing more than chance. That is, there is no reason other than the 'luck of the draw' for becoming sick.

Those explanations can be very different from the scientific explanatory model that is the basis of most clinical healthcare (Allshouse 1993). Healthcare is disease oriented, based on understanding of pathophysiology and psychopathology. Understanding a disease from this scientific perspective is based on notions of objectivity that are generalised to all people. Illness, on the other hand, is what a patient experiences (i.e. from a subjective perspective). The former is *case knowledge,* while the latter encompasses both *patient* and *person knowledge* (see Ch 1).

Currently, the Australian healthcare system is monocultural, with Western ideology being dominant and even 'imposed' on patients (Blackford & Street 2000). This ideology is based on the autonomous individual, with high value placed on independence and self-agency (Cioffi 2003). This orientation may not accommodate people from cultures in which collective identity and interdependence take precedence over individual autonomy and independence.

The culture of individual nurses as well as the culture of the healthcare system does have an influence on interpretation of patient behaviour and their responses to patients (Cioffi 2003). A failure to appreciate the cultural differences between patients and healthcare professionals has been shown to negatively impact on the quality of care and patient satisfaction (Flores et al 2002). In addition, cultural and language differences between patients and healthcare professionals have been shown to limit patient access to care (Bolton et al 2004). A lack of understanding of a patient's culture can result in negative patient outcomes and patient harm (Green-Hernandez et al 2004).

Patients' personal, subjective experiences of illness are imbued with cultural meaning, which may or may not fit biomedical explanations of ill health. For example, a family might share the belief that wearing warm undergarments in winter wards off colds and flu; a 'scientific' explanation of colds and flu is that viruses cause them. Indigenous peoples of Australia believe that disharmony and discontinuity cause ill health and healing seeks to reintegrate people with one another and with the environment (Short et al 1998 p 156). Knowledge developed in the field of biomedical science does not accommodate such understandings.

Nurses from social and cultural backgrounds that are different from the patient may not understand cultural meanings of health and illness, especially if they operate from an exclusively biomedical orientation (an ethnocentric view). Likewise, patients whose health beliefs are different from those supported by the biomedical model may be reluctant to share these beliefs with nurses (Allshouse 1993).

Differences in illness-related behaviour may occur because of disparity between biomedical thinking and cultural beliefs. An individual nurse's background can create barriers to understanding cultural practices that are unfamiliar. For example, some social groups hold strong beliefs that members who are well have an obligation to pay respects to the sick and to attend to their needs. Family and friends are expected to visit the sick, provide them with home-cooked food, help them to rest and regain their health. The sick, in turn, have an obligation to accept these attentions. Making brave attempts to care for oneself, and indicating that such attentions are not needed, may be regarded as ill-mannered.

The approaches of the above-described groups contrast with those who place a high value on independence and avoidance of relying on others beyond what is absolutely necessary. Attempts to get well quickly and to resume normal roles are admired and praised by other members of such groups. In these cultures, people who are sick have an obligation to make every effort to minimise the time that they are dependent on others. Nurses who, due to their own cultural backgrounds, value such independence may have trouble understanding the patients who do very little for themselves in relation to healthcare.

In some countries, hospitalisation is beyond the financial means of most people, and patients are admitted only when they are severely ill. A logical consequence of this situation is a view of hospitals as places where patients are very likely to die. It is, therefore, quite understandable that patients from such countries may be terrified by the prospect of admission to hospital. Health professionals without an understanding of the basis of that fear may regard these patients as irrationally anxious.

Differences related to patients' relationships with healthcare workers also vary across cultures. While in some cultures attitudes towards health professionals are largely deferential and it is rare for patients to question diagnosis or treatment, in other cultures people take a more critical view of healthcare. Some people often actively 'shop around' for the doctor who suits them best, while others may not only hesitate to do so, but believe that such behaviour demonstrates an overly critical and disrespectful attitude towards healthcare professionals.

Differences in healthcare practices can lead to serious misunderstanding between patients and healthcare professionals. For example, there are traditional Vietnamese healing methods that include 'coin rubbing' to dispel poisons believed to be responsible for colds and flus. This practice may result in marks and breaks on the skin, which could be interpreted as child abuse when the practice is used by a parent or grandparent (Suh 2004, Wolf & Calmes 2004).

The results of a recent Australian study (Cioffi 2006) revealed that both patients and nurses experienced tension in their interactions when they were from different cultures. Their perceived differences posed difficulties in achieving mutual understanding, thus creating misunderstandings. More importantly, there was recognition that it was difficult to develop a relationship beyond a superficial level (i.e. the instrumental/clinical level of involvement) (see Ch 2).

In another study, nurses were concerned with their lack of cultural sensitivity when children were dying in an intensive care unit (McKinley & Blackford 2001). They recognised a tendency to base their care on their own beliefs and cultural values, rather than those of the patient's family and cultural group. They recognised and described systems in which they controlled and dominated the care.

Not only should nurses be aware of their own cultural heritage, but they should also be aware of the healthcare culture in which they practise. Awareness is the first step in delivering care that is culturally congruent with the patient.

Culturally congruent care

Culturally congruent care is respectful of and responsive to the patient's culturally based values and beliefs. It is based on mutual understanding between nurse and patient. There are four elements to this care: an appreciation of cultural diversity, an awareness of individual patient's cultural values and beliefs, sensitivity to differences between and within different cultures, and skilled know-how when interacting with patients, especially when nurse and patient come from different cultural backgrounds (Schim et al 2007). In providing culturally congruent care, nurses must be receptive to learning from patients, as it is the patient who can best explain their values and beliefs.

There are two approaches to conceptualising culturally congruent care (Fuller 2003). The first is based on learning the customs and particular aspects of identified cultures. This approach is essential when nurses work with specifically identified cultural groups. However, relying on lists of characteristics of specific cultures can lead to superficial understandings that are based on stereotypes. Additionally, this approach is limited in its practical application, as it is difficult for nurses to anticipate the variety of cultures that they may encounter.

The second approach to culturally congruent care is through the development of 'cultural humility' (Kleinman 1988, cited in Fuller 2003 p 783). Cultural humility means that the nurses appreciate that their culture, both as an individual and as reflected by healthcare culture, is not the yardstick by which patients should be evaluated; this is the opposite of an ethnocentric view. Rather than relying on a set of cultural attributes or adhering to popular beliefs about a culture, culturally humble nurses will inquire into the individual patient's personal interpretations and beliefs (Kleiman 2006).

The development of cultural humility is an ongoing process of awareness and reflection (see Ch 3). Nurses who are 'culturally humble' will not impose their value system on a patient, but rather enter the relationship with openness to different ways of seeing the world. They are ready to learn from the patient and negotiate care that is based on the patient's cultural belief systems (Coffman 2004).

Cultural safety

Although necessary, awareness of cultural diversity is not sufficient for professional nursing practice that is culturally congruent. Nurses are morally and professionally bound to provide care that is safe. The notion of safety extends beyond physical and psychological parameters to include care that is culturally safe (Richardson 2004, Polaschek 1998, Ramsden 1993). Cultural safety is more than simply learning about cultural practices and beliefs; it is an ethical standard that recognises the position of cultural groups and how they are perceived. Likewise, unsafe practice is any action that demeans or diminishes cultural identity and wellbeing (Polaschek 1998). Imposing a biomedical perspective on illness while dismissing beliefs that do not fit a biomedical model is an example of culturally unsafe practice.

Unlike notions of 'cultural awareness' or 'cultural sensitivity', which can be evaluated by professional standards, cultural safety can only be judged by the patient or recipient of care (Richardson 2004). Cultural safety does not mean that all recipients of care are treated the same, as is often touted as the key to cultural awareness and sensitivity. Rather, the tenets of cultural safety imply that nurses adjust their care in accordance with the cultural sensitivities of each individual patient.

Cultural safety is more than recognition of the uniqueness of cultural identity and the need for equity in healthcare. Cultural safety also includes recognition of social structures that disempower cultural groups. It is a means by which nurses examine healthcare structures that disadvantage some people, rendering them powerless in that structure (Richardson 2004).

Culturally safe nurses recognise social structures that account, in part, for lack of access to adequate healthcare for some cultural groups. Culturally safe nurses accommodate and respect a diverse range of views on health and healing. They are not set in one particular pattern of thinking about illness, be it a biomedical orientation or one that derives from their own cultural background.

Cultural competence

Cultural competence is a multidimensional concept currently used to describe the conditions necessary for appropriate delivery of healthcare that is culturally congruent. Cultural competence encompasses awareness, knowledge, understanding, sensitivity, tolerance and skill (Schim et al 2007, Suh 2004, Wolf & Calmes 2004, Rosenjack Burchum 2002). It is directly related to the capacity to understand fully a patient's perspective and, more importantly, to provide healthcare that incorporates this perspective.

Culturally competent practitioners will have the desire and motivation to seek cultural encounters to obtain further knowledge and skill (Campinha-Bacote 2003). That is, cultural competence is an ongoing process in which nurses continually strive to deepen their understanding and appreciation of cultural diversity (Schim et al 2007, Green-Hernandez et al 2004). Like cultural safety, cultural competence extends beyond the individual nurse, and includes the development of healthcare systems that are culturally congruent to the population being served.

Nurses who work with a specific population of people should make every effort to learn of that group's cultural beliefs, values and healthcare practices. For example, Australian Aboriginal cultures, although having much diversity within them, hold a tradition of not using a deceased person's name because doing so calls their spirit back to earth (McGrath & Phillips 2008). A nurse could inadvertently disturb this sensibility by asking for specifics of family members' names when collecting healthcare information. Culturally competent nurses would know not to do so. When nurses routinely care for a population of patients whose language is different from their own, their cultural competence will include making an effort to learn a few key words or phrases in the language that is used by that population. Doing so can not only prevent misunderstandings, but also demonstrates a sincere desire to be 'for' the patient.

Language differences

In certain situations it is likely that patients will have difficulty understanding the language used by nurses. At such times it is common for nurses to use a third person to act as an intermediary.

Where the difficulty is related to the non-English speaking background of the patient, a member of a medical interpreter service may be brought in to translate. If this is not possible, a member of the patient's family who does speak English may act as an interpreter, but this has potential problems.

Where the interaction difficulty is related to the age of the patient (e.g. a young child) or to specific communication problems (e.g. an intellectual disability), members of the family or individuals who are familiar with the patient are commonly used. It should always be remembered that interacting through a third person increases the likelihood of misinterpretation or reinterpretation of the content. This may be due to the filtering process associated with a third person, and the interpretations and meanings attached to the content by that person. In addition, the intermediary may make a conscious decision to alter the meaning by omitting, adding or distorting the content of the message, or patients may withhold information because of the personal relationship that exists between themselves and the intermediary.

All of the alterations to the content mentioned in the previous paragraph are more likely to occur in situations where the topic under discussion creates a high level of discomfort for those involved in the interaction (e.g. if a male adolescent is asked to interpret while his mother's personal and obstetric history is taken, or an unfamiliar, middle-aged male is interpreting for a female adolescent patient who is being questioned about her sexual activity).

The following situation illustrates problems that may occur when an untrained interpreter is used:

> A Lebanese cleaner was asked to interpret for a couple who had given birth to an infant with Down syndrome or 'mongolism'. The cleaner told the parents that they had given birth to a 'Chinese baby', a literal translation. This caused a great deal of conflict between the husband and wife and was not cleared up for many months. This situation would have been avoided if a trained healthcare interpreter had been used.

Australian healthcare systems have established health-interpreter programs to meet the need for interpreters with the expertise required to work within health-related areas. If it is necessary to use an untrained interpreter in an emergency situation, a professional interpreter should be employed as soon as possible to check on the understanding of the patient and the family. Working effectively with an interpreter is a skilled activity, and there are enormous advantages in making the effort to acquire the skill.

Interpreters who are trained to work in the healthcare system are able to translate medical terminology accurately and have proven useful in bridging gaps between the culture of the health professional and that of the patient. Misunderstandings arising both from language barriers and from differences in cultural beliefs and practices may, therefore, be prevented or minimised with the help of a trained interpreter. Whenever important or sensitive discussion is needed, or when complex information is sought or given, it is important that an interpreter, bound by the ethic of confidentiality that applies to all healthcare professionals, is involved.

Activity 4.2 WORKING WITH AN INTERPRETER ➡301

PROCESS

1 Form as many groups of three as possible where two members of the group are fluent in the same language, which should not be English. The remaining participants are observers.

2 Using the given situations, one foreign language speaker plays the role of a nurse and the other an interpreter. The third person plays the role of the patient. If there is more than one group, different groups can play each situation. Alternatively, the same group can play the two situations consecutively.

3 The role play is set in the Accident and Emergency Unit where a patient has been admitted with severe asthma. Emergency treatment has been instituted and the patient is now breathing more comfortably. The nurse has arranged for an interpreter to help collect information for a nursing history. For the purpose of this role play, any nursing history format may be used.

Situation A - The nurse and interpreter face each other and the nurse directs questions to the interpreter using the third person. For example, 'Has he/she ever been in hospital before?' 'When did he/she have his/her last meal?'; 'Is he/she allergic to any medications?' The role play ends when the history is completed.

Situation B - The nurse introduces the interpreter to the patient. The interpreter sits next to the patient. The nurse addresses questions directly to the patient. After the history is completed, the nurse asks the patient if they have any questions about any aspect of treatment or care. Answers are directed to the patient, not to the interpreter. After the interview, the nurse is the first to leave while the interpreter stays and chats briefly with the patient before leaving.

DISCUSSION

1 How did it feel to be the 'patient' in situation A? How did it feel to be the 'patient' in situation B?

2 What difficulties did the 'nurses' in situation A experience? What difficulties did the 'nurses' in situation B experience?

3 What principles should be observed when working with an interpreter? Compare your answers with the following text about using interpreters.

Guidelines when using an interpreter

Prior to the interview, it is important that the interpreter is briefed about the purpose of the interview. The interpreter should have the opportunity to meet the patient, explain the purpose of the interview and establish a level of rapport. This is especially important if there is to be a discussion of sensitive and private matters. In instances when sexual or personal details must be discussed, it may be important that the interpreter be of the same gender as the patient. There is a general tendency for people of all cultural backgrounds to feel more comfortable discussing personal matters with a person of the same sex.

During the interview, the interpreter should be seated next to the patient. This allows the interpreter to take on the role of the patient's ally so the patient is less likely to feel outnumbered and disadvantaged. The nurse should maintain eye contact with and speak directly to the patient, not to the interpreter. This helps the nurse to develop a relationship with the patient, as well as facilitate observation of the patient's non-verbal communication.

The interaction usually works best if the interpreter is able to interpret the words simultaneously, *as they are spoken*. This is the 'trailing' method of interpreting and is most likely to promote a good rapport between the patient and the nurse. In the other type of interpreting, *consecutive interpreting*, the patient completes a whole sentence or phrase before it is translated. On completion of the interview, the nurse should leave the room first, allowing an opportunity for the interpreter to chat with the patient. It is important to avoid engaging the interpreter in lengthy discussions in which the patient is not involved. Further discussion between the nurse and the interpreter should be left for another time, as the interpreter should be seen to be aligned with the patient, not the nurse.

While an interpreter should be used whenever there is important information to convey, it is often necessary to manage without an interpreter when interacting with a patient who has limited English. At times, there may not be an interpreter who is immediately available. Therefore, it is important for nurses to prepare for such times by learning key phrases for the population that is being served. In addition, a list of basic words in the patient's language should be compiled for use by all staff.

COMMUNICATING WITHOUT LANGUAGE

With patience and care, it is possible to convey simple information to a person who has minimal English. It is important to speak slowly and clearly. Avoid using jargon and phrases that can be readily misunderstood, such as 'that wound seems to be breaking down; we had better keep an eye on it'. It is best to use plain, correct English, avoiding ambiguities and, above all, avoiding forms of 'pidgin' English, which is used to simplify language but may actually make it more confusing. For example, a nurse may ask a patient, 'When you see doctor, what he say?' Ambiguity in tense may cause patients with little English to wonder if the interaction under discussion was in the past or is to occur in the future.

Many migrant patients are proud of their English, and may be offended by the patronising stance of the nurse who speaks to them loudly or in 'pidgin'. They may even misunderstand the intent and believe that the nurse has a poor command of English. It may be difficult for patients to extend respect to such nurses and to accept them as professional people. In addition to focusing on the verbal components of interactions, remember to make full use of all forms of non-verbal communication. Write down instructions. Non-verbal, supportive feedback can show that the nurse is listening and has understood. Try not to look impatient with the patient's attempts to speak English.

When nurses have given information or instructions, it is vital that they check patients' comprehension by asking them to display their understanding of what has been said (see Ch 8). It is important that patients do not simply repeat the nurse's words, but that they use their own words to demonstrate that they truly understand. Patients may be able to repeat the words but may be too embarrassed to admit that they do not understand what they mean. It is important to remember that phrases familiar to nurses may be confusing to patients who are unfamiliar with them (e.g. 'light diet'). Failure to check patients' understanding can result in unnecessary confusion and possible mishaps.

Activity 4.3 COMMUNICATING WITHOUT LANGUAGE ➡302

PROCESS

1 Form a pair with two members in the group, one of whom speaks a language other than English and who plays the role of a nurse who is trying to take a nursing history. The other person plays the patient. Make as many pairs as there are foreign-language speakers. The remainder of the group act as observers.

2 Half the pairs use instruction A and the other half use instruction B.

Instruction A - You are feeling annoyed that you have to obtain a nursing history from a person who does not understand your language and there is no available interpreter. Your annoyance is obvious to the patient, and you behave rather impatiently, speaking in a voice louder than usual, hoping that this will help the patient better understand. No English is to be used.

Instruction B - You have to obtain a nursing history from a person who does not understand your language and there is no available interpreter. You are very patient with the person and use every means at your disposal to help the person understand what you are saying. You speak slowly, in a soft tone, and use gestures, facial expressions, drawings, diagrams or whatever is necessary to convey your meaning. No English is to be used.

DISCUSSION

1 Compare the amount of information that was obtained for each set of instructions.

2 How did it feel to be the 'patient' in instruction A? How did it feel to be the 'nurse' in instruction A?

3 How did it feel to be the 'patient' in instruction B? How did it feel to be the 'nurse' in instruction B?

4 Have you ever been in a situation (e.g. in a class or in a bank) where you were not able to make yourself understood? How did you feel? How could you have been helped to convey your message?

5 What did you learn from this exercise about interacting with non-English speaking patients?

THE IMPORTANCE OF NON-VERBAL COMMUNICATION

Non-verbal behaviours form an integral component of the communication process, irrespective of the verbal content. Actually, when inconsistencies exist between the verbal and non-verbal content of the message, there is a general tendency for the non-verbal aspects to be viewed as the more accurate or honest of the two.

As the opportunity for, and/or adequacy of, verbal content decreases, non-verbal communication becomes increasingly important. Throughout the human lifespan, the significance of non-verbal behaviours may in fact go full circle— from the only form of communication available in infancy, into partnership with verbal communication as language develops, and back to a relatively more significant position for those who experience deterioration of hearing and/or other senses.

In terms of individuals who, for one of any number of reasons, do not have adequate language skills (e.g. hearing impairments or non-English speaking backgrounds), non-verbal communication is an even more critical element in everyday life. To a neonate the message, 'the world is not such a bad place' is conveyed by a comforting voice and a warm touch; to a patient with a hearing impairment the words, 'I'm here to help you through this' may be replaced by a confident, inspiring manner and an encouraging smile.

Activity 4.4 NON-VERBAL COMMUNICATION: TOUCH

PROCESS

1 Form into groups of four to six members. All members of each group should think of a situation or a 'type' of patient whereby they would find it relatively easy to touch the patient. Share and explain this choice to others within the group.

  a Are there any commonalities between the patients or situations chosen by individual members? If so, what are they?

  b What do you think governs individual choices?

2 Group members should now think of a situation or 'type' of patient whereby they would find it difficult to physically touch the patient.

3 As individuals, rank the patients or situations (chosen by individual members) from the easiest to the most difficult to touch.

4 Share and explain your choice within the group.

DISCUSSION

1 How much do the lists of individual group members coincide?

2 Try to come to a group consensus on the ranking exercise.

3 Why is it easy to touch certain patients and not others?

4 Should nurses attempt to overcome or camouflage their difficulties in this area? If so, how?

The development of appropriate non-verbal communication skills is, therefore, of fundamental importance to the nurse. While the non-verbal component is a normal part of interpersonal interactions, conscious development of particular non-verbal behaviours and their judicious use increases significantly nurses' ability to relate effectively.

The use of an appropriate tone, pitch and rhythm will help convey or stress the importance of the content of verbal messages. An unsteady or wavering voice when discussing a required procedure, for example, will hinder attempts to convey a sense of confidence and may leave patients feeling vulnerable and distressed. Once patients become emotionally upset, the verbal part of the message may become meaningless. A nurse wishing to comfort distressed patients would be more successful if a soothing vocal tone was employed. Touch is an especially important means of non-verbal communication.

Nurses' actions or behaviours can convey a sense of concern, empathy, tolerance of differences, respect, admiration or competence. A self-confident demeanour may help patients feel less concerned about a painful or technically difficult procedure; a thoughtful touch may help dispel fear; and the maintenance of eye contact should encourage patients to truly believe what is being told to them.

In order to minimise their patients' and their own discomfort, nurses need to be aware of the messages they are sending through their actions. Insight into messages associated with particular actions allows nurses to monitor and adjust behaviours for the best possible outcomes. For example, if nurses are trying to convey a sense of acceptance and a matter-of-fact attitude when undertaking particularly repulsive dressings, their behaviours and facial expressions can play a pivotal role. The nature of some of the work undertaken by nurses commonly makes interactions with patients distressing and/or embarrassing. It is difficult, for instance, to conceal negative feelings associated with the ongoing invasion of personal space, or the feelings of repugnance that accompany some of the more unpleasant activities shared by the patient and nurse (Lawler 1991).

Taking the time to mentally rehearse the activity (e.g. the dressing), and what it will look, smell and feel like, as well as practising any specific skills, may be beneficial. In addition, thought may be given to strategies for putting the patient at ease. These may include making a mental list of topics that could be of interest to patients (nursing histories may provide valuable clues) or developing a number of age-appropriate stories or riddles for use with children.

A poignant reminder that non-verbal messages are open to misinterpretation is provided in the following account of the hospitalisation experience of a 12-week-old infant:

> A victim of child abuse, Gary, a 12-week-old infant, was admitted to a large children's hospital with a fractured left femur, seven fractured ribs and extensive bruising. Over the first 2 days of his hospitalisation he was given very few doses of an intramuscular narcotic for pain. As a result of his unrelieved pain, Gary became withdrawn and unresponsive. Instead of alerting the staff who were caring for him to the fact that he was in pain, Gary's behaviour was interpreted as a sign that he was pain-free. 'He wouldn't be so quiet if he was in pain.' When the attending doctor changed the analgesia orders to paracetamol on the third day after admission, not one member of the nursing staff challenged the assumption that Gary's pain was resolving and therefore that the change in medication orders was appropriate.

It may be argued that interpreting Gary's somewhat ambiguous behaviour as benign is in the 'best' interests of nurses who need to protect themselves from potentially overwhelming feelings. In other words, by interpreting Gary's quietness as a sign that he was pain-free, those caring for him avoided the psychological distress that would be associated with caring for a severely abused infant.

It is perceived that one of the most common problems with non-verbal behaviour is the notion that the behaviour may be interpreted in a way that matches with the needs and worldview of the observer; however, this may or may not be an accurate interpretation. Nurses' worldviews, among other things, can also have implications for the types of cultural stereotypes that nurses are likely to apply to patients.

CHAPTER SUMMARY

As societies become increasingly culturally diverse, nurses are challenged to appreciate and accommodate the multiple perspectives on health that cultural diversity brings. This chapter is a beginning step in developing such appreciation and accommodation. Material in the chapter has focused on the importance of understanding cultural diversity and developing nursing practice that is culturally safe. In addition, the chapter has enabled nurses to consider some of the impediments to such understanding (e.g. cultural stereotyping). Some of the challenges of working with interpreters and communicating non-verbally have also been reviewed. Readers should bear in mind that this chapter represents a very brief introduction to the challenges of cross-cultural communication.

REFERENCES

Allshouse K 1993 Treating patients as individuals. In: Gerteis M, Edgman-Levitan S, Daley J, Delbanco TL (eds), Through the patients' eyes: understanding and promoting patient-centered care, pp. 19–44. Jossey-Bass, San Francisco, CA

Blackford J, Street A 2000 Nurses of NESB working in a multicultural community. Contemporary Nurse 6(1):15–21

Bolton LB, Giger JN, Georges A 2004 Structural and racial barriers to health care. Annual Review of Nursing Research 22:39–58

Campinha-Bacote J 2003 The process of cultural competence in the delivery of health-care service: a culturally competent model of care, 4th edn. Transcultural CARE Associates, Cincinnati, OH

Cioffi J 2003 Communicating with culturally and linguistically diverse patients in an acute care setting: nurses' experiences. International Journal of Nursing Studies 40:299–306

Cioffi J 2006 Culturally diverse patient–nurse interaction on acute care wards. International Journal of Nursing Practice 12:319–325

Coffman MJ 2004 Cultural caring in nursing practice: a meta-synthesis of qualitative research. Journal of Cultural Diversity 11(3):100–109

Flores G, Rabke-Verani BA, Pine W, Sabharwal A 2002 The importance of cultural and linguistic issues in the emergency care of children. Pediatric Emergency Care 18:271–284

Fuller J 2003 Intercultural health care as reflective negotiated practice. Western Journal of Nursing Research 25(7):781–797

Green-Hernandez C, Denman-Vitale S, Judge-Ellis T 2004 Making nursing care culturally competent. Holistic Nursing Practice 18(4):215–218

Kleiman S 2006 Discovering cultural aspects of nurse–patient relationships. Journal of Cultural Diversity 13(2):83–86

Lawler J 1991 Behind the screens: nursing, somology and the problem of the body. Churchill Livingstone, Melbourne

McGrath P, Phillips E 2008 Australian findings on Aboriginal cultural practices associated with clothing, hair, possessions and the use of name of deceased persons. International Journal of Nursing Practice 14(1):57–66

McKinley D, Blackford J 2001 Nurses' experiences of caring for culturally and linguistically diverse families when their child dies. International Journal of Nursing Practice 7:251–256

Polaschek NR 1998 Cultural safety: a new concept in nursing people of different ethnicities. Journal of Advanced Nursing 27:452–457

Ramsden I 1993 Kawa Whakaruruhau: cultural safety in nursing education in Aotearoa (New Zealand). Nursing Praxis 8(3):4–10

Richardson S 2004 Aotearoa/NewZealand nursing: from eugenics to cultural safety. Nursing Inquiry 11(1):35–42

Rosenjack Burchum JLR 2002 Cultural competence: an evolutionary perspective. Nursing Forum 37(14):5–15

Schim SM, Doorenbos A, Benkert R, Miller J 2007 Culturally congruent care: putting the puzzle together. Journal of Transcultural Nursing 18 (2):103–110

Short S, Sharman E, Speedy S 1998 Sociology for nurses: an Australian introduction, 2nd edn. Macmillan Education Australia, Melbourne

Suh EE 2004 The model of cultural competence through an evolutional concept analysis. Journal of Transcultural Nursing 15(2):93–102

Wolf KE, Calmes D 2004 Cultural competence in the emergency department. Topics in Emergency Medicine 26(1):9–13

Part II
The skills

This part of the book explores specific interpersonal skills that nurses must develop in order to interact with patients effectively. In Chapters 5–7, there is a focus on the individual skill sets of listening, understanding and exploring. While there are numerous references to how each set relates to other sets, separating them by chapter enables readers to develop skills within manageable learning segments. Chapter 8 offers insight and guidance to nurses as they move from understanding patients' situations to taking meaningful action to comfort, support and enable patients. The numerous learning activities that appear throughout these chapters serve to deepen readers' understanding of the skills and how to use them effectively.

CHAPTER 5

Encouraging interaction: listening

INTRODUCTION

'It wasn't much; I mean, I really didn't do anything to help. All I did was to listen.' Comments such as these, especially when expressed by nurses, fail to acknowledge or demonstrate an appreciation for the complexity and power of effective listening. 'Just listening' seems so simple, as if no effort is required, and no expertise is needed. Listening is powerful because it encourages patients to share their experiences; it validates patients as people with something to say; it promotes understanding between nurse and patient; and it provides the nurse with information on which to act.

It is not nearly as 'simple' as it sounds on the surface. Quite a lot is happening when nurses 'just' listen. When nurses listen, *just* listen, they pay careful attention to what they hear and observe, they focus on what is explicitly expressed by the patient and they try to determine what the patient is meaning. Effective listening requires receptivity, sustained concentration and astute observation. All of this can hardly be summed up as 'not doing anything'.

Nursing care is based on an understanding of patients' personal experiences of health and their responses to illness. In order to reach this level of understanding, nurses must first listen to patients' stories. The skills of listening are fundamental and crucial to patient–nurse relationships. Listening permeates the entire relationship; if meaningful interpersonal connections are to occur, listening must be engaged in throughout every interaction.

Listening actively demonstrates nurses' presence with and interest in patients. Through listening, nurses orient themselves towards patients as people who 'are there'. Listening encourages patients to express themselves, because it provides the necessary time and space for such expression. Listening enables patients to experience being heard and accepted by nurses. Listening enables nurses to understand and appreciate patients' experiences. As such, it sets the stage for effective helping. Nurses base their responses to patients on what is perceived through listening. Once the stage is set, the players can enact their roles (the one helping and the one helped), but it is vital that the stage remains set throughout the relationship.

Chapter overview

This chapter begins with a description of the process of effective listening, highlighting its complexity. Then the benefits of listening within the context of patient–nurse relationships are discussed. Because nurses need to listen with 'nursing ears', listening goals within the nursing-care context are explored next. The following section on mental preparation—the readiness to listen—focuses on how to become more receptive to patients by reducing potential interferences and distractions. A discussion of the skills of listening follows. These include attending, observing, perceiving, interpreting and recalling. The chapter concludes with a description of how to evaluate whether listening has been effective.

THE LISTENING PROCESS

Listening is a complex process that encompasses the skills of reception, perception and interpretation of input. The process begins with input. Sights, sounds, smells, tastes and tactile sensations are received through the sensory organs. The initial step in the listening process is the reception of this input, predominantly through the eyes and ears. The ability to receive the input is dependent upon the listener's state of readiness, when receivers are 'turned on' and 'tuned in'. Next, the received input must be noticed as important; it must be actively perceived. During this stage of the process, external and internal distractions often interfere with accurate perception and create filters, which partially or completely block the input. Almost as soon as the input is perceived, the listener attaches meaning to it—an interpretation is made.

The meaning attached to a particular piece of sensory input is connected to the listener's memory, previous experience, expectations, desires, wants, needs, and current thoughts and feelings. For example, nurses working in a hospital unit know when they hear a particular buzz and see a light over a doorway to a patient's room (sensory input received and perceived) that the patient in that room has turned on the call light, requesting assistance (interpretation). To an outsider, the sound and sight of the call light activation may be received and noticed, but no particular meaning is derived unless there is a familiarity with how hospital units are equipped. If they are busy, nurses who notice the call light may interpret the patient's request for assistance as a nuisance (interpretation based on needs). Likewise, a nurse may decide that the patient requesting assistance is not in immediate need if this particular patient turns on the call light for minor reasons (interpretation based on experience and expectations).

Effective listening encompasses not only receiving sensory input, but also perceiving it and interpreting its meaning. When nurses correctly interpret what patients are expressing, listening has been effective.

Hearing and listening

Listening and hearing are not the same. Any person with the apparatus for detecting audible tones can hear, but may or may not be capable of listening. People without hearing capabilities may be able to listen, while those with hearing capabilities may fail to listen. Listening involves paying active attention to what is being said; it is more than simply receiving sensory input.

Active and passive listening

Effective listening, the active process of taking in, absorbing and eventually understanding what is being expressed, requires energy and concentration on the part of the listener. Have you ever been in a conversation with somebody who claimed to be listening to you but was attending to another matter (e.g. watching television or reading)? No matter how much this person may try to convince you that they are listening, it is not likely you will believe it because they are not offering their full attention.

Hearing, without fully concentrating and attending, is passive listening. Active listening is listening for the purpose of understanding. Not only does it require the reception of sensory input, but also astute observation, undivided attention and the processing or interpretation of what is heard. While some people may be capable of listening to background music while reading or studying, this type of passive reception does not serve listeners well during engaged interpersonal interaction. Effective listening is only achieved in an active and involved manner. It cannot be done passively.

The distinction between hearing and listening has been highlighted in a synthesis of nursing research related to the topics of presence, touch and listening (Fredriksson 1999). Hearing involves 'being there' for patients, while listening involves 'being with' patients. Hearing promotes interpersonal contact between patient and nurse, with the emphasis on task-related activities. Listening promotes interpersonal connection between patient and nurse at a deeper level of commitment. The patient's desire for contact or connection is important to consider, and this reinforces the negotiated aspects of the level of involvement in the relationship (see Ch 2).

BENEFITS OF LISTENING

It is important that nurses understand the benefits of effective listening in order to more fully appreciate its power and helpfulness. Although considered essential to effective communication and relationship building, there is little empirical evidence in the nursing literature on the subject of listening (Kagan 2008b). The benefits are described as those for the patient, those for the nurse and those for the relationship between them.

For the patient

Effective listening is consistent with the concept that nurses care about patients. When nurses take and make time to listen to what patients are expressing, they demonstrate genuine interest in and regard for patients. Listening is one of the clearest ways for nurses to convey respect for and acceptance of patients. By listening, nurses actively demonstrate to patients that what they have to say matters—that patients matter. Nurses give of themselves when they listen. Patients feel worthwhile because they have been given the nurse's time, energy and attention.

Listening reinforces the inherent worth of patients and, as a result, patients feel comforted because they feel valued. Their sense of wellbeing and mental ease are enhanced when nurses are fully present and available to interact because they feel acknowledged and validated as a person (Kagan 2008a, Finfgeld-Connett 2006, Jonas-Simpson 2003, Doona et al 1999). Patients report that listening is an important aspect of what they want in a nurse (Webb & Hope 1995). Likewise, patients associate nurses' caring with their capacity to be fully present and available to them (Nyström et al 2003). In contrast, 'not being listened to' has negative effects on their sense of wellbeing and healthcare (Courts et al 2004).

For the nurse

Any verbal response that nurses make is based on what is perceived through listening to the patient. Listening to patients enables nurses to receive information about patients, collect data on which to base nursing-care activities and reach deeper levels of understanding with patients. Being fully present with a patient, as would be evidenced through listening, has been linked to effective clinical decision making in nursing (Doona et al 1999, 1997).

Theoretical understanding of a particular clinical situation offers possibilities and probabilities, but listening to an individual patient's experience offers concrete, personally unique data on which to base responsive nursing care. For example, chronic illness often affects a patient's sense of self-worth (a theoretical possibility). But by listening to an individual patient's experience of and reactions to chronic illness, the nurse comes to understand concretely and specifically how this particular patient's sense of self-worth is, or is not, affected by the experience. Listening encourages patients to open up and tell their stories and, as a result, nurses are in a better position to understand patients more personally.

For the relationship

Listening encourages further interaction between patient and nurse. It is a catalyst in promoting trust in their relationship, because patients will come to know that they can rely on the nurse to 'be there'. When patients feel listened to, they feel a sense of connection with nurses, thus enabling the relationship to progress (Kagan 2008a, Jonas-Simpson et al 2006, Gilbert 2004, Doona et al 1999).

At times, listening with understanding is all that is needed in an interaction; it is an end in itself. For example, listening to a patient's expression of sadness in response to a loss may be just what the nurse needs to do in order to be of help. At other times, listening is a means to another end—a responsive nursing action based on understanding that is achieved through listening. For example, as a result of listening to a patient express a lack of understanding about a current medication regimen, the nurse can explain why it is important (e.g. to take medication prior to eating).

LISTENING WITH NURSING EARS

The general benefits of listening in the nursing-care context are important to appreciate; however, the benefits refer primarily to how meaningful interaction between patient and nurse is enhanced. What about the content of listening in the nursing-care context? When nurses listen, they need to listen for aspects of the patient's experience that are significant in the context of nursing care. What should be the focus when listening to patients? What kinds of meanings and understandings are specific to the clinical practice of nursing? What particular aspects of patients' experiences are most relevant to nurses? Listening with 'nursing ears' is listening for specific nursing-related meanings, and an understanding of these meanings forms the basis of listening goals within the nursing context.

Activity 5.1 poses challenges because it suggests that certain limitations can be imposed on listening. Does listening with 'nursing ears' mean that nurses should ignore, avoid or filter out aspects that are not directly related to nursing concerns? The answer is no, as it implies partial listening. While it is important for nurses to recognise what concerns them *as nurses*, there is potential danger when listening goals are overemphasised. When this occurs, goals for listening become barriers.

Activity 5.1 LISTENING GOALS IN NURSING

PROCESS

1 Form small groups of about five participants.

2 Discuss the answers to the following questions:
   a 'What do I need to know and understand about patients in order to care effectively for them?'
   b 'When I am listening to patients, what is most significant for me to notice about what they are expressing?'

3 Record and compare your answers with other small groups.

DISCUSSION

1 Do the answers to the questions provide any focus for listening in nursing? If so, what is the focus?

2 Are there aspects of patients' experiences that are more significant to nursing than other aspects? What are these?

3 What are the major goals of listening in the nursing context? List them.

4 Listening with nursing ears means focusing on goals. Compare your list in step 3 with the following goals (presented in question form):
   a What effects do patients' current health status have on their daily living?
   b How do patients interpret their health status?
   c How are patients reacting to the healthcare they are receiving?
   d How are patients reacting to your nursing approach in particular?
   e How much do patients understand about their health status and healthcare? How much do they want to understand?
   f Who or what is most important to patients? What do they value the most in life?
   g What is worrying patients the most about their health status and healthcare?

Rather than perceiving these goals as limitations, it is better to think of them as focusing lenses through which to view patients. To take the analogy further, imagine looking through the lens of a camera and focusing on a particular subject within a scene. While the entire landscape is in view, the camera lens brings some aspects of the picture into sharper focus than others. Such is the case when using listening goals in the nursing context. While the entire 'picture' (i.e. the patient) is in view (received), some aspects are brought more sharply in focus (perceived), because these aspects have direct relevance to nursing care.

Another way to employ listening goals in nursing is to use them as orienting and guiding frameworks during the interpretation of received messages. Attention needs to be paid to the patient's entire message; however, the message is interpreted in light of the goals of listening. The message is perceived as is, but the meaning is interpreted using a nursing framework. This framework, or orientation to listening, is then viewed as enhancing rather than limiting because it provides direction to the nurse's listening. Consider the following story:

> When he first met James Nott, Matthew, an experienced cardiac nurse, was completing the usual admission procedure onto the cardiac surgical ward. He had to complete all the necessary observations of James' physical condition but, more importantly, he needed to get to know James as a person. As Matthew listened to his story of a lifelong problem with his mitral valve, he realised that James understood the implications of his scheduled valve replacement surgery. James told Matthew that he knew that the surgery would need to be done someday.
>
> Naturally, James was concerned about the surgery itself, but he reassured himself with the knowledge that he was in the capable hands of an experienced cardiac surgery team. As he listened, Matthew began to realise the potential impact of the surgery on James' life. He was employed as a night-shift supervisor of a large coal preparation plant, a position he worked hard to obtain and an achievement of which he was proud. Nevertheless, his job involved a great deal of walking around the plant and James noted his increasing inability 'to get around like I used to'. He was afraid that he might become disabled after the surgery, unable to continue in a job he obviously enjoyed. He understood the details of the surgery, recognised that it was necessary, and accepted it. Yet he was worried about what it might mean for his future.

In focusing on James' concern about the potential impact of the surgery, of what it might mean in terms of his daily life, Matthew was listening with 'nursing ears'.

READINESS TO LISTEN

Effective listening requires a certain amount of mental preparation in order to achieve a state of readiness. A nurse's 'readiness to listen' is as important as the act of perceiving actively and fully what a patient is expressing. Even before messages are received, the conditions necessary for the reception of input must be realised. Firstly, nurses must have the intent and desire to listen to patients. Positive intentions and desires alone, however, are not enough; they need to be conveyed to the patient.

Activity 5.2 highlights characteristics of effective listeners, namely:
- availability to interact
- having the time to listen
- not interrupting the speaker
- not judging, evaluating, advising or imposing their own ideas on the speaker
- not merely listening for what they want to hear, and
- openness to whatever is being expressed.

Effective listeners demonstrate the readiness to listen through these attitudes and behaviours.

Activity 5.2 INDICATORS OF LISTENING

PROCESS

1 Think of someone in your life who really listens to you. Visualise this person. Reflect on your reasons for choosing this person. Why do you think of this person as one who listens? What does this person do that leads you to believe that they listen?

2 Record your thoughts and reflections about this person.

3 Now think of someone in your life who does not seem to listen to you. Visualise this person. Reflect on your reasons for choosing this person. Why do you think of this person as one who does not listen to you? What does this person do that leads you to believe that they do not listen?

4 Record your thoughts and reflections about this person.

DISCUSSION

1 Compare your recordings of each person, the listener and the non-listener. What differences do you note?

2 Summarise the major differences between people who listen and people who do not.

3 If working in a group, compare your summary with the summaries of other participants.

People who are inpatients in acute care hospital settings have reported that nurses often appear 'too busy' with the completion of tasks, and therefore did not have the time to interact with patients (Chang et al 2005, Shattell 2005, McCabe 2004). It may be that nurses are feeling overwhelmed by their workload as they attend to the numerous tasks that occupy their workday, but this may communicate to patients that there is little time available to listen. When this happens, nurses cannot convey a readiness to listen. Focusing on tasks reflects a value that the tasks are more important than the people who are the patients. Patients are left with the feeling that the nurse's time is too precious to interrupt.

When the desire to help is present, yet there is a perception that there is no time to listen, nurses are placed in a bind. There is a fear that the demands of current healthcare systems on nurses increasingly are distracting them from interacting with patients (Corbin 2008). Lack of time and competing demands can prevent nurses from being fully present and available to listen (Doona et al 1999). A recent study uncovered that a shortage of supplies and an inability to get to know patients and their families led to difficult encounters in the nurse–patient relationship (Macdonald 2007). That is, when there is little time for nurses and patients to connect, care can become diminished.

Receptivity

In order for a television set to receive a signal or transmission, the set has to be tuned into the correct frequency so the signal can be processed. This analogy is useful in understanding the readiness to listen. Nurses must 'tune into' patients' signals and adjust their receivers so that the messages are not only audible, but also comprehensible. This involves the mental preparation of focusing concentration on a patient's messages and developing antennae to notice what a patient is expressing.

Tuning in to a patient's message is hard work. Some signals are easier to receive than others. At times, there is so much interference that the signal cannot be received at all.

Activity 5.3 EASY OR HARD TO LISTEN TO

PROCESS

1 In small groups of about five to six participants, think about the subjects, topics, feelings and experiences that patients bring up with nurses. Consider as many as possible. List these.

2 Review the list and discuss whether the item is easy to listen to or hard to listen to, and mark each accordingly.

3 In small groups, compare lists and discuss similarities and differences.

DISCUSSION

1 Were there any general areas that were assessed as difficult? As easy? What are they?

2 On what basis were assessments of easy or hard made?

3 Are there any general trends and themes present? What are these themes? Divide these into easy and hard categories.

4 How might this assessment of easy and hard enhance or interfere with effective listening?

Reducing interference

Interference stems from distractions that draw attention away from the patient and prevent clear reception of a message. Such distractions originate externally (from outside of the nurse) and internally (from within the nurse).

External interference

It is important to pay careful attention to the external environment when attempting to listen. For example, the sights and sounds of a busy, bustling hospital setting often present many potential sources of external interference. The ringing of telephones, a variety of healthcare personnel coming and going, and patients being transported from one area to another, are potential distractions. When nurses visit patients in their home setting, distractions such as the playful noise of small children and a radio or television may be sources of interference. It is not always possible to eliminate external sights, sounds and other stimuli, but attempts should be made to reduce them as much as possible when listening to patients.

In a hospital setting, drawing the curtains around a patient's bed not only provides a degree of privacy, but also decreases the number of external distractions and potential interferences. This simple act is effective in reducing the amount of visual distractions, but may not reduce the audible ones. Also, it sends a clear message to others that a meaningful activity is occurring.

Interruptions from other staff members can be particularly distracting—even the fear of being interrupted is a potential distraction. Nurses working together in a clinical setting need to be mindful of this; they should assess the need to distract another nurse who is engaged in an interaction with a patient.

Sometimes, there are aspects of patients themselves that are sources of external interference. Examples of this kind of interference include: patients who speak in accents that are distracting to a nurse; patients who express themselves in a disjointed, rambling manner; and patients whose speech is barely audible and halting. In these instances, nurses can reduce the interference by attempting to put aside the distractions and concentrating carefully on what the patient is expressing.

In general, the reduction of external interference occurs whenever attempts are made to exclude the outside world. This is done by placing barriers between the outside world and the patient and nurse, or by consciously tuning out external noise.

Internal interference

When nurses are ready to listen, they are able to forget themselves for the moment. They allow themselves to be engrossed in the interaction with a patient and to notice and perceive what the patient is expressing. Internal interference, the nurse's own thoughts, feelings, preoccupations or value judgments, are often more difficult to control than external interference. A noisy television set (an external interference) can simply be switched off in order to eliminate it as a source of distraction. Internal interferences cannot simply be switched off.

Thoughts as internal interference One common preoccupation that interferes with listening is the worry a nurse often feels about how to respond to the patient. 'What am I going to say to this patient?' 'What am I going to do for this patient?' Thoughts such as these are often related to a self-expectation that nurses must 'do something' in order to help patients. As a result, nurses become so preoccupied with their own anxieties that they fail to listen and perceive what the patient is expressing. An internal reminder that something is being done—'I am listening to what this patient is expressing'—can help to draw nurses' focus away from their own thoughts and onto the patient. If something else can be done, it will become evident *after* the nurse listens with understanding to what the patient is expressing.

Other thoughts that potentially interfere with listening include any preoccupations that a nurse may have at any given moment. These range from 'Have I remembered to defrost something to eat for dinner tonight?' to 'There is a waiting room full of mothers and babies and I am not going to have time to see each of them' to 'Ms Holmes will need pre-op medications soon. I wonder how long this conversation is going to last. How can I bring it to a close?'

Sometimes these thoughts can be excluded from conscious awareness, while at other times they signal the need to attend to another matter, and then return to the interaction at hand. At yet other times, such thoughts are impossible to exclude from conscious awareness, but nurses pretend to be listening. It is far better to cease the interaction until such time that undivided attention can be given to a patient than to feign listening.

Value judgments as internal interference The natural tendency to judge what is heard as right or wrong, good or bad, interesting or boring is one of the greatest sources of internal interference when attempting to listen. This tendency is considered natural because it happens automatically, often without conscious awareness. 'That is a stupid way to react.' 'I don't think he should be feeling that way.' 'What's she going on about—it's really nothing.' Such thoughts are judgmental, because they channel the patient's message through the nurse's personal interpretive filter. They interfere with listening because they close off possibilities that do not match the nurse's internal frame of reference.

What is heard may be evaluated negatively and rejected outright as unacceptable. Even if what is heard is evaluated in a positive light, it interferes with a nurse's ability to fully appreciate and understand the uniqueness of a patient's experience, because the nurse is still relying on a personal frame of reference.

While it is almost impossible to prevent valuative thoughts, aware nurses recognise them as stemming from a personal value system, and therefore are able to separate their own value system from the patient's value system. Personal judgments, once separated, can then be held in suspense, deferred and kept peripheral to the patient. Being non-judgmental is a near impossible goal to achieve; however, keeping one's value system separate and suspended is achievable. The most critical aspect of suspending judgment is the nurse's self-understanding (see Ch 3).

Feelings as internal interference Sometimes, internal interference stems from a nurse's lack of ability to cope with what the patient is expressing; for example, a feeling of despondency might overwhelm a nurse listening to the sorrow of a young mother dying of cancer. Nurses may fail to listen because of their own anxieties, and they may, unwittingly or unknowingly, either change the subject or avoid interacting with the patient altogether. There are times when nurses' own circumstances create a sense of vulnerability that prevents them from being fully present with a patient. When emotional demands are high, nurses are at risk of 'switching off' in an effort to protect themselves (Barrett et al 2005).

The majority of times, nurses fail to listen to patients' stories that are distressing out of fear of not knowing what to say or how to respond. Not listening or even avoiding a patient for these reasons potentially compounds the patient's distress because it isolates and distances a patient from the nurse, thus disabling the relationship.

Nurses must remind themselves that listening to a patient's distress, no matter how disturbing, is comforting simply because it shows they are fully present and genuinely interested in the patient. Words spoken by nurses in an attempt to comfort may actually intrude. Listening is 'being there' with these patients. Often, patients do not want or need words in these extreme situations. The caring of another human being is more than adequate, and helps to make the 'unbearable bearable' (Doona et al 1999).

When nurses become overwhelmed, and perhaps paralysed, by their own feelings as a result of what patients are expressing and experiencing, seeking support from other nurses is preferable to avoiding or emotionally abandoning the patient (see Ch 11).

Once the state of readiness to listen is achieved, a nurse is available to be fully present during an interaction with a patient. Attention is focused and undivided, perceptual filters are open, antennae are up and interference is reduced. This state of readiness, when maintained throughout the interaction, not only enables nurses to listen, but also encourages further interaction.

THE SKILLS OF LISTENING

The groundwork involved in achieving the readiness to listen is an inward process initiated by nurses as they prepare both themselves and the environment. Readiness alone, however, is not sufficient for effective listening because two-way communication with a patient has not yet begun. This section explores the interactive nature of listening because the skills of listening are enacted through interchange with another person. The skills of listening are divided into five areas: attending, observing, perceiving, interpreting and recalling.

Attending

Attending behaviour is the outward, physical manifestation of a nurse's readiness to listen. It communicates to the patient that the nurse is available to listen and accessible to interact. The outward behaviour of attending conveys the message, 'Go ahead, you have my attention, I'm here with you now.' Patients find it valuable when nurses give of their time to be available to patients and associate such attending behaviour with helpful communication (McCabe 2004).

The messages of attending are sent through non-verbal channels, predominantly body posture and eye contact. For example, a nurse checking a patient's healthcare record for recent documentation (no matter how casually), while attempting to listen, is not fully communicating their intent because they are not demonstrating attending behaviour to the patient.

Attending behaviour has two key elements: the spatial position of the nurse in relation to the patient and the maintenance of eye contact. During Activity 5.4, the Bs will probably alter their non-verbal behaviour by leaning forward and looking directly at the As when the conversation becomes more 'interesting'. They will assume the posture of attending.

| Activity 5.4 PHYSICAL ATTENDING | ➥302 |

PROCESS

1 Divide the large group into three groups. Designate one of the three groups as As, one as Bs and one as Cs.

2 Distribute instructions to As, Bs and Cs. (These instructions can be found in the appendix.) Do not share the instructions with participants who are not in the same group.

3 As and Bs should seat themselves according to the instructions. Allow enough room between each B so that they will not disturb other groups during the activity.

4 Cs should stand around the edge of the room and act as observers during the activity. Cs should follow the guidelines for observing as outlined in their instructions.

5 As and Bs now have a quiet conversation, following the instructions.

6 After 5 minutes, As and Bs stop the conversation and show each other their instructions.

7 Cs report their observations.

DISCUSSION

1 How did the Bs' non-verbal behaviour change during the conversation?

2 What did the Cs notice about the change in the Bs' non-verbal behaviour about 2 minutes into the conversation?

3 What did the As notice about the Bs' non-verbal behaviour during the conversation?

4 What did the Bs notice about their own non-verbal behaviour during the conversation?

While attending, nurses physically place themselves in a manner that promotes interaction between themselves and patients. Attending behaviour demonstrates active interest in the patient. Egan (2007) presents general guidelines for attending using the acronym SOLER, which stands for:

S Squarely facing the person in a front-on presentation

O Open posture, conveying an acceptance and openness to the other person

L Leaning forward, demonstrating active interest

E Eye contact maintained, including being at the same eye level as the other person

R Relaxed posture, demonstrating an ease with self, the other and the situation.

Attending promotes active engagement between nurses and patients, and encourages patients to continue expressing themselves.

Attending encourages further interaction between patient and nurse, while non-attending is discouraging. In Activity 5.5, person A will probably not wish to continue the conversation after person B begins non-attending. No matter how intent a nurse may be on listening, without attending a patient will not be encouraged to continue.

Activity 5.5 ATTENDING AND NON-ATTENDING ➡302

PROCESS

1 Divide into pairs and designate one person as A and the other as B.

Instructions to A

2 Tell a story to B about something exciting or interesting that has happened to you. Talk for about 5 minutes on the subject.

Instructions to B

3 Begin the interaction by assuming the attending posture (i.e. face A, maintain eye contact, lean forward and remain relaxed and open). After about a minute or two, start to lean back, fold your arms and look away from A. Focus on something other than what A is saying (e.g. stare out the window, clean your nails, flip through a book). Do anything to violate the rules of attending. Remain silent, do not interrupt or change the subject, but do try to keep listening.

4 Stop the conversation after about 5 minutes.

DISCUSSION

1 How did A feel during the interaction? What happened to A when B began non-attending?

2 How did B feel during the interaction? What happened to B when they began non-attending?

3 How did the conversation change when B no longer appeared interested?

Some words of caution about attending

The intensity of attending is not always appropriate, because it is not always warranted by the topic at hand. Try assuming the posture during a conversation about the weather. You will note that intense attending feels awkward when the subject of the conversation is of little consequence. A discussion about the weather, unless there has recently been a significant event related to the weather, does not warrant such an intense listening response. This is important for nurses to bear in mind. There are times when patients discuss subjects that do not require the intensity of attending and for a nurse to assume the posture is not only awkward, but inappropriate.

The attending guideline about maintaining eye contact is another area that presents some difficulty, and caution needs to be exercised when applying this guideline. Unbroken eye contact is unnatural, awkward and even threatening because of the discomfort it creates. The head-on position of attending is criticised (Shea & Maloney 1998) because it forces eye contact that is then difficult to break. When nurses are attending, it is important to bear in mind that occasional breaks in eye contact are not only natural, but also desirable in maintaining comfort and ease during the interaction.

Finally, an attending posture, which focuses on eye contact as one of its central aspects, may not be appropriate in some cultures. Maintaining eye contact can be a sign of disrespect when there are cultural norms about status. Looking directly into the eyes of a person who is of a higher status is unacceptable when these cultural norms are operating. Likewise, eye contact may vary with age and gender. Nurses need to be sensitive to how patients are responding to their attempts to encourage interaction through attending behaviour and a large part of this sensitivity is awareness of age-related and cultural variances (see Chs 4 and 10). For example, in some cultures it is considered rude to look a person in authority (as nurses are often viewed) directly in the eye (i.e. to make eye contact with them).

Attending within the clinical nursing context

In nursing, it is sometimes difficult to assume the classic attending posture. Nurses must learn to adapt the attending posture to the realities of their particular clinical setting. It is not always possible to face the patient squarely. In a hospital, when patients are lying in bed and the nurse is standing nearby, the attending mandate of squarely facing the other may be impossible to achieve. How can attending be demonstrated under these circumstances? Nurses need to physically situate themselves in such a manner to establish eye contact, maintain a relaxed stance and be close enough to interact in a meaningful manner, but far enough away to maintain comfort.

Standing at the side of the bed is preferable to standing at the foot of the bed. Although the foot position would allow a nurse to squarely face a patient, it may actually discourage interaction because it leaves too much distance between patient and nurse, and places the nurse in an authoritarian stance. By placing themselves at the side of the bed, nurses are almost facing the same direction as the patient. Shea and Maloney (1998) believe this position is actually preferable to the 'squarely facing' one, because it demonstrates that a nurse is attempting to view the world *with* the patient, sharing a common perspective.

While standing at the side of the bed, nurses are faced with the challenge of lowering themselves to the eye level of the patient, unless the height of the bed is at a level that places the patient at the same eye level as the nurse. Having a seat is the most logical way to meet this challenge. This also sends the message to the patient that the nurse intends to remain there—to interact. While seated, nurses are obviously accessible and available to patients.

Awareness that being seated is preferable can pose a dilemma for nurses. There may be a shortage of chairs. If they seat themselves, they may be reprimanded or frowned upon by other nurses for not working hard enough. The hard work of listening to patients is often unrecognised and unacknowledged, especially in the hospital setting where so much 'other work' needs to be accomplished. In long-term residential settings, such as nursing homes, it is vital for nurses to lower themselves to the level of the patient and establish eye contact in an effort to gain their attention.

Silence

Obviously, when nurses are attending and listening to patients, they are silent. Silence plays a major part in effective listening, and its value is important to recognise. To be silent and not interrupt patients who are expressing themselves is a sign of respect and interest.

Silence can also go further in its helpfulness. Both patient and nurse may be silent for short periods of time. Silent moments are useful because they allow patient and nurse time to collect their thoughts and reflect on what has been expressed; they provide an opportunity for either patient or nurse to change the direction of the conversation; and they slow the pace of the interaction. Nevertheless, nurses frequently experience difficulty in remaining silent because of a felt need to say or do something.

There are times when silently being with a patient, fully attending and being fully present is quite helpful. Patients who are in severe physical pain may not wish to talk or be spoken to, but would like to have a nurse present. Patients who are psychologically depressed may feel pressured to interact, and would benefit from a nurse's silent, undemanding presence. These two situations provide examples of contexts in which the silent presence of nurses is appropriate and helpful.

During a verbal interaction, it is important to ascertain when to allow the silence to proceed and when it is better to break the silence with speech or action. Nurses can employ some general guidelines when they are faced with the decision. First and foremost, silence should not be used as a substitute or excuse for not knowing how to respond or what to say. When used in this way, silence could be interpreted by the patient as rejection or lack of interest on the part of the nurse. It is better for nurses to admit to feeling 'at a loss for words' under these circumstances. Silence is also ineffective if the patient expects or wants a verbal response from the nurse. Careful attention to the flow and direction of the interaction allows nurses to 'check its pulse' and perceive patient cues that indicate discomfort with the silence.

Silent periods also have limitations if they last longer than about 10–15 seconds. When silence progresses beyond these time limits, the flow of the interaction may be stifled, rather than enhanced. Try this experiment the next time you are interacting with a patient: when a silent period ensues, check your watch and time it. You may be surprised how long a 10–15-second period of silence actually feels. Next, evaluate whether or not the silence is of benefit to the interaction. Repeated experiments of this kind enable nurses to judge the length and usefulness of silent moments during interactions with patients.

Observing

Effective listening includes astute observation of the patient. A large part of listening is not only paying careful attention to what is expressed, but also how it is expressed. During listening, nurses have a good opportunity to observe the non-verbal aspects of the patient's expressions. Subtle and obvious cues about patients' experiences are better understood when nurses perceive patients' non-verbal behaviour. Non-verbal cues often shed light on the feeling aspects of a patient's experience. Feelings are most often expressed through facial expression, eye contact, body posture and movements, and other non-verbal behaviour. Such patient cues are signals for further exploration (see Ch 7), but the nurse must first notice the cues. The noticing of cues and their initial interpretation occur in the context of listening.

No doubt, participants in Activity 5.6 will experience a heightened awareness of the non-verbal indicators of feelings, because they are asked to determine what feelings other participants are expressing. Their perceptual antennae are ready for the reception of non-verbal input. It is beneficial for nurses to develop and maintain this degree of heightened perceptual awareness when interacting with patients. Heightened perceptual awareness enables nurses to be more astute in their observations. It makes them notice the way in which a patient is relaying messages.

The inherent difficulty in accurately interpreting non-verbal messages is also demonstrated in Activity 5.6. This highlights and reinforces the need for nurses to check their perceptions through exploration (see Ch 7). Noticing and

Activity 5.6 NON-VERBAL EXPRESSIONS OF FEELINGS

PROCESS

1 Form groups of five to six participants and decide on a topic for discussion. The chosen topic can be of any nature, but it needs to be one about which participants *can* express emotions. Controversial topics are most effective (e.g. euthanasia, abortion, IVF, rights of smokers).

2 Participants should reflect on their feelings or emotions in relation to the selected topic. Each participant records this feeling or emotion on a slip of paper. These slips of paper are not shared with other participants.

3 Participants should reflect on how they usually express their chosen emotion non-verbally.

4 In small groups, now discuss the chosen topic. Throughout the discussion, each participant expresses their chosen feeling through non-verbal means only. Participants are not to express their chosen feeling in a verbal manner (i.e. they cannot *say* how they feel).

5 Stop the discussion after about 10 minutes.

6 Each member of a small group should record what feeling they believe was being expressed by each of the other members, as well as the non-verbal behaviour that led to this conclusion. Participants do not consult with any other members at this point.

7 Each group member takes a turn asking other members what feeling they thought they were expressing. After each states their conclusion, the member whose feeling was being discussed shows the other members the feeling recorded during step 2. Continue around the small group until each member's feeling expression is discussed.

DISCUSSION

1 On what basis did participants determine what feeling was being expressed? Would this differ between cultural groups, age groups or gender groups?

2 How accurate were the guesses about what feeling was being expressed? What discrepancies existed between what others interpreted and what the participant intended to convey? Why?

3 What does this say about the valid interpretation of non-verbal messages?

observing non-verbal cues of patients is significant in the context of listening. The cues must then be validated by the patient as to their correct meaning because listening enables nurses to observe them, but not necessarily to interpret them accurately.

Perceiving messages

Attending demonstrates nurses' interest in listening to the patient and observing enables nurses to notice non-verbal cues presented by patients. Patients are now encouraged and free to tell their story to an actively interested nurse, and the nurse is in a position to receive the patient's messages.

There are many facets to patients' stories, including the actual content of the story, the related feelings and the general theme of the story. Each facet comes together to create a picture of the patient—the whole story. While it is vital that the nurse receives the entire story, knowledge of the various facets of messages guides a nurse's perception throughout the listening process.

The following story, related by a female resident of a nursing home, serves as an example of the various facets of a story:

> Michael, the diversional therapist, never pushes you to participate in his activities. He takes one look at you and knows whether you feel like participating that day. He'll say, 'Come along, and just watch today, okay?' He always has so many activities going, but you really don't have to do anything you don't feel like doing. That is what's so good about this place.

The content of this story revolves around the activities conducted by the diversional therapist. The feelings expressed are of contentment and satisfaction at not being forced to participate in these activities. The resident uses her discussion of the diversional therapy program as an illustration of the general manner in which residents of the nursing home are treated. The general theme is one of feeling respected by the way she is treated. The content (the diversional therapy activities) and its related feelings (happy and satisfied) come together to form the theme—the importance of having her wishes respected by others.

Notice how the resident speaks of herself in the second person, using the personal pronoun 'you' to indicate herself. When listening to patients it is important that nurses recognise use of the pronoun 'you' in patients' direct reference to themselves. In doing so, they are relating information about themselves, not another person. Perceptive nurses, who are in tune with patients' expressions, notice this use of language and can more fully understand the themes of patients' stories as a result.

At times, patients directly express the content, feeling and thematic facets of their stories, as in the example about the diversional therapist. At other times, however, any or all of the facets are expressed indirectly, through implications, hints and cues. Either way, the various facets of the patient's story must be received and perceived by the nurse who is listening.

Perceiving content

The content of a message contains the objective, factual data about the topic being discussed and includes what is being discussed, who it involves, and when and where an event occurred. The content of a message is the story line. The following example, related by a female patient on an orthopaedic ward of a hospital, serves as an illustration:

> I had these pains in my Achilles tendon. I think it had something to do with playing tennis every day. At first I tried to ignore the pain, but it became so bad that I knew I had to do something. When I saw my local GP, he suggested cortisone injections, so I took the advice and had the injections. That was when the real trouble started. First my right leg started to give way, buckling on me. I fell a few times, and then the final time I fell, I really hurt myself. Now I'm told the right tendon has snapped, and here I am, needing to have it repaired. The whole thing has been going on for about 6 months now.

The content of this patient's story includes pain, falling, the local GP, cortisone injections, an injured Achilles tendon, the need to have the tendon repaired and a time frame of the past 6 months.

Activity 5.7 highlights some of the difficulties inherent in listening. Firstly, there is a tendency for the listener to add elements that are not directly stated. For example, the assumption is often made that the person speaking in story II is the mother of the child. It could be a primary caregiver of any relationship.

Activity 5.7 LISTENING FOR CONTENT ➡302

PROCESS

1 This activity lists six patients' stories, as told by them. Read each one *once* only. Then cover it up and try to recall the content of the story. If possible, have someone else read the stories to you aloud (once only).

2 Record as much of the content of the message as you can recall. In recalling content, think about the following: 'who' is being discussed; 'what' is being discussed; 'when' and 'where' did the 'what' occur; and 'why' it is being discussed. Record the content on a piece of paper using the headings who, what, when, where and why.

Patient story I – I felt something really strange in my hip when I stood up yesterday. It began to really hurt and I was having trouble walking properly. Because it was Sunday afternoon, I didn't want to bother anybody. So I took some aspirin, took it easy and went to bed early. Today when I woke up, I rang my doctor. She said to go and have the hip X-rayed before I do anything else.

Patient story II – The day started off as usual. I fed him breakfast, and got him ready to go to kindy. I was getting ready to go to work, when he suddenly began rolling on the floor, clutching his stomach and writhing in pain. It took me a while to work out what was happening, and I felt panicked inside, although I didn't let on. I knew it was something major, but had no idea what was happening. I rang my GP's surgery, and the receptionist said to come in straight away. I got into the car immediately and drove there.

Patient story III – I was outside doing the gardening when I suddenly realised I could not move my left arm. I looked at it, saw it was still there, but could not make it move an inch. My beautiful left arm was just hanging there. I walked towards the house, not knowing exactly what I was going to do. I sat down on the sofa to think, when I realised that I could move my arm again. Then I really didn't know what to do.

Patient story IV – I have been really worried about him. He hasn't been himself for months. When he comes home from work, he has dinner and then just sits in front of the television. I can tell he is not really paying attention to it because he just stares. He doesn't even laugh at the funny bits of his favourite show. When I ask what's wrong, he just shrugs his shoulders.

Patient story V – I know I should have regular pap smears, but I never seem to find the time. What with the kids, my job and everything, I can't fit in a trip to my GP. Anyway, there is no cancer in my family. Maybe doing all those tests is just a way for the doctors to make money.

Patient story VI – All that chemo and radiotherapy really takes it out of me. I try so hard not to give in to feeling so tired. I go to my room and think, 'Oh, I'll just go close my eyes for a few minutes', and the next thing you know I have been asleep for a few hours. It's not fair on my kids because they need me to be there for them.

(Note: Suggested answers to this activity can be found at the end of this chapter.)

DISCUSSION

1 In each story, which part of the content was easiest to recall? Which was most difficult? What difficulties did you experience in recalling the content of the stories?

2 How accurate was your recall of content, when you compare your results with those provided at the end of the chapter? (Do not become overly concerned if your answers do not match exactly the ones provided.)

3 Did you discover you 'read into' the stories, and added content that was not originally there? Were there aspects of the content that you deleted? Or distorted?

4 What methods did you find yourself using as you attempted to recall the content of the stories?

Source: Adapted from Carkhuff (1983).

When nurses are listening, there is a tendency to make assumptions about what the patient is discussing. Sometimes, these assumptions are accepted and even acted upon as if they were fact. When listening, it is important that nurses keep this tendency under check and recognise that further interaction is necessary to validate these initial assumptions (see Ch 7).

Perceiving feelings

When listening, the nurse must perceive the feeling aspects of the patient's story, the emotional reactions and subjective responses that accompany the content. Patients often have strong emotional reactions to their health status and healthcare, and the importance of emotions in coping with demands such as those created by health events is increasingly recognised as central to understanding (Lazarus 2006). The connection of feelings to content begins to complete the picture that is the patient's experience. At times, patients express their feelings directly. For example:

- 'I'm really worried about the surgery.'
- 'I am so pleased with the results of that MRI test.'
- 'I'm feeling a bit down and blue today.'

When expressed in a straightforward manner, patients' feelings are easy to perceive, as long as nurses are ready to listen and receive input. More often, feelings are not expressed so openly and directly. Feeling expression follows a more circuitous route, unlike content, which is often expressed in a straightforward manner. Feelings are often hinted at, implied, inferred and talked around, rather than talked about. It could be that patients are reluctant to share their feelings because of uncertainty about how the nurse will react. This is especially true when trust has not yet been established. It could be that patients are unaware of, and out of touch with, their feelings. These are possible explanations for why feelings are expressed indirectly.

A more probable reason is that adults often try to conceal emotions, because they have learnt, through socialisation, which emotions are appropriate to express in various situations (Nelson-Jones 2005). It may be that patients believe it is not appropriate to share their feelings with nurses. But, no matter how much patients try to disguise or hide their feelings, their indirect expression is received by nurses whose perceptual antennae are ready to receive feeling messages.

There is, however, a word of caution about focusing on feelings. Research demonstrates that when nurses are perceptive to patients' feelings, the patients' distress increases (Reid-Ponte 1992). This could be because patients were encouraged to express emotions to nurses who were good listeners. There is evidence that nurses tend to overestimate the degree of emotional distress patients are experiencing, when compared to what patients report (Hegedus 1999, Farrell 1991). That is, patients often do not perceive their feelings to be as significant as nurses think they are. The interpersonal dynamics at play are important to bear in mind when listening for feelings.

In listening for feelings, it is vital for nurses to suspend their personal judgments about what is acceptable and appropriate. Feelings, by their very nature, are often irrational, illogical and difficult to control. In order for nurses to be open to the perception of patients' feelings, they must hold the view that feelings are acceptable.

Open perception of feeling messages poses a challenge to nurses, not only because of the natural tendency to judge them, but also because of the way in which they are indirectly expressed. As described in the section on observing, feelings are often expressed non-verbally, and an observant nurse will pick up these non-verbal cues. Feelings are also expressed indirectly, through verbal means, and the perceptive nurse will notice them.

While there is a tendency to jump to conclusions and make assumptions when listening for content, there is an even greater danger of this when listening for feelings. Listeners tend to project their own opinions about what feelings are being expressed. This is partly because feelings are subjective by nature. The tendency is for listeners to perceive feelings on the basis of what they would feel, given a similar set of circumstances. As with suspending judgment, nurses need to rely on their self-awareness and emotional intelligence (Ch 3) in order to keep this tendency in check.

Activity 5.8 LISTENING FOR FEELINGS   ➡303

PROCESS

1 Participants in a group take turns reading each patient statement aloud. Before each participant reads the statement they should think about a feeling to be conveyed along with the statement and then read it with the non-verbal cues that depict that feeling. Each participant records what they think the person reading the statement is feeling.

   a 'I'm dying, aren't I?'

   b 'Are you sure you know what you are doing?'

c 'That right leg won't ever be as strong as it used to be, no matter how hard I try.'
d 'I just wish I could be like I was before.'
e 'I've had enough. I just want to die.'
f 'Why can't anybody show me how to get out of this bed without pain?'
g 'I don't think my back will ever stop aching.'
h 'You have to be tough to be a nurse, don't you?'
i 'The surgery didn't go the way I expected.'
j 'Have you ever done this procedure before?'
k 'I'm not sure I should be taking all those tablets.'
l 'I should have known better than to leave the cleaning liquid sitting out on the bench top. Now look what's happened.'

(Note: The answers to this activity can be found at the end of this chapter.)

DISCUSSION

1 Refer to the end of the chapter and compare your answers with those provided. Reflect on the differences between your answers and the ones provided.

2 If you are working in a group, compare your answers with other participants' following the reading of each patient statement. Discuss any differences in perception of feelings and try to determine why they are different.

Interpreting: listening for themes

The content of a patient's story and its accompanying feelings come together to form the general theme. Themes are the general point of the story, the consequences and implications of the content and feelings. It could be said that an understanding of the theme is the ultimate goal of listening, as once the point of each story is understood, the patient's entire experience comes into sharper focus. Nurses come to understand the theme of a patient's story by asking the following questions:

- How is the patient experiencing a health event in terms of thoughts/content and feelings?
- What seems to be the most frequent topic/content brought up by the patient?
- What emotions are associated with the topic?
- What is 'triggering' the patient to bring up this topic at this time?
- How is this experience affecting the patient at the moment?
- What are the consequences of what the patient is experiencing?
- What are the implications for the patient in relation to effects of the health event on the patient's life?

Understanding themes requires interpretation. This is always tentative at first and needs to be validated with the patient. After nurses have listened and attempted to understand, they are ready to respond. Perhaps the nurse's current understanding, achieved through listening, needs to be clarified, explored and/or reflected back to the patient through paraphrasing. The skills needed to achieve any of these are covered in Chapters 6 and 7.

During Activity 5.9, it will probably be easier for the listeners to identify the theme if they have had a similar experience (i.e. when the story has a sense of familiarity about it). Repeated listening and identification of themes enables nurses to attain a sense of familiarity with common patient experiences. Listening with understanding becomes a valuable learning experience in accurately perceiving patients' stories.

Activity 5.9 LISTENING FOR THEMES   ➥303

PROCESS

1 Form pairs for this activity. Each member of a pair is to relate a story of something that has recently happened in their life. The story need not be earth shattering, but it should be meaningful to the person telling the story.

2 The other person is to listen, attend and say little during the telling of the story. At the completion, the listener states what they think is the theme. The person telling the story then validates (or invalidates) what the listener has interpreted as the theme.

3 Discuss any differences in interpretation.

DISCUSSION

1 How accurate were the interpretations of the theme? What accounted for any inaccuracies?

2 What interfered with listening? What enhanced it?

Recalling messages

Sometimes, the greatest challenge in listening is to recall what patients have said. Accurate recall is important if understanding is to occur. Themes often become apparent only after numerous interactions with a patient. Nurses must rely on their ability to recall previous interactions and put them together with current ones.

Patients' stories are usually not as complicated as the one told in Activity 5.10. Nevertheless, this activity does highlight how easily stories become diminished, embellished and/or distorted. Recalling patients' stories takes concentration and effort. If nurses find themselves asking patients to retell their stories many times, patients may not believe that they have listened in the first place. When nurses listen and remember what they have heard, patients are comforted to know that somebody has taken the time to understand them.

Activity 5.10 RECALLING MESSAGES

PROCESS

1 Four volunteers are needed for this activity. They will participate in the relating of an incident that occurred during the night shift at a hospital. The details of the incident are provided below.

2 Two of the volunteers are to leave the room. The other two are to seat themselves in a place where all other participants can hear their conversation.

3 All other participants act as observers. They are to make notes of what is added, deleted and distorted each time the incident is reported.

4 The two volunteers who are in the room are to pretend they are in a handover report at the end of a night shift. One of them relates the following incident to the other by reading it aloud:

At about 2 a.m., Mr Smithers became confused and agitated. He got out of bed, went into the next room, over to Mrs Blue's bed and began to tell her about how to grow azaleas. Mrs Blue became frightened, rang her husband on the phone, and asked him to come in immediately. She was so loud on the phone that all the other patients in the room were awakened. There was a recently admitted patient in bed 18. She reacted to Mrs Blue, tried to get out of bed and fell to the floor. In the meantime, Mr Smithers made his way off the ward and was heading towards the lift. Fortunately, another nurse was getting out of the lift and escorted him back to the ward. We contacted the RMO to come and see the new admission and Mr Smithers. He ordered X-rays for the new admission and a sedative for Mr Smithers. Now everybody is settled and back in bed. There were no major injuries, but it was a real circus here for a while. In the midst of all of the chaos, Mr Blue arrived, in response to his wife's request. We let him visit her for about 20 minutes and now he's returned home. The incident report was completed and sent.

5 One of the volunteers, who is out of the room, is now called back in. The volunteer who received the report relates the incident to the volunteer who has come into the room, by retelling the story without reading it. No assistance is offered to the volunteer who is relating the story; they must rely on memory to recount the incident.

6 The remaining volunteer (who is still outside of the room) is brought back into the room, and the previous volunteer relates the incident to them by retelling the story. Again, no assistance is offered to this volunteer in retelling the story.

7 Each time the incident is retold, the observers are to record any additions, deletions and distortions made to the original story.

8 The incident report is now read aloud, as it was told originally.

DISCUSSION

1 The participants who observed the activity should now relate what was added to the original story. What was deleted? What was distorted when the story was retold?

2 What accounted for the alterations that were made to the original story?

3 Volunteers should report their reactions to having to retell such a complex story.

EVALUATION OF LISTENING

In the final analysis, nurses listen in order to respond in a manner that matches the patient's experience. Listening is considered effective when the nurse's response reflects understanding of what the patient is expressing. This is not to say that initial understanding (achieved through listening) will be entirely accurate. The nurse's interpretation is always tentative, awaiting correction, validation or further explication from the patient. Responses that shift the focus, change the subject or miss the point entirely do not indicate active listening.

Activity 5.11 RESPONSES THAT INDICATE LISTENING ➡303

PROCESS

1 Each of the following patient statements has a variety of possible responses. Evaluate each response in terms of whether it indicates that the nurse making the response has listened. Record on a piece of paper a YES or NO on the basis of your evaluation. Do not evaluate how good or bad the response seems to you, or base your decision on whether or not you would make the same response. Judge the response *only* in terms of listening, by asking yourself, 'Does the listener's response indicate that the listener has heard the patient?' 'Does the response indicate an understanding of what the patient has expressed?'

a *Patient*

I don't think I'm going to make it. Am I going to die?

Responses

  i The power of positive thinking can really help a lot. Many people in your situation have survived because they refused to give up. Keep fighting. Where there is life, there is hope.

  ii What has happened to make you worried about it?

  iii I can't really say. You'll have to ask your doctor this question.

  iv We are all going to die sometime, but it's a frightening prospect when it stares us in the face.

b *Patient*

Why is my blood pressure being taken so often?

Responses

  i We have to check your blood pressure frequently.

  ii It's doctor's orders.

  iii It is a general observation to keep a check on your vital signs.

  iv Is it worrying you?

c *Patient*

How long will I be in here?

Responses

  i As long as we think you need to be.

  ii Let's discuss it with the doctor. If you think you're ready to go home, and the doctor is happy for you to go, you can be discharged.

  iii People who have the operation you are having usually stay in hospital about 3 days. That's the usual routine, if there are no complications.

  iv What has your doctor said about this?

d *Patient*

Why me? Why do I have to be the one who suffers like this?

Responses

  i It is a part of the usual course of this disease. If you tell me when you feel worse and better, I can help with the pain.

  ii We all suffer some kind of pain during our lifetime.

    iii It is just a bit of misfortune. You'll have better luck next time, I'm sure.

    iv I wish I could answer that question. I'm not sure there always is a reason.

e *Patient*
I have contemplated suicide because I've hit rock bottom.
Responses

    i Are you thinking about suicide right now?

    ii Things can't be that bad.

    iii What's happened to you that you have hit rock bottom?

    iv What exactly have you contemplated?

f *Patient*
What's going to happen when I come out of the operation?
Responses

    i We will look after you.

    ii There's nothing to worry about. You will feel better than you did before.

    iii Have you had a general anaesthetic before?

    iv You'll be drowsy for a few hours and, depending on your level of pain, you will receive regular pain relief.

g *Patient*
I'm not sick, and yet I have to take all of these tablets every day.
Responses

    i It does seem a bit silly, doesn't it?

    ii It could be that you don't feel sick because you *are* taking the tablets.

    iii Which tablets are you taking?

    iv How long have you been taking the tablets?

2 Now review each response for which you recorded a YES. Evaluate each in terms of the major goal of listening—that is, the encouragement of patients to continue expressing their experiences. How encouraging is each?

3 Compare your answers with the ones provided at the end of the chapter.

(Note: The answers to this activity can be found at the end of this chapter.)

CHAPTER SUMMARY

Meanings are derived and initial understanding is achieved through active listening. Listening enables nurses to perceive the patient's reality—the world as the patient is experiencing it. After listening effectively, nurses are in a position to respond according to what is perceived. Listening engages both the nurse and patient. It is an essential and fundamental process in establishing effective relationships in nursing practice and actively demonstrating that nurses care about patients' wellbeing.

Answers to activities

Activity 5.7 LISTENING FOR CONTENT

PATIENT STORY I

WHO: self (speaker), doctor
WHAT: something happened to hip, difficulty walking
WHEN: Sunday afternoon
WHERE: not stated
WHY: reason for having the X-ray

PATIENT STORY II

WHO: speaker, child, GP's receptionist
WHAT: serious stomach pain, rang GP, drove to GP's surgery
WHEN: beginning of a day
WHERE: GP's surgery
WHY: explain the story, but not entirely clear

PATIENT STORY III

WHO: speaker
WHAT: unable to move left arm
WHEN: not stated
WHERE: garden, then house
WHY: don't know what to do

PATIENT STORY IV

WHO: speaker, 'him'
WHAT: he is not himself
WHEN: 'for months'
WHERE: home, in front of television
WHY: worried about 'him'

PATIENT STORY V

WHO: speaker, GP
WHAT: no time to have regular pap smears
WHEN: not stated
WHERE: not stated
WHY: questioning whether regular pap smears are necessary

PATIENT STORY VI

WHO: speaker
WHAT: chemo and radiotherapy, feeling tired
WHEN: now
WHERE: speaker's room
WHY: can't attend to children

Activity 5.8 LISTENING FOR FEELINGS

a fear, anxiety, worry
b fear, anxiety, worry
c frustration, anger, resignation
d sadness, anger, frustration
e sadness, anger, resignation
f anger, frustration
g sadness, anger
h fear, anxiety, apprehension
i disappointment, frustration
j apprehension, anxiety, fear
k uncertainty
l regret, guilt

Activity 5.11 RESPONSES THAT INDICATE LISTENING

The answer NO indicates that the nurse responding has not understood/acknowledged what the patient is saying, while the answer YES indicates active reception of what the patient has said.

1 a *Patient:* I don't think I'm going to make it. Am I going to die?

    i NO The power of positive thinking can really help a lot. Many people in your situation have survived because they refused to give up. Keep fighting. Where there is life, there is hope.

    ii YES What has happened to make you worried about it?

    iii NO I can't really say. You'll have to ask your doctor this question.

    iv YES We are all going to die sometime, but it's a frightening prospect when it stares us in the face.

 b *Patient:* Why is my blood pressure being taken so often?

    i NO We have to check your blood pressure frequently.

    ii NO It's doctor's orders.

    iii YES It is a general observation to keep a check on your vital signs.

    iv YES Is it worrying you?

 c *Patient:* How long will I be in here?

    i NO As long as we think you need to be.

    ii YES Let's discuss it with the doctor. If you think you're ready to go home, and the doctor is happy for you to go, you can be discharged.

    iii YES People who have the operation you are having usually stay in hospital about 3 days. That's the usual routine, if there are no complications.

    iv YES What has your doctor said about this?

 d *Patient:* Why me? Why do I have to be the one who suffers like this?

    i NO It is a part of the usual course of this disease. If you tell me when you feel worse and better, I can help with the pain.

    ii NO We all suffer some kind of pain during our lifetime.

iii NO It is just a bit of misfortune. You'll have better luck next time, I'm sure.

iv YES I wish I could answer that question. I'm not sure there always is a reason.

e *Patient:* I have contemplated suicide because I've hit rock bottom.

i YES Are you thinking about suicide right now?

ii NO Things can't be that bad.

iii YES What's happened to you that you have hit rock bottom?

iv YES What exactly have you contemplated?

f *Patient:* What's going to happen when I come out of the operation?

i NO We will look after you.

ii NO There's nothing to worry about. You will feel better than you did before.

iii NO Have you had a general anaesthetic before?

iv YES You'll be drowsy for a few hours and, depending on your level of pain, you will receive regular pain relief.

g *Patient:* I'm not sick, and yet I have to take all of these tablets every day.

i NO It does seem a bit silly, doesn't it?

ii NO It could be that you don't feel sick because you *are* taking the tablets.

iii YES Which tablets are you taking?

iv YES How long have you been taking the tablets?

REFERENCES

Barrett C, Borthwick A, Bugeja S, Parker A, Vis R, Hurworth R 2005 Emotional labour: listening to the patient's story. Practice Development in Health Care 4(4):213–223

Carkhuff RR 1983 The student workbook for the art of helping, 2nd edn. Human Resource Press, Amherst, MA

Chang T, Lin Y-P, Change H-J, Lin C-C 2005 Cancer patient and staff ratings of caring behaviors. Cancer Nursing 28(5):331–339

Corbin J 2008 Is caring a lost art in nursing? International Journal of Nursing Studies 45: 163–165

Courts NF, Bechanan EM, Werstlein PO 2004 Focus groups: the lived experience of participants with multiple sclerosis. Journal of Neuroscience Nursing 36(1):42–47

Doona ME, Haggerty LA, Chase SK 1997 Nursing presence: an existential exploration of the concept. Scholarly Inquiry for Nursing Practice: An International Journal 11(1):3–16

Doona ME, Haggerty LA, Chase SK 1999 Nursing presence: as real as a Milky Way bar. Journal of Holistic Nursing 17(1):54–70

Egan G 2007 The skilled helper, 8th edn. Brooks Cole/Thomas Learning, Boston, MA

Farrell GA 1991 How accurately do nurses perceive patients' needs? A comparison of general and psychiatric settings. Journal of Advanced Nursing 16:1062–1070

Finfgeld-Connett D 2006 Meta-synthesis of presence in nursing. Journal of Advanced Nursing 55:708–714

Fredriksson L 1999 Modes of relating in a caring conversation: a research synthesis on presence, touch and listening. Journal of Advanced Nursing 30:1167–1176

Gilbert DA 2004 Coordination in nurses' listening activities and communication about patient–nurse relationships. Research in Nursing and Health 27:447–457

Hegedus KS 1999 Providers' and consumers' perspectives of nurses' caring behaviours. Journal of Advanced Nursing 30:1090–1096

Jonas-Simpson CM 2003 The experience of being listened to: a human becoming study with music. Nursing Science Quarterly 16(3):232–238

Jonas-Simpson CM, Mitchell GJ, Fisher A, Jones G, Linscott J 2006 The experience of being listened to: a qualitative study of older adults in long-term care settings. Journal of Gerontological Nursing 32(1):46–53

Kagan PN 2008a Feeling listened to: a lived experience of human becoming. Nursing Science Quarterly 21(1):59–67

Kagan PN 2008b Listening: selected perspectives in theory and research. Nursing Science Quarterly 21(2):105–110

Lazarus RS 2006 Emotions and interpersonal relationships: toward a person-centered conceptualization of emotions and coping. Journal of Personality 74(1):9–46

Macdonald M 2007 Origins of difficulty in the nurse–patient encounter. Nursing Ethics 14(4):510–521

McCabe C 2004 Nurse–patient communication: an exploration of patients' experiences. Journal of Clinical Nursing 13:41–49

Nelson-Jones R 2005 Practical counselling and helping skills, 5th edn. Sage, London

Nyström M, Dahlberg K, Carlsson G 2003 Non-caring encounters at an emergency care unit—a life-world hermeneutic analysis of an efficiency-driven organization. International Journal of Nursing Studies 40:761–769

Reid-Ponte P 1992 Distress in cancer patients and primary nurses' empathy skills. Cancer Nursing 15(4):283–292

Shattell M 2005 Nurse bait: strategies hospitalized patients use to entice nurses within the context of the interpersonal relationship. Issues in Mental Health Nursing 26:205–223

Shea SC, Maloney M 1998 Psychiatric interviewing: the art of understanding. Saunders, Philadelphia, PA

Webb C, Hope K 1995 What kind of nurses do patients want? Journal of Clinical Nursing 4(2):101–108

CHAPTER 6

Building meaning: understanding

INTRODUCTION

Understanding a patient's experience (i.e. viewing the world from the patient's perspective) is one of the most central aspects of interacting and building relationships in nursing. Mutual understanding is the basis of meaningful interaction and, in the patient–nurse relationship, it is the nurse's responsibility to facilitate this understanding. Mutual understanding requires time, effort, commitment and skill. It is challenging for one person to understand and appreciate another person's reality.

Effective attending and listening opens doors and aids the nurse's entry into the patient's world. The stage is set for a meaningful relationship because interpersonal contact has been established. Listening enables the nurse to develop an initial understanding of the patient's experience. It is important to recognise that this understanding remains tentative until it is either validated or corrected and altered through further interaction with the patient. The impressions formed in the process of listening are often partial, inaccurate and superficial. The nurse who acts immediately, without further interaction to check the accuracy of these impressions, risks attempting to build a relationship that lacks mutual understanding and providing help that is not necessarily congruent with the patient's needs. Taking time to understand a patient's experiences enables nurses to ground nursing care within the patient's reality.

Listening is largely an absorptive activity, as nurses take in and process patients' stories. But at some point during an interaction, verbal responses must be uttered; the nurse usually has to say something. A variety of verbal responses are possible; however, a response that promotes greater understanding between patient and nurse is most beneficial, especially in the early stages of the relationship. Responses that promote understanding not only demonstrate that the nurse has listened, but they also convey a desire to comprehend the patient's experience more fully.

Effective listening demonstrates open acceptance of the patient, and encourages the patient to interact. Effective understanding encourages further interaction because it openly acknowledges the patient's experience, confirming its reality. Understanding responses check how effectively the nurse's perceptions and interpretations correspond to the patient's meaning. Because they build meaning, understanding responses deepen the relationship between patient and nurse.

Chapter overview

This chapter begins with an overview of the ways in which nurses can verbally respond to patients. The various ways of responding are explained in depth, in order to demonstrate how they differ in intent and impact on the patient–nurse relationship. Understanding is shown to be the most appropriate way to respond when building this relationship. Understanding is viewed as the basis of the relationship, and the importance of understanding between patient and nurse is highlighted. The skills of understanding are covered next in the discussion. The skill of paraphrasing is the major skill of understanding, and therefore is treated more extensively than the other skills. The other skills include seeking clarification, reflecting feelings, connecting and summarising.

Empathy is presented as a central concept in understanding. The concept of empathy is explained, and how this concept is integrated into nursing practice is delineated. An analysis of how empathy is conceptualised in nursing assists in the comparison of empathy with other related concepts such as sympathy.

VERBAL RESPONDING

After actively listening to a patient and forming an initial impression, it is natural for a nurse to respond verbally. While it is important that responses be spontaneous and sincere, it is equally important that they be thoughtful, developed with intention and skilfully employed. The nurse's initial verbal responses set the direction for further interaction. Because there is a variety of possible ways to respond, nurses must ensure that their verbal responses move the relationship in a desired and intended direction. Choice of a response is based on insight into how it may affect the patient, the interaction and the relationship. A nurse who has this insight and awareness is in the best position to respond in a manner that both matches the current situation and realises the response's desired intent. In regard to intent, nurses should consider what they need to know about patients and why they need to know it.

The initial phase of the relationship between patient and nurse is a particularly sensitive and critical time for responding, because, more than likely, the trust required for full patient disclosure is not yet firmly established. Responses that work best at this time are those that validate patients by acknowledging their experiences. Validating and acknowledging responses convey the nurse's willingness to understand the patient. Patients will come to trust those nurses who can be relied on to understand. Inadvertently, nurses may respond in a manner that suggests a lack of desire to understand. The following response, which denies the patient's experience, is an example:

Patient: I'm worried about how my family is going to manage without me.
Nurse: No need to worry, they'll survive without you. It'll do them good to realise how much you do for them.

While the nurse may have wished to encourage the patient with this response, it is likely that the response indicates a rejection of the patient's perception of the situation. By failing to acknowledge the patient's reality, responses such as these engender the feeling that the nurse does not want to understand. Compare the preceding example with the following:

Patient: I'm worried about how my family is going to manage without me.
Nurse: What is worrying you most about how they will manage?

Here the nurse provides acknowledgment and confirmation of the patient's reality. Responses such as this deepen interpersonal engagement and promote understanding between patient and nurse; as such, they build trust.

Most nurses develop habitual, routine and even stylised ways of responding to patients. The intent is usually to be of help or assistance to patients, but this intent may not be fully realised if nurses overuse one type of response and/or lack awareness of the impact of their responses. Goodwill and desire alone are not sufficient in the absence of awareness and direction.

Activity 6.1 YOUR USUAL STYLE OF RESPONDING I

PROCESS

1 For each of the following statements/questions (a–o), write a response. Do not spend too much time pondering your response, but do try to be helpful to the person speaking. Record a response that is typical of how you would usually respond.

    a A resident of a nursing home: 'I miss my wife. I don't know where she is. Where is she? Can you tell me?'

    b A relative of an unconscious patient hospitalised in intensive care: 'Mum is really going to be upset when she wakes up. She is going to kill us for letting her be in here.'

    c An adolescent patient during a routine health check-up: 'My folks keep pressuring me about the future. I don't have a clue about what I want to do.'

    d A first-time mother about to be discharged from a postnatal unit: 'How am I ever going to be able to manage this baby on my own?'

    e A client to a community nurse during a home visit: 'I am so glad to see you. I have not been at all well lately.'

    f A patient, a young man, who is having haemodialysis at home: 'My girlfriend left me because she's afraid she might catch something and my best mate doesn't visit me any more because he hates the sight of blood.'

    g A resident of a hostel for the elderly: 'It's really boring in here. The days are so long and there's no one to talk to except the nurses, and they are always so busy.'

    h A mother during a routine visit at an early childhood centre: 'My husband left and I am having so much trouble managing on my own.'

    i A resident of a nursing home: 'It's hard when you grow old and your friends and family start to die. My children are great, but they have their own lives.'

i A patient, a woman, during an outpatient clinic visit for a routine pap smear: 'I am not really sure about having any more children. I'm 39 now and reckon I've pushed my luck far enough. I have two healthy children. Perhaps I should just leave it at that.'

k A patient during a postoperative clinic visit: 'You know, I just take one day at a time. It's been 2 months since my surgery and I'm still not sure if I'll ever feel like my old self again.'

l A patient during an admission interview in hospital: 'I've lived with arthritis for years, but lately I'm having more trouble than usual. I can hardly get out of bed in the morning and the pain is becoming unbearable.'

m A resident of a hostel for the elderly: 'You can't possibly understand what it feels like. You never had this problem. How would you understand?'

n A client, a pregnant woman, during an antenatal visit: 'People are kind and concerned, but no one really knows what it is like to lose a child. It's the most painful experience imaginable. You never get over it.'

o A patient, a man hospitalised for a myocardial infarction: 'I'm really worried about how my family will cope without my help. I have three small children, my wife works and we share all the household chores. Now that I've had this heart attack, I'm not sure how much assistance I can offer.'

2 Reflect on each of your responses:
- What is your intention?
- What do you hope to achieve by responding in this way?
- How do you hope the patient will react to your response?

3 If you are working in groups, form pairs. One person now reads the statement or question and the other person reads their recorded response. The *patient* reflects after each response:
- What is your impression of the nurse? And of the response?
- How has the response affected you?
- How encouraged are you to continue the interaction?
- How much do you think the nurse understands your situation?

The *patient* then shares these reflections with the *nurse*.

4 The *nurse* now shares their intention (step 2 of the process) with the *patient*. Make a note of the following:
- How congruent is the nurse's intention with the effect on the *patient*?

5 Continue to read each statement or question followed by its response and share the reflections.

6 Switch roles and complete steps 3, 4 and 5.

DISCUSSION

1 What differences are there between the *nurses'* intentions and the *patients'* impressions of the responses? How do you account for this?

2 Were some responses more encouraging than others? Which ones were encouraging? And discouraging?

3 Which responses resulted in a negative impression on the *patient* (e.g. 'the nurse does not understand', 'does not really care' or 'does not wish to discuss the topic')?

WAYS OF RESPONDING

This section explores the various types of responses nurses might have to patients based on categories developed by Johnson (2009). In this scheme, responses are categorised according to their intent—what they are designed to do or their purpose. On this basis, the majority of responses fit into one of the following categories:

- advising and evaluating
- analysing and interpreting
- reassuring and supporting
- questioning and probing, and
- paraphrasing and understanding.

The categories include those responses that are significant—ones with the potential to have a critical impact on the interaction and the relationship. There are other possible responses that would not fit into any of these categories (e.g. small talk about the weather). They are not included because they are of less consequence to the overall relationship.

Each way of responding may be helpful in its own right and can be effectively employed within the context of the patient–nurse relationship. Nevertheless, each has a different intent, suggests a different type of relationship between patient and nurse, and therefore has a different impact on their interactions, especially in the sensitive early stages. Some responses facilitate interaction better than others, so timing and an awareness of each type of response are crucial.

Advising and evaluating

This category includes responses that offer an opinion or advice, ranging from a mild suggestion to a directive about what the patient should do. Such responses are based on the nurse's opinions and ideas and therefore have an evaluative edge. Examples in this category include:

- 'It's best not to dwell too much on such things.'
- 'Try to relax and stop worrying so much; it doesn't really help.'
- 'Ask the doctor these questions.'
- 'Just tell your mother it's your life and you'll do with it what you want.'

Responses such as these are among the most common made by people who are trying to help. When nurses use this type of response, they convey the message that they 'know best' and are in a position that is superior to the patient (Johnson 2009). Advice and evaluation carry the implication that patients are unable to know what to do, thus increasing their sense of vulnerability. For this reason, advising and evaluating responses run the risk of being met with a defensive reaction or a rejection of the advice. Have you ever told a friend what you think they should do to resolve a problem, only to be met with 'Yes, but …', or 'That's easy for you to say', or 'I already tried that and it didn't work'. When given as an initial response, advice rarely works because of its potential to produce a sense of inadequacy in the patient and the patient's need to defend against this feeling.

Responses that advise offer solutions about what ought to be done. As a general rule, it is better to reach a sound understanding of a patient's situation before launching into solutions. An advising response gives the impression that a patient's difficulties and problems are easily solved—that there is a 'quick fix'. Some situations are easily resolved but, more often than not, further elaboration is needed before answers are found (if any *can* be found). Advice giving is better left until the nurse fully understands the patient's experience.

Just as it is difficult to listen without judging, it is equally difficult to curtail the tendency to evaluate and advise. The tendency of nurses to give advice reflects the perception of many nurses that their role involves possessing knowledge and expertise. This perception often leads nurses to attempt to help patients by telling them what to do and providing answers.

While there are times when nurses offer expert advice to the patient, it is important that the patient's need and desire for such advice is established beforehand. Likewise, if advice is to be effective, it must be based on a clear understanding of the patient's experience. For example, explaining the usual course of events following anaesthesia and advising how to cope with 'waking up' is advice based on understanding of the situation. This is an objective 'case knowledge' (see Ch 1), which does not necessarily require interaction with the patient. In a more subjective situation, such as anxiety about impending surgery, telling a patient to relax is of little use unless the nurse takes the time to understand the nature of the patient's worry. Advice given without understanding runs the risk of being ill-timed or irrelevant.

Advising versus sharing information

Giving advice is sometimes confused with sharing information. While they are similar, sharing information is not the same as telling patients what to do. When they share information (see Ch 8), nurses provide knowledge, alternatives and facts. When they offer advice, nurses provide specific actions to perform. Advice also involves reliance on the nurse's personal value judgments, while sharing information is free of such judgments.

Analysing and interpreting

A response that analyses and interprets reaches beyond what the patient has expressed into a deeper level of meaning. An interpretive response reads into patients' messages, giving the impression that the nurse knows how patients *really* feel or what they *really* think. Interpretations imply that a nurse knows more about patients than they know themselves (Johnson 2009). Examples of analysing and interpreting responses include:

- 'You really don't want to assume responsibility for your own health.'
- 'You are acting like most new mothers, worrying too much and being overprotective of your baby.'
- 'You are afraid that if you tell the surgeon how you feel about the operation, he will reject you entirely and drop you as a patient.'

Responses such as these delve beneath the surface and open up areas that the patient has not expressed directly. As with advising, interpreting may have a legitimate place, but as an initial response it is often too threatening to be effective in building the relationship. An interpretation, regardless of its accuracy, can be threatening because it confronts patients with another reality—one that they may not be willing or able to face. Because such interpretations have a confronting edge, they are better left until the relationship has been established and the nurse has 'earned the right' to challenge in this way (see Ch 8).

Patients are more likely to accept interpretations from a nurse who has taken the time to fully understand their situation. It is unlikely that a nurse would know a patient well enough to make interpretations early in the course of their relationship. As an initial response, interpretations are intrusive and invasive and may impede the development of trust.

Reassuring and supporting

There is a definite place for realistic reassurance and support (see Ch 8) in the course of patient–nurse relationships, and a nurse's approach needs to convey an overall attitude of support whenever interacting with patients. Nevertheless, a falsely reassuring response (the type discussed here) is one that glosses over and minimises the importance of the patient's experience before that experience is entirely acknowledged and understood. In this respect, a falsely reassuring response is one that attempts to smooth the patient's discomfort by making everything sound 'all right', regardless of the objective or subjective reality of the situation. It may convey a patronising attitude or present the patient with a sense of unrealistic assurance. Examples of responses that falsely reassure and support include:

- 'A good night's sleep will do wonders for you.'
- 'There is nothing to worry about. It is only a minor procedure.'
- 'Don't be silly, Mrs Jones, nothing will go wrong.'
- 'You'll feel better after the operation and will get well soon.'

False reassurance may sound good on the surface but, more often than not, it is dismissive of the patient's reality; it lacks understanding. Reflect for a moment on how you feel whenever someone tells you not to worry about something that is causing you concern. Do you have an impression that this person is genuinely interested? Does this person demonstrate a desire to understand your concern?

The use of clichés is another example of responses that attempt to support and reassure. Some examples include:

- 'It's always darkest just before a storm.'
- 'Every cloud has a silver lining.'

Responses such as these, often said whenever patients express anxieties and concerns, fail to acknowledge the subjective reality of patients' experiences. They carry an implied judgment that patients' concerns are unfounded, and even foolish. Because they discount the validity and significance of patients' feelings and perceptions, falsely reassuring responses sound as if the nurse is not really interested. Like premature advice, reassuring responses and clichés attempt to 'fix things' before they are fully clarified and understood.

Questioning and probing

A response that questions and probes is one that attempts to gather more information and explore the situation further. It indicates a need for elaboration and may ultimately lead to greater understanding. Examples of this type of response include:

- 'What is worrying you most about the operation?'
- 'Where is your pain?'
- 'What methods have you tried to get to sleep?'
- 'What do you think?'

Responses that question and probe indicate that nurses are trying to understand, but need more information to do so. Early in the course of the relationship, the nurse frequently employs questions in an effort to get to know the patient. Throughout the course of the relationship, questions are further employed to develop an even greater understanding of the patient's experience. Unless they are overused, responses that question and probe are quite useful if they are stated correctly and timed appropriately. There are other ways to explore aside from questioning and probing, and effective exploration involves the use of a variety of skills (see Ch 7).

Paraphrasing and understanding

When nurses paraphrase, they share their understanding with patients by rephrasing what patients have expressed, using their own words instead of patients' words. Responses that paraphrase what the patient has expressed demonstrate that the nurse's intention is to understand the patient more fully. Examples in this category include:

- 'You are unable to sleep because of your uncertainty about the future.'
- 'You are feeling more relaxed now that you are in your own home.'
- 'It seems strange to you that you should have to keep asking the same questions over and over again.'

Responses that demonstrate understanding confirm and validate what patients have expressed, thus communicating nurses' genuine interest in and acceptance of patients. Through the use of the paraphrase, nurses share their understanding of patients' messages in order to ensure this understanding is correct. Paraphrasing and understanding responses demonstrate that the nurse wants to follow the patient's meaning and will check to ensure this happens. They convey the message, 'I won't assume I know what you mean or what you need until I am certain I know—and only you can tell me'. Early in the course of the relationship, this type of response is especially effective because it places patient and nurse on equal footing and helps to build trust.

All other categories of responses, except questioning and probing, are based on an assumption that nurses know what patients are experiencing and what is best for them. An understanding response attempts to validate or invalidate these assumptions. The meaning a nurse constructs from what a patient has expressed may not be what the patient actually meant. An understanding response is of value in preventing such lack of congruency; it addresses one of the most common problems in communication, which occurs when people do not realise there is sometimes a difference between what is meant and what is said and consequently misunderstand what is meant.

Activity 6.2 RECOGNITION OF THE TYPES OF RESPONSES ➡304

PROCESS

1 For each statement below (a–l), five possible responses are provided. Read all five responses to the statement and decide on the response that most closely matches what you would say under the circumstances.

2 For each set of five responses, determine which of the following categories best represents each response (record your answer on a separate sheet of paper):
E Advising and evaluating
I Analysing and interpreting
S Reassuring and supporting

P Questioning and probing
U Paraphrasing and understanding
There is a response from each category in each set.

a 'I'm just so fed up with being sick and in pain. I'm tired of having to rely on the nurses all the time.'

Responses

  i 'It's okay to rely on us. That's why we are here.'

  ii 'You are an independent type of person who prefers to do things for yourself.'

  iii 'All of this is really starting to get you down.'

  iv 'Just relax and let us help you.'

  v 'What is bothering you the most?'

b 'I never really looked after myself. Now look how I am suffering.'

Responses

  i 'I don't know what you mean.'

  ii 'Lots of people say the same thing.'

  iii 'Well, you would have looked after yourself if it mattered to you.'

  iv 'It's hard to look back with regrets, isn't it?'

  v 'Sounds as if you're angry at yourself.'

c 'Don't bother with me. I am going to die anyway.'

Responses

  i 'That sounds sad and depressing.'

  ii 'Don't talk like that. You are not going to die.'

  iii 'What makes you say that?'

  iv 'It's not a bother to look after you. I am here because I want to help you.'

  v 'You have given up hope because you are getting on in age.'

d 'I'm in so much pain all the time. I manage to get through the day all right, because I keep busy, but my backache prevents me from getting a good night's sleep. So I keep busy during the day, end up really tired, but then can't get the rest that I need. I'm getting more and more tired all the time.'

Responses

  i 'Why don't you try some relaxation exercises to get to sleep?'

  ii 'How often do you have a bad night?'

  iii 'Keeping busy during the day helps with the pain, but getting enough sleep at night is more of a worry for you right now.'

  iv 'Sounds as if you are letting the pain control your life.'

  v 'I'm sure you'll be able to work something out once you become accustomed to living with the pain.'

e 'People think they want to live a long time, but I'm telling you, don't ever grow old. You'll end up in a place like this. It's boring and depressing. Look at everybody here. Do they look happy to you?'

Responses

  i 'Everybody feels a bit blue sometimes. Things will get better—you'll see.'

  ii 'Come on, let's go for a walk. It's a beautiful day today.'

  iii 'What's so boring and depressing about this place?'

  iv 'You are approaching things with a negative attitude so, naturally, the whole world looks grim.'

  v 'You're really not happy about being here, are you?'

f 'My wife died recently. I don't want to talk about it.'
Responses
  i 'It does help to talk about these things.'
  ii 'What do you want to talk about?'
  iii 'You'll get over it in time, I am sure.'
  iv 'Maybe you are the type of person who has difficulty letting people help you.'
  v 'You don't feel like talking to me?'

g 'I know I should change my diet and alter my lifestyle. The doctor said I am a high risk for a heart attack. I've always been a bit of a go-getter—take after Dad in that respect. He had a heart attack at 50, so I guess I should do something—but I really don't know where to start.'
Responses
  i 'Sounds as if you have been avoiding the inevitable. You know what to do, but don't want to face it. You could change if you really wanted to.'
  ii 'Just try a bit harder to slow down and eat the right foods.'
  iii 'You have an idea about what you should do, but are having trouble getting started.'
  iv 'What do you think you should change first?'
  v 'Worrying about it will only make things worse. I'm sure you can change.'

h 'I get so tired looking after David day after day. There is all the physical care, but I think the mental strain is the worst. I worry constantly about where he is and what he is doing. I think he gets a bit annoyed with my constant hovering over him. The worst thing is that I get no relief—it's so constant.'
Responses
  i 'The constant worry is really getting to you and wearing you down. You just can't seem to get away from it.'
  ii 'People in your situation often feel this way. It's a difficult problem to come to terms with.'
  iii 'Try to put the worry out of your mind at least once each day. Make yourself a cup of tea, sit down and just relax.'
  iv 'Is there ever an opportunity for you to get away?'
  v 'There may be a bit of guilt in what you are saying. You probably keep thinking about the times in the past when you could have been more understanding and supportive towards David.'

i 'The least they could have done was warn me that Dad was going to be sedated. Those doctors didn't even tell me beforehand so I could have a quick visit with him. Now I need to leave the hospital without even speaking to Dad.'
Responses
  i 'You sound like one of those people who likes to be in control.'
  ii 'The doctors were really busy. Otherwise, I am sure they would have told you.'
  iii 'I can see you are frustrated and angry about not getting to talk to your Dad.'
  iv 'If this happens again, I would say something if I were you.'
  v 'What exactly did they tell you?'

j 'Mum was always there to look after us when we needed something. Now that she's sick, I guess it's our turn to look after her. It feels so strange and I'm not sure she will even let us do much for her.'

Responses

  i 'Because you always had her to look after you, you wonder if she will let you look after her.'

  ii 'Of course she will. Your mother is a sensible woman.'

  iii 'You feel scared that you won't be able to switch roles with your Mum.'

  iv 'Tell me more about it.'

  v 'Just tell her she needs you now and she will have to let you take care of her.'

k 'What will happen to me if John dies. I don't know what I would do. I couldn't go on without him.'

Responses

  i 'No need to worry about things before they happen.'

  ii 'You're scared because you have allowed yourself to become too dependent on John and can't see how you'll make it on your own.'

  iii 'What makes you think he won't make it?'

  iv 'I suppose it's frightening to think you can't survive without John.'

  v 'There is plenty of help around. You can join a social club in your area.'

l 'That surgeon explained everything about the operation, but I could not understand what was being said. I didn't even know what to ask.'

Responses

  i 'You're scared to ask questions of the doctors because they are so powerful.'

  ii 'So the surgeon's explanation was not quite enough for you to understand.'

  iii 'What questions do you still have?'

  iv 'The next time you see the surgeon, tell him you want some answers.'

  v 'Don't worry too much. Most people don't really understand the technical aspects of surgery.'

(Note: The answers to this activity can be found at the end of the chapter.)

DISCUSSION

1 Compare your answers with those provided at the end of the chapter. Are there any types of responses that were difficult to recognise? Which are they? Review the section of the text that pertains to these.

2 In groups of five to six participants, discuss your answers. Are there any types of responses that other members had difficulty recognising? Which are they? Discuss these until understanding of each type of response is achieved.

3 Review your responses to step 1 of the process and determine whether there are some types of response you seem to provide naturally. Compare these results with the other participants in the group.

4 Discuss the reason(s) you tend to provide some types of response more than others.

Activity 6.3 YOUR USUAL STYLE OF RESPONDING II

PROCESS

1 Refer to the responses that you recorded for Activity 6.1, 'Your usual style of responding I'.

2 For each of your responses, determine which type of response you used (i.e. advising and evaluating; analysing and interpreting; reassuring and supporting; questioning and probing; or paraphrasing and understanding) and mark each accordingly. You may have used more than one category in a given response. If this is the case, include all categories used.

3 Tally the total number of times you used each type of response. Is there one type you used more than others? Reflect on the reasons for your apparent preference.

4 Have someone else determine which types of responses you used. Discuss any discrepancies and make a final determination about which type of response was used.

DISCUSSION

1 Compare your tally with other participants. Is there a type of response that was preferred by a majority of participants? Discuss the results.

2 Which ways of responding seem to fit the perceived role of the nurse? Which do not?

3 How frequently was the paraphrasing and understanding response used? Discuss why this is the case.

The advising and evaluating type of response is one of the most frequently used when people are trying to be helpful (Johnson 2009). This is probably due to people's natural tendency to make judgments and offer opinions, especially when they are trying to be of help. There are times when being directive and prescriptive will be of help to patients, but there are risks if this approach is used exclusively or too extensively. When using advising and evaluating responses, nurses place themselves in the position of expert and fail to acknowledge patients' expertise and capabilities in managing their own lives. Patients are not encouraged to seek solutions that fit their unique experience, but rather are offered solutions and answers.

Nurses often show a strong preference for the reassuring and supporting type of response. This is understandable because nursing care is best given in a reassuring and supportive atmosphere. Nevertheless, a truly reassuring and supportive manner differs from glossing over the patient's experience with a reassuring cliché. Falsely reassuring statements may negate the reality of patients' experiences. Because of their failure to acknowledge and affirm the patient, such responses interfere with effective interaction between patient and nurse.

Two studies demonstrate how nurses respond to patients' anxiety. The most common responses were trying to cheer the patient up (reassuring and supporting) and offering an explanation about the symptoms (advising and evaluating). The least frequent response was understanding (Motyka et al 1997, Whyte et al 1997). For more detail on these studies, see Chapter 8, 'Ways of responding revisited'.

It is important to recognise that none of the categories is inherently good or bad. Each is appropriate at different times in the relationship and under different circumstances. The ultimate aim is for each nurse to develop as wide a repertoire as possible, and to use each type of response with awareness of its appropriateness and consequence. (Subsequent chapters cover the various types of responses, except the understanding type, which is the subject of this chapter.)

Understanding responses are most appropriate for building a relationship based on mutual meaning. They are effective in the early stages of the relationship and are also used throughout as a natural reaction to active listening (see Ch 5). Regardless of how effectively a nurse has suspended judgment during listening, the patient's messages still are processed through personal, interpretative filters. In processing patients' messages, nurses form impressions and reach conclusions about what patients are expressing and experiencing. These interpretations may not be entirely correct. If a nurse's interpretation of what a patient is saying is not shared actively and openly with the patient, potential misunderstandings are likely to go unchecked. In giving an understanding response, nurses share their interpretations so that they can be validated or corrected. Such responses enable nurses to build meaning that is congruent with a patient's experience.

THE IMPORTANCE OF UNDERSTANDING

In order to be of help to patients, it is best if nurses operate from a vantage point within patients' experiences. When responding with understanding, nurses attempt to view the world from the patient's point of view. Nurses reach for meaning by asking. 'What is this patient experiencing?' 'What is the meaning of the experience for the patient?' 'Am I following … do I get the drift?' Understanding responses check the answers to such questions. The following scenario serves as an illustration:

Patient: It doesn't seem right that I am still in so much pain. My hip surgery was 6 weeks ago, and I still can't seem to get comfortable. Is it just me? I asked my doctor and she said, 'No, this is not unusual, so don't worry.' But I really don't know.
Nurse: It doesn't seem right to you that you are still in so much pain 6 weeks after the surgery.
Patient: Yes and no, because I really didn't know exactly what to expect.
Nurse: So, it's more that you don't know the usual course of events following hip surgery.
Patient: Yes, I mean the only thing the doctor said was this is not *unusual,* so I'm still in the dark. I think I'm getting a bit neurotic about the whole thing.
Nurse: So, what you really want to know is how much pain is reasonable and to be expected 6 weeks after the surgery.
Patient: Yes, if I knew for sure that this is expected, I wouldn't be so worried. What do you think?

Because understanding is achieved, the nurse can now proceed to act. The nurse can provide the patient with concrete information (see Ch 8) about recovery after hip surgery. Exploration (see Ch 7) into the exact nature of the patient's pain also may be warranted. Perhaps support (see Ch 8) in pain management can be provided. The key is that the nurse is guided by the understanding that, for *this* patient, fear of the unknown is the central meaning in the expression.

Notice how the nurse's initial understanding response was not entirely accurate. The patient took the opportunity to clarify the meaning because the nurse's response indicated a desire to understand. The patient's final question, 'What do you think?', is indicative of the beginning of trust in the nurse. The patient feels able to rely on this nurse because the nurse has taken the time to understand the situation.

Because each patient's experience is unique, another patient may have expressed similar thoughts for an entirely different reason. Here is a similar scenario, with a different patient:

Patient:	It doesn't seem right that I am still in so much pain. My hip surgery was 6 weeks ago, and I still can't seem to get comfortable. Is it just me? I asked my doctor and she said, 'No, this is not unusual, so don't worry.' But I really don't know.
Nurse:	It doesn't seem right to you that you are still in so much pain 6 weeks after the surgery.
Patient:	It's not the pain so much, but the amount of medication I'm taking.
Nurse:	You think it might be too much.
Patient:	Well, yes, I take those tablets every 4 hours. Could I be taking too many?

As with the first scenario, the nurse may need to explore this situation further, or offer concrete information about the likelihood of taking too much pain medication. The illustrations show how different patients experience the same event. These scenarios exemplify the importance of achieving understanding that is based on the patient's view of the situation. While the situation is similar, each patient's experience of it is different. In each scenario, the nurse listens to the patient's view, comes to understand it and is then able to operate from a vantage point within the patient's experience. The nurse can now offer help, in the form of advice, information or reassurance that is specific to the patient.

Internal and external understanding

The understanding that is emphasised here is termed internal because it is grounded in the patient's subjective world and personal view of a situation. External understanding, on the other hand, is an objective view of a situation. In nursing, these external understandings are based on clinical information that is devoid of any specific patient (e.g. a textbook case, referred to as case knowledge: see Ch 1).

Nurses often become so focused on having the answers that they rely exclusively on an external understanding of the situation. An overconcern with 'What can I do?' often prevents nurses from asking, 'What is this like for this patient?' This keeps nurses externally focused. There is a danger that nursing care based solely on external understanding will be misguided and will not take into account the uniqueness of the patient. In the scenarios given earlier, the nurse could have relied on an informed understanding of recovery following hip surgery, and not taken the time to understand this patient's experience of recovery.

Focusing externally can lead to premature and automatic solutions that look to results and outcomes. Focusing internally meets patients where they are and offers a way of operating from within their experiences before moving to solutions and outcomes. Advising, evaluating, interpreting and falsely reassuring, in the absence of internal understanding, usually arise from an externally focused approach. Both external and internal understandings are necessary. They can be combined to provide guidance in appreciating what is appropriate in caring for a particular patient.

Barriers to understanding

Many potential barriers exist when nurses are trying to understand a patient's perspective and frame of reference. The interferences that affect listening (see Ch 5) are still active. The natural tendency to judge and evaluate must still be kept in abeyance. An even greater barrier that exists is the tendency to jump to conclusions about what the patient is experiencing. Unless the patient validates these conclusions, they remain assumptions. Unshared assumptions lead to unshared meaning.

THE SKILLS OF UNDERSTANDING

An interpersonal capability to build meaning through skilled interaction is as significant as an awareness of the importance of understanding. The skills of understanding are presented here in a particular order. Paraphrasing, seeking clarification and reflecting feelings are used prior to connecting and summarising. The final skill, expressing empathy, is viewed as the sum total of all other understanding skills (see Fig 6.1). The point at which the nurse can accurately express empathy is the point at which mutual understanding is achieved.

FIGURE 6.1 Hierarchy of understanding skills

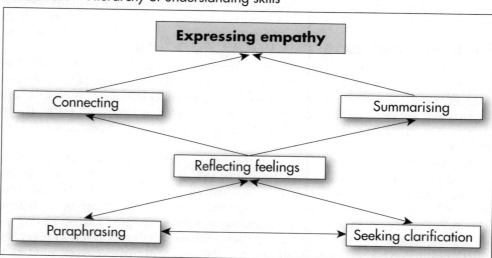

Paraphrasing

Paraphrasing is the backbone of understanding skills. When nurses paraphrase, they restate what the patient has expressed, but instead of using the patient's words, nurses rephrase the patient's message in their own words and mode of expression. A paraphrase is a translation from the patient's language and manner of expression into the nurse's. Through the use of the paraphrase, nurses share their understanding of what patients have expressed.

Paraphrases acknowledge what the patient has said and demonstrate that the nurse has listened. They encourage further patient expression because they are confirming and accepting. Paraphrases, although statements, contain an implied question, 'Is my understanding of what you are saying the same as what you mean to say?' They often begin with phrases such as:

- 'So, what you are saying is …'
- 'Would I be correct in saying that you …'
- 'In other words …'
- 'Let me see if I understand correctly …'

Beginning a paraphrase with phrases such as these brings the implied question into the open. However, it is not essential that paraphrases begin in this manner. A nurse may simply rephrase what the patient has expressed.

The value of the paraphrase is its ability to check the accuracy of the nurse's understanding of what the patient means against the patient's intended meaning. Use of the paraphrase is an effective way to prevent misunderstandings. Because patients hear the nurse's interpretation, they are afforded an opportunity to confirm or deny its accuracy.

Interchangeable responses

When paraphrasing, the nurse attempts to produce a response that is interchangeable with what the patient has expressed. An effective paraphrase neither adds to (additive response) nor detracts from (detractive response) what the patient has said.

Additive responses include comments on, explanations of, and opinions about what the patient is expressing. Analysing and interpreting responses are examples of additive responses. Although quite helpful when the goal is to increase the patient's awareness, additive responses do not necessarily facilitate the nurse's understanding.

Responses that detract are those that shift the focus away from the patient or focus only on what the *nurse* thinks is important. Offering premature solutions and advice are examples of detractive responses. Paraphrases neither add nor detract; they are interchangeable with what the patient has expressed, and do not attempt to alter the meaning of that expression.

Accuracy in paraphrasing

Even though nurses attempt to make paraphrases interchangeable, there is still no guarantee that they will be entirely accurate. The meaning a nurse derives from the patient's expression may not be what the patient intended. This does not signal failure, because an inaccurate paraphrase allows the patient to correct the nurse's misinterpretation before progressing further in the interaction. In responding to a paraphrase, the patient has an opportunity to restate the meaning of an expression, amplify it or reiterate what was originally expressed. As long as nurses do not detract completely from the meaning, understanding can still be achieved through further interaction.

For this reason, it is important to state a paraphrase in a tentative manner and closely observe the patient's response to it. Even when it is inaccurate, a paraphrase still conveys the nurse's desire to understand and a willingness to engage in interactions that build meaning. The ultimate aim is to achieve congruence between what the patient means and what the nurse understands the patient to mean. This requires effort, time and the use of responses that work towards this aim. Mutual understanding must be negotiated between patient and nurse. The paraphrase works towards the goal of mutual understanding, because it enables meaning to be negotiated.

Activity 6.4 PARAPHRASING: HAVE I GOT IT RIGHT? ➡304

PROCESS

1 Form pairs for this activity, and designate one person as A and the other as B.

2 A makes a statement about a recent interaction with a patient that was significant.

3 B responds with a paraphrase and begins with, 'So, in other words, what you are saying is …' B is not to advise, judge, evaluate or probe. At the end of the paraphrase, B asks, 'Have I got it right?'

4 A confirms or denies B's paraphrase and then continues to discuss the situation. B continues to paraphrase each of A's statements, asking each time, 'Have I got it right?' This process continues until A is able to say to B, 'Yes, you have got it right, that's exactly what I mean.'

5 Reverse roles, with B relating a story and A paraphrasing.

DISCUSSION

1 How accurate were the initial paraphrases? What was the response to an inaccurate paraphrase? How long did it take to achieve accuracy?

2 What were the effects of the use of the paraphrase on the interaction? How did each participant feel during the interaction?

3 How was listening affected when you knew you had to paraphrase?

The paraphrase is effective in building meaning and, when used to this end, it results in greater understanding between patient and nurse. As with any skill, nurses must pay careful attention to how patients respond to paraphrasing. When the paraphrase encourages patients to elaborate on their experiences, thus enabling nurses to understand these experiences more fully, it is working towards its desired end.

Overuse of the paraphrase

Overuse of the paraphrase, in the absence of other skills, can be frustrating for a patient because the interaction may seem to be going in circles, with little forward progress. Continuous rephrasing of what the patient has said gives the impression that the interaction is 'going nowhere'. To prevent this, paraphrases need to be used with a mixture of other skills.

The aim and intention of the paraphrase must be borne in mind. An accurate paraphrase is a direct acknowledgment of what a patient has expressed. It serves as confirmation of the patient's reality. It conveys that the nurse is willing and able to view the patient's experience from the patient's frame of reference. All of this is done in order to deepen the relationship and encourage further interaction. When paraphrases stifle interaction, they do not meet their intended aim.

Reluctance to use paraphrasing

Despite the value of the paraphrase in building and negotiating meaning, there is sometimes a lack of appreciation of its use. Nurses are sometimes reluctant to employ the paraphrase out of a fear of appearing inept or poorly informed. They often think they 'should' automatically understand what patients are experiencing, and may feel foolish in not knowing. It is virtually impossible for nurses to fully appreciate what patients are experiencing until an effort is made to understand. Each patient's experience is unique, and subjective. To believe there is an objective reality that is applicable to all patients is unrealistic.

At other times, reluctance to employ the paraphrase stems from a fear of reinforcing a patient's negative state. For example, when patients express unpleasant emotions or self-destructive thoughts, nurses may fear that restating such negative experiences elevates them, giving them more status than they deserve. Nurses may believe that it is better to deny or dismiss them, avoid further discussion of them or try to talk the patient out of them. But avoidance alienates patients, giving the impression that nurses do not really care.

The paraphrase acknowledges the patient's reality, demonstrates acceptance of it and conveys the nurse's desire to understand that reality. This is not the same as agreement and reinforcement; eventually, a nurse may challenge a patient and encourage the adoption of an alternative perspective (see Ch 8). Another perspective cannot be introduced until the nurse shares the patient's current perspective and paraphrases work towards this shared understanding.

Seeking clarification

The skills of clarification are used whenever nurses are uncertain or unsure about what patients are saying. Under these circumstances, paraphrasing is not possible, because the nurse is unable to get an adequate sense of what the patient means. Through clarification, nurses convey that they are trying to understand, and will not proceed until they are able to do so. Statements that clarify could begin with:

- 'I'm not sure I follow you …'
- 'That's not clear to me …'
- 'Run that by me again …'
- 'I'm not certain what you mean …'
- 'I don't follow what you are saying …'
- 'I'm having difficulty understanding that …'
- 'I'm a bit confused about …'

Notice how the nurse takes responsibility for the lack of clarity and understanding. The intent and effect would be very different if statements such as 'You're not expressing yourself clearly' or 'That's not clear' were made. A properly phrased clarification is focused on a desire to receive a clearer message from the patient—a rephrase, an illustration and/or amplification. It should not put patients on the defensive or lead to discomfort by creating the feeling that they have to justify themselves or provide rational explanations to nurses.

Clarification through questioning

Clarification is often achieved through the use of probing skills (see Ch 7); however, the intention is not focused as much on exploration as it is on clearing up an area of confusion or ambiguity. An open question, such as 'What do you mean?', is a direct clarification. Nurses must use such a question with care and caution because of its potential to sound critical and accusatory (it could imply, 'You are not making sense'). Intonation and other non-verbal aspects make the difference.

Restatement

At times a restatement of what a patient has said is an effective means of clarifying. The nurse simply parrots the patient's exact words, usually switching from the first person to the second person. The accompanying non-verbal intonation should indicate that the restatement is really a prompt, which is aimed at further amplification. Restatement is similar to one-word or phrase accents (see Ch 7) except that, in restatement, the entire message is reiterated. An example of a restatement is:

Patient: I can't move my right arm.
Nurse: You can't move your right arm?

Sometimes, nurses overuse restatement because they do not know what else to say. Overuse of parroting can lead to frustration on the part of the patient, so its use should be kept to a minimum. It should be used with the intention of reaching greater clarity and understanding, not as a substitute for lack of words.

Clarification through self-disclosure

At times, nurses clarify what a patient has said by sharing how they might feel, think and perceive the situation if they were the patient. An example is: 'I'm not sure I entirely follow what it's like for you, but if I were you I'd be …' Care must be exercised when using self-disclosure, because of the potential to shift the focus from the patient to the nurse. In using self-disclosure in this manner, the nurse is attempting to clear an area of confusion, not detract from what the patient is expressing.

Reflecting feelings

Reflection is the mirroring of feelings expressed by patients. Because feelings are often expressed indirectly, nurses translate the feeling aspects of a patient's message into other words. In this sense, reflecting feelings is similar to the paraphrase. Instead of rephrasing the actual words of the patient, the nurse rephrases an indirectly expressed emotion. An example of reflecting feelings is:

Patient: This darn leg won't get any stronger, despite all the physio.
Nurse: That leg is frustrating you, isn't it?

Reflecting feelings is useful because it conveys the nurse's recognition of feelings and confirms the existence of emotions. More than any other area of the patient's experience, feelings must be accepted as valid and real. Like the paraphrase, the reflection of feelings must be stated tentatively, awaiting feedback from the patient, which either confirms or denies the accuracy of the nurse's perception.

Reflecting feelings is verbalising what a patient has implied, but this is not the same as interpreting the patient's feelings. An interpretation involves adding to the patient's expression, rather than bringing into the open what was expressed indirectly. The nurse is still working with what the patient has communicated, not providing an explanation of, or judgment about, the patient's feelings.

In reflecting feelings, as in paraphrasing, nurses attempt to respond interchangeably with what patients have expressed. An interchangeable feeling reflection matches both the type of feeling and its intensity. Frustration is different from anger; feeling a bit blue is not the same as feeling despondent; happiness is not equivalent to elation. Making the distinction between different emotions and feelings requires an extensive vocabulary. A major difficulty in reflecting feelings is a limitation of the language the nurse possesses for describing feelings. Activity 6.5 is designed to increase your feeling-word vocabulary.

Activity 6.5 BUILDING A FEELING-WORD VOCABULARY

PROCESS

1 Divide a blank piece of paper into seven vertical columns. Place the following 'feeling' categories at the top of the columns:
   Happy Sad Angry Confused Scared Weak Strong

2 In each column, record as many words as you can that express the emotion. Phrases such as 'over the moon' can also be used.

3 Form groups of five to six participants and compare lists. Add words from other participants' lists that you have not already recorded.

4 Evaluate each feeling word on the list according to its intensity. Label each as *high*, *medium* or *low* intensity. For example: elated = high; happy = medium; pleased = low.

DISCUSSION

1 In which feeling category(ies) was it easy to develop words and phrases? Which were difficult? Why are some categories easier to describe than others?

2 Which feeling category has the most words and phrases? Which the least? What do you make of this?

3 Compare the feeling categories that were hard and easy with the ones that have the most and least words and phrases. Is there any relationship? Explain.

4 Look at the language used in each of the categories. Are some feeling words and phrases more appropriate with patients in different age groups and from different cultural backgrounds?

5 What role does culture play in the evaluation of feeling-word intensity?

6 Are there some words and phrases that you would not personally use under certain circumstances? What are they and why would you not use them?

Source: Adapted from Carkhuff (1983).

When nurses are reflecting feelings, they must first identify the appropriate feeling category. Most feelings will fit into one of the categories used in Activity 6.5. Secondly, the intensity of the feeling expressed must be determined. Once the correct feeling and its intensity have been decided, a word or phrase that accurately describes the feeling is selected. The choice of words must suit the age (see Ch 10) and cultural background (see Ch 4) of the patient.

A nurse's feeling-word vocabulary can be further built through interactions with patients by paying careful attention to the language used when patients express various emotions and feelings.

Because feelings are often expressed indirectly, through non-verbal means, inference and innuendo, nurses may first need to check their perceptions (see Ch 7) of how a patient is feeling before attempting to reflect the feeling accurately. Frequently, it is better to check perceptions of feelings before proceeding to reflect them.

Activity 6.6 REFLECTING FEELINGS

PROCESS

1 Refer to patient statements from Activity 5.8, 'Listening for feelings'. For each statement, develop a response that reflects the expressed feeling. Refer to the list of words and phrases developed in Activity 6.5, 'Building a feeling-word vocabulary'.

DISCUSSION

1 Which feelings were easy to reflect? Which were difficult? What do you make of this?

2 Are there any feeling reflections you would find personally difficult to express? Why?

A word of caution about reflecting feelings

Some patients are more comfortable than others in discussing their feelings. Additionally, a discussion of feelings may enhance a patient's sense of vulnerability, because feelings are difficult to control and contain. When a patient is working hard at containing emotions, and prefers to keep doing so, it is insensitive for a nurse to proceed into a discussion that uncovers these feelings and focuses on them. Nurses must pay careful attention to a patient's reaction to the discussion of feelings.

Likewise, discussion of feelings should be left until trust has formed between patient and nurse. The extent to which a patient is relaxed and at ease with a discussion of feelings demonstrates the degree of trust that has been established. The nurse can use a feeling discussion as a means of determining how much trust has been established. This requires acute awareness and sensitivity to the patient's response.

Connecting thoughts and feelings

Chapter 5, on listening, differentiated listening for content and listening for feelings. In this chapter, the skill of paraphrasing is used predominantly to respond to content, while reflecting feelings responds to emotional states. While it is possible to perceive them separately, and even respond to them separately, patients' experiences include both content and feelings. Initially, nurses may choose to focus on one or the other when responding. Eventually, thoughts (content) and feelings (emotion) must be put together. Connecting skills are used for this purpose. When connecting, nurses can use the following format: 'You feel … when …'

Connecting thoughts and feelings adds depth to the nurse's understanding and moves the interaction in a forward direction. Through this response, a nurse is moving into the area of fully understanding a patient's experience. Listening attentively and clarifying enables nurses to make the connection between patients' thoughts and their feelings. Again, it is necessary for the nurse to await feedback from the patient, which confirms, denies or expands on the nurse's understanding.

Activity 6.7 CONNECTING THOUGHTS AND FEELINGS ➡304

PROCESS

1 Refer to each patient statement in Activity 6.2, 'Recognition of the types of responses'. Ignore the responses that are provided and develop one of your own that connects the patients' expressed thoughts to their feelings. Use the format: 'You feel … when …' as a guide. Refer to your feeling-word vocabulary, developed in Activity 6.5, for ways to describe feelings.

2 Compare your responses with those of other participants.

DISCUSSION

1 What differences are there in responses developed by various participants? Were there some responses that were the same?

2 In comparing connecting responses, how similar are the feeling portions? How different are they?

3 In comparing the connections between feelings and content, did some participants focus on content that was different from that of other participants?

Summarising

Summarising is the skill of responding in a way that reviews what has been discussed between patient and nurse. It is a brief, concise collection of paraphrases and feeling reflections that are accurately connected. Like other skills of understanding, a summary allows the nurse to check understanding by verbalising it, then awaiting feedback from the patient. Summaries often begin with:

- 'So, to sum it up …'
- 'We have discussed so much, let me see if I can pull it together …'
- 'Overall, I get the picture that …'

Summarising is used most often to bring closure to an interaction, and serves as a final check of the nurse's understanding. When nurses use summarising to bring closure to an interaction, it is important that they allow adequate time for patients to respond. As with other understanding skills, the patient needs an opportunity to clarify, expand on an idea or correct the nurse's misinterpretation.

There is an even more important reason for allowing adequate time following a summary. Frequently, patients present the most significant aspect of their experience just as the time draws near to close an interaction. In this case, the patient perceives the nurse's summary as a signal that time is of the essence, and uses the remaining time as a final opportunity for expression. This is not at all uncommon during patient–nurse interactions. An aware nurse recognises and accepts this interpersonal dynamic, and allows time for its occurrence.

While closure is the most common reason to summarise, a summary is also effectively used either in the middle or the beginning of an interaction. When used in the middle of an interaction, a summary serves to open new areas of discussion, by clearing the way for new ideas (Brammer & MacDonald 1996). When it is used at this point, summarising serves as an exploration skill that encourages patients to bring forward new thoughts and feelings. When it is used at the beginning of an interaction, summarising serves to orient both patient and nurse to the current interaction by reviewing previous interactions.

EXPRESSION OF UNDERSTANDING: EMPATHY

When nurses employ the skills of understanding (paraphrasing, seeking clarification, reflecting feelings, connecting and summarising), in conjunction with effective exploration (see Ch 7), they are in a position to know what a patient is experiencing from the personal perspective of the patient. This inside understanding involves knowing what is happening to that person, and even feeling what it is like to be that person. Knowing and feeling through vicarious experiences such as these are often referred to as empathy.

Empathy is the ability to perceive the world from another person's view, and take on the perspective of another, while not losing one's own perspective (Rogers 1961). In stressing the notion of not losing one's self, Rogers is referring to the sense of otherness that characterises a professional helping relationship (see Ch 2). For this reason, empathy relies on a strong sense of self, for without awareness of one's own perspective, attempts to enter another person's world may result in becoming lost in the world of the other.

The strong sense of self that is required to fully appreciate the reality of another is related to emotional intelligence and therapeutic agency (see Ch 3). The ability to understand others (i.e. to be empathic) is a core dimension of emotional intelligence (Goleman 1998), and is one process that enables people to be competent communicators.

Empathy is the process that enables nurses to know the patient as a patient and a person (see 'Knowing the patient' in Ch 1). As such, it is often considered a prerequisite for nursing practice, as it is difficult to comprehend how a person who is attempting to help another person can do so without a clear understanding of how the person in need of help perceives their situation and the circumstances surrounding it, including what they want to happen (Reynolds & Scott 2000).

Empathy in nursing

Nurses have long embraced the process of empathy as essential to caring practices (Kunyk & Olson 2001, Reynolds & Scott 1999, White 1997, Wiseman 1996, Olsen 1991, Pike 1990). As a result of being empathic, the nurse comes to know and understand the patient's experience. This absorption of the patient's reality is one way that empathy is realised in nursing. Some of the first nursing theorists to discuss empathy (Travelbee 1971, Triplett 1969, Zderad 1969) emphasised the purpose of empathy as the promotion of rapport between patient and nurse. Rapport is essential to building and maintaining a relationship with the patient that is based on mutual understanding. It is a reciprocal process of give and take, and it is important that patients feel understood by nurses, not just that nurses believe that they feel empathic. Therefore, nursing theorists who first discussed empathy also stressed the importance of the nurse communicating their understanding to the patient (Gagan 1983, Kalisch 1973, Zderad 1969). In addition, it is important that the patients perceive that nurses do indeed understand their health-related circumstances.

It is important that nurses be able to express empathic understanding because its use in nursing practice involves the ability to perceive the feelings of the other and the self. That is, empathy facilitates awareness and organises perceptions in addition to promoting mutual understanding. It is not simply the ability to label and name feelings in a rote fashion (Halpern 2003). Empathy involves the ability to actually know what it feels like to experience a particular emotion. It is a perceptual activity—that is, empathy is not simply an intellectual activity or an interpersonal skill. It is a form of interaction that involves attitudes and perceptual skill (Reynolds & Scott 1999).

Effects of empathy on the relationship

When communicating empathy, nurses respond with a direct, clear and accurate statement that reflects the core of the patient's experience. Doing so promotes trust because patients are put at ease to disclose when they experience emotional attunement with the nurse (Halpern 2003). Expressing empathy is a skill that involves nurses sharing openly with patients that they understand their perspectives. Expressing empathy communicates this understanding, conveying both acceptance and confirmation of the reality of the patient's experience. In addition, empathy contributes to mutuality (described in Ch 2).

Empathic statements capture the essence of the patient's experience and move the relationship into a more intimate zone (Shea & Maloney 1998). For this reason, empathy expression, especially in relation to patients' feelings, can be intrusive and prematurely intimate. Yet empathy expression in nursing is often equated with emotions. For example, White (1997) and Wiseman (1996) consider critical attributes of empathy to be recognition and understanding of the patient's feelings. Nevertheless, knowing the patient (see Ch 1) in such an intimate way may not be appropriate or desirable.

An empathic statement exposes patients, laying their reality in the open. It can expose areas of weakness, uncertainty and vulnerability. A patient may not want this exposure, and sensitivity to the patient's reaction to an empathic statement is needed. If the patient wants to appear strong or maintain control, the nurse who is sensitive will accept this and move out of the intimacy that empathy can bring.

This move into intimacy is one reason that there are cautions in the nursing literature against a wholehearted, unquestioning embrace of empathy. Gould (1990) warns that it may be unrealistic and idealistic to expect nurses to be empathic with all patients. Diers (1990) says that empathy may not be always appropriate to the patient's situation. Gordon (1987) cautions against a danger in nurses projecting their own perceptions onto patients in an effort to be empathic.

It is for these reasons that timing is crucial when expressing empathy. If a nurse moves too quickly into empathic expression, a patient may feel invaded and inhibited. For these reasons, all the other skills of understanding should be used first in order to establish understanding and build the relationship. When the patient demonstrates comfort with discussing feelings, has validated the nurse's paraphrases, confirms the connections made between thoughts and feelings, and agrees with the summary, then the relationship is ready to move into the intimate zone of empathy. The point at which a nurse truly understands is the time to express empathy.

Another purpose of empathy: counselling

In addition to the promotion of rapport and understanding, empathy in nursing is considered a means of promoting personal change and growth within the patient (Pike 1990). This purpose of empathy relies on the nurse's objective analysis of the patient's experience and is based on a counselling model of helping, which promotes the development of more effective ways of living.

The counselling view of empathy in the nursing literature is based primarily on the work of Carl Rogers (Thompson 1996, Morse et al 1992, Gould 1990). Rogers, a psychologist who pioneered client-centred therapy, considered empathy to be an essential feature of the therapeutic counselling relationship (Rogers 1961, 1957). The humanistic philosophy that underpins Rogers' theory of counselling is consistent with patient-centred nursing care and the development of a therapeutic patient–nurse relationship as central to that care. Therefore, it is understandable that nurses who first conceptualised the therapeutic nature of the patient–nurse relationship were influenced by the work of Carl Rogers.

Nevertheless, there is critique in the nursing literature that conceptualisations of empathy in nursing that have been based on theory borrowed from and developed for another discipline and therefore is inappropriate (Walker & Alligood 2001, Alligood & May 2000, Baille 1996, Morse et al 1992, Gould 1990). A counselling view of empathy, with its focus on encouraging a patient's personal growth, may not always be appropriate in a nursing situation unless the nurse is also a psychotherapist. Although nurses often interact with people who are experiencing change and transition, not all patients are in the process of personal growth. Nurses need to understand a patient's personal experience of illness (one purpose of empathy), but not necessarily focus on encouraging psychological growth and personality change (another purpose of empathy).

There are times when nurses do promote change in a patient—for example, assisting patients in developing new skills, such as teaching self-injections for Type 1 diabetes. However, care is not necessarily focused on bringing about change in the patient's way of being and living. Nurses often support and assist people as they experience transitions in health and illness, acting as partners in the patient journey; and change is inevitable with transition (see Ch 9). However, rather than guide the change for the patient, nurses help by standing alongside and comforting, supporting and enabling patients along their journey (see Ch 8).

Description of empathy in nursing literature

In addition to empathy being recommended for different purposes, many authors claim empathy is poorly described in the nursing literature (Morse et al 2006, Kunyk & Olson 2001, White 1997, Wiseman 1996, Gould 1990). The result is a weak theoretical understanding. Part of the difficulty lies in the fact that empathy is a complex concept. It 'may be seen as ability, a communication style, a trait, a response, a skill, a process, or an experience' (Wheeler & Barrett 1994 p 234).

In their review of the nursing literature on empathy, Morse et al (1992) identify four components of empathy, which were reinforced by a subsequent review (Reynolds & Scott 1999). First is emotional empathy, which involves the subjective sharing of feelings. Next is cognitive empathy, which involves the ability to comprehend another's feelings from an objective stance. Third is moral empathy, or the inherent motivation to comprehend the experience of another. Fourth is behavioural empathy, which involves conveying understanding of another's perspective through communicating. The more recent literature review confirms this multidimensional nature of empathy.

The four aspects of empathy that were identified by Morse et al (1992) can be compared to those described in Alligood's (1992) analysis of empathy. Alligood identifies two types of empathy: basic and trained. Basic empathy is an innate capacity to apprehend another's perspective, and can be likened to the emotional and moral components of empathy. Unlike basic empathy, trained empathy is learned. Trained empathy involves the cognitive and behavioural aspects of empathy, which is standing back and analysing the patient's situation and communicating that understanding to the patient.

The most recent concept analysis of empathy, in which five concepts are identified (Kunyk & Olson 2001), confirms the findings of these earlier reviews. The five main concepts are that empathy is: a human trait that is natural and instinctive; a professional state that is learned, objective and has clear boundaries; a communication process that involves expressed and received understanding (and encompassing the first two concepts); the equivalent of caring in which nursing actions of 'being with' patients and offering physical care and emotional comfort are central; and a special relationship in which patients are empowered to cope as a result of being understood.

Empathy that is considered to be therapeutic most often includes the cognitive and behavioural components (Morse et al 2006)—that is, trained empathy (Alligood 1992). Although empathy is a skill that can be taught (Wheeler & Barrett 1994), there is evidence that 'trained empathy'—that is, the learnt skills of reflecting understanding to a patient—is not really sustained over time (Evans et al 1998). While the communicative aspects of empathy can be taught, empathy as a trait is inherent. Nurses need self-awareness of their innate capacity for empathy so that they can build on their basic empathy and learn to express it through a personal style rather than a textbook formula.

Halpern (2003) critiques the term 'clinical empathy', or what has been termed a professional state (Kunyk & Olson 2001), which is promoted as a way of intellectualising patients' feelings, rather than perceiving and experiencing them in an affective/feeling manner. She questions traditional views that the desired type of empathy in healthcare is one that stands apart and 'sees into' the patient's experience, in favour of an empathy that 'feels into' the experience. Halpern (2003) challenges a long-held view in medical care that emotional detachment is necessary in medical decision making, and claims that grasping another's emotional state through empathic understanding and involvement enhances medical diagnosis.

One question that has yet to be answered by research is whether nurse empathy makes a difference to patient outcomes. An empirical study in a residential aged care setting (Hollinger-Samson & Pearson 2000) sheds some light on the answer to this question. In this study, empathy was investigated and measured along three dimensions: empathy as emotional resonance with the patient, likened to an innate ability to feel the emotions of another (a human trait); empathy as expressed through communicating and relating (an interpersonal process); and empathy as perceived by the recipient of empathic expression (the perception of the patient).

While the third dimension has not received much focus in nursing literature, the perception of 'feeling understood' was the only dimension associated with a reduced level of depressed mood in the residents who participated in this study. The findings suggest that, no matter how perceptive a nurse may be to a person's feelings, without the reciprocated acknowledgment from that person as to the accuracy of the perceptions, there is little to be gained by simply expressing emotional understanding through empathy.

Empathy and sympathy

Often, a distinction is made between empathy and sympathy. Sympathy is viewed as 'feeling for' another person and empathy as 'feeling with' the other. Sympathy is often considered less desirable because nurses need to put their own concerns to one side and focus on the patient (Pike 1990, Kalisch 1973); these authors consider sympathetic responses to be focused on the nurse. In contrast Morse et al (2006) assert that because a sympathetic response is focused on the other (i.e. the patient), responses such as sympathy and pity may be as comforting for patients as empathy. Florence Nightingale encouraged nurses to be sympathetic; so did Travelbee (1971). Still, nurses are encouraged to be empathetic, not sympathetic. What is the difference between sympathy and empathy?

Wispé's (1986) analysis of the distinction between empathy and sympathy assists in answering this question. She asserts that in empathy we consider what it would be like *if* we were the other person; in sympathy, we automatically (reflexively) know what it would be like *to be* the other person. In empathy, we 'reach out' to that person; in sympathy, we are 'moved by' the other. Sympathy urges action to alleviate the suffering of the other; empathy urges efforts to comprehend the consciousness of the other. Sympathy is a way of relating, while empathy is a way of knowing. We can send a sympathy card as an action; we do not send empathy cards.

Despite the useful analysis, the attempt to differentiate sympathy and empathy remains troublesome. The results of Baille's (1996) research into empathy have been critiqued as confusing empathy with sympathy (Yegdich 1999), as the nurses in Baille's 1996 study described empathy as familiarity with the patient's situation because they had similar experiences. Perhaps what is at issue is not delineating one from the other, but recognising that both sympathy and empathy have a place in nursing. Just because they can be distinguished from each other does not mean one is more beneficial to patients than the other. In nursing, empathy is often touted as more beneficial even though its effects on patient outcome have not been fully researched. There is evidence that empathy decreases patient distress (Olson 1995, Reid-Ponte 1992), but other responses such as commiseration, pity and consolation serve to comfort patients (Morse et al 2006). More importantly, such responses engage the patient more than the learnt response of behavioural and cognitive styles of empathy that rely on objective analysis.

In their analysis, Morse et al (2006) use the criteria of engagement with the patient and focus on the patient as a way of determining what type of nursing response is of comfort to the patient. In a way, this approach sidesteps the sympathy–empathy distinction, but offers a useful way of determining the purpose of responses intended to be helpful and understanding. Those responses that engage patients and focus on them (as compared to responses that focus on the nurse and disengage the patient) are considered to be helpful because they are comforting.

Omdahl and O'Donnell (1999) differentiated emotional contagion from empathic concern, with the former involving taking on the emotions of the other and the latter being the capacity to understand the subjective experiences of the other without taking on the emotions. Emotional contagion does prompt action, but this can be focused on the self, while empathic concern is focused on the wellbeing of the other. Nurses who experience high levels of contagion are more prone to job stress than those who can express empathic concern and have the ability to discuss emotional and sensitive topics (Omdahl & O'Donnell 1999).

Expressing empathy

The purpose of expressing empathy should be borne in mind. Empathy is used to encourage the patient to continue expression, to provide direction to the nurse, to decrease the patient's sense of isolation and to bond the patient and nurse in understanding. Often support and reassurance, direct aid and assistance, or advice or challenge, follow the expression of empathy. At other times, empathy expression is an end in itself; it offers comfort and solace to patients—they know they are not alone because they are understood. (See Ch 8, 'Comforting', for further discussion of empathy.)

The frequency of empathy expression is also crucial. Short, precise empathic statements should be employed whenever nurses think understanding has been achieved. Too much empathy expression, especially early in the relationship, can sound paternalistic and superficial (Shea & Maloney 1998). Lack of empathy expression leaves patients with a sense of isolation, as if nurses do not care to receive their world.

The most congruent and compelling goal of empathy in nursing—that is, for nurses to come to understand a patient's experience—is that nurses' actions are based on their understanding of the patient's situation. In nursing, there is an obligation to act, not simply to understand, and acting without understanding may result in actions that are not helpful to patients. This is one possible explanation about why more experienced nurses in Reid-Ponte's (1992) study were less empathic than their less experienced colleagues. Clinical experience provides the knowledge to act; therefore, experienced nurses may need to spend less time being verbally empathic in order to understand patient needs.

As a moral position, empathy demonstrates a commitment to understanding patients. In this regard, its benefits are without question. What is questionable is whether cognitive and behavioural aspects of empathy should be given more credence because they are considered 'therapeutic'. They also have the potential to create greater intimacy than is warranted by the patient's situation (e.g. the clinical/instrumental relationship described in Ch 2), or disengage the patient because they are mechanical and objective when empathy is expressed in a formulaic manner, such as 'I hear what you are saying'. Beginning nurses should bear these considerations in mind when employing the skills of understanding.

Reluctance to express empathy

At first, it feels awkward for nurses to express to patients what patients are experiencing. The awkwardness is based on a false notion that it is presumptuous and arrogant, if not downright impolite, to openly state what another person is experiencing. When empathy is expressed with an attitude of 'let me tell you what you are experiencing', its basic nature has been violated. When employed in this manner, attempts at empathy expression will be met with defensiveness on the patient's part and will work against an effective relationship. Empathy expression is a confirmation, not an accusation. The nurse must remain sensitive and open to correction. When stated with too much certainty, empathy expression alienates rather than engages the patient.

Activity 6.8 EXPRESSING EMPATHY

PROCESS

1 Refer to Activity 6.1, 'Your usual style of responding I'.

2 For each statement or question, develop a response that expresses empathy with the 'patient's' experience. Assume you have validated your understanding and have accurately understood the patient.

3 Compare these responses with the ones you originally developed when completing Activity 6.1.

DISCUSSION

1 What differences are there between the responses you originally developed and the ones you have now developed?

2 Which took more time to develop?

3 What risks are there in expressing empathy to patients?

4 What benefits are there in expressing empathy?

CHAPTER SUMMARY

Understanding responses are used after nurses have received meaningful input from patients during the process of listening. Once initial impressions are formed, understanding responses are employed to build meaning between patients and nurses. The skills of understanding are used to bring nurses in touch with patients' private and personal worlds. They allow nurses to be 'in tune' with patients.

Attending and listening to patients' reactions to understanding responses is essential, and highlights the need for constant listening. Patients may react to an understanding response by validating it, denying it, altering it or expanding on it. Each of these patient reactions provides an opportunity for nurses to deepen their level of understanding.

It requires time and effort to truly understand another's reality. Nurses need to allow themselves time to think and reflect on how effectively they are understanding patients' experiences. They need to allow themselves enough time to respond with understanding to patients. This may also involve 'letting go' of familiar ways of responding, in favour of responses that reflect understanding.

Answers to activity

Activity 6.2 RECOGNITION OF THE TYPES OF RESPONSES

2 a i S (reassuring and supporting)
  ii I (analysing and interpreting)
  iii U (paraphrasing and understanding)
  iv E (advising and evaluating)
  v P (questioning and probing)

b i P (questioning and probing)
  ii S (reassuring and supporting)
  iii E (advising and evaluating)
  iv U (paraphrasing and understanding)
  v I (analysing and interpreting)

c i U (paraphrasing and understanding)
  ii E (advising and evaluating)
  iii P (questioning and probing)
  iv S (reassuring and supporting)
  v I (analysing and interpreting)

d i E (advising and evaluating)
  ii P (questioning and probing)
  iii U (paraphrasing and understanding)
  iv I (analysing and interpreting)
  v S (reassuring and supporting)

e i S (reassuring and supporting)
  ii E (advising and evaluating)
  iii P (questioning and probing)
  iv I (analysing and interpreting)
  v U (paraphrasing and understanding)

f i E (advising and evaluating)
  ii P (questioning and probing)
  iii S (reassuring and supporting)
  iv I (analysing and interpreting)
  v U (paraphrasing and understanding)

g i I (analysing and interpreting)
ii E (advising and evaluating)
iii U (paraphrasing and understanding)
iv P (questioning and probing)
v S (reassuring and supporting)

h i U (paraphrasing and understanding)
ii S (reassuring and supporting)
iii E (advising and evaluating)
iv P (questioning and probing)
v I (analysing and interpreting)

i i I (analysing and interpreting)
ii S (reassuring and supporting)
iii U (paraphrasing and understanding)
iv E (advising and evaluating)
v P (questioning and probing)

j i U (paraphrasing and understanding)
ii S (reassuring and supporting)
iii I (analysing and interpreting)
iv P (questioning and probing)
v E (advising and evaluating)

k i S (reassuring and supporting)
ii I (analysing and interpreting)
iii P (questioning and probing)
iv U (paraphrasing and understanding)
v E (advising and evaluating)

l i I (analysing and interpreting)
ii U (paraphrasing and understanding)
iii P (questioning and probing)
iv E (advising and evaluating)
v S (reassuring and supporting)

REFERENCES

Alligood MR 1992 Empathy: the importance of recognising two types. Journal of Psychosocial Nursing 30(3):14–17

Alligood MR, May BA 2000 A nursing theory of personal system empathy: interpreting a conceptualization of empathy in King's interacting systems. Nursing Science Quarterly 13(3):243–247

Baille L 1996 A phenomenological study of the nature of empathy. Journal of Advanced Nursing 24:1300–1308

Brammer LM MacDonald G 1996 The helping relationship: process and skills, 6th edn. Allyn and Bacon, Boston, MA

Carkhuff RR 1983 The student workbook for the art of helping, 2nd edn. Human Resource Press, Amherst, MA

Diers D 1990 Response to 'On the nature and place of empathy in clinical nursing practice'. Journal of Professional Nursing 6(4):240–241

Evans GW, Wilt DL, Alligood MR, O'Neil M 1998 Empathy: a study of two types. Issues in Mental Health Nursing 19:453–461

Gagan JM 1983 Methodological notes on empathy. Advances in Nursing Science 5(2):65–72

Goleman D 1998 Working with emotional intelligence. Bloomsbury, London

Gordon M 1987 Nursing diagnosis: process and application, 2nd edn. McGraw-Hill, New York

Gould D 1990 Empathy: a review of the literature with suggestions for an alternative research strategy. Journal of Advanced Nursing 15:1167–1174

Halpern J 2003 What is clinical empathy? Journal of General Internal Medicine 18:670–674

Hollinger-Samson N, Pearson JL 2000 The relationship between staff empathy and depressive symptoms in nursing home residents. Aging and Mental Health 4(1):56–65

Johnson DW 2009 Reaching out: interpersonal effectiveness and self actualization, 10th edn. Allyn and Bacon/Merrill, Boston, MA

Kalisch BJ 1973 What is empathy? American Journal of Nursing 73:1548–1552

Kunyk D, Olson JK 2001 Clarification of conceptualization of empathy. Journal of Advanced Nursing 35(3):317–325

Morse JM, Anderson G, Bottoroff JL, Younge O, O'Brien B, Solberg M, Mellveen KH 1992 Exploring empathy: a conceptual fit for nursing practice? Image: Journal of Nursing Scholarship 24(4):273–280

Morse JM, Bottoroff J, Anderson G, O'Brien B, Solberg S 2006 (originally 1992) Beyond empathy: expanding expressions of caring. Journal of Advanced Nursing 53(1):75–90

Motyka M, Motyka H, Wsolek R 1997 Elements of psychological support in nursing care. Journal of Advanced Nursing 26:909–912

Olsen DP 1991 Empathy as an ethical and philosophical basis for nursing. Advances in Nursing Science 14(1):65–75

Olson JK 1995 Relationship between nurse-expressed empathy and patient-perceived empathy and patient distress. Image: Journal of Nursing Scholarship 27(4):317–322

Omdahl BL, O'Donnell C 1999 Emotional contagion, empathic concern and communicative responsiveness as variables affecting nurses' stress and occupational commitment. Journal of Advanced Nursing 29:1351–1359

Pike AW 1990 On the nature and place of empathy in clinical nursing practice. Journal of Professional Nursing 6(4):235–340

Reid-Ponte P 1992 Distress in cancer patients and primary nurses' empathy skills. Cancer Nursing 15(4):283–292

Reynolds WJ, Scott B 1999 Empathy: a crucial component of the helping relationship. Journal of Psychiatric and Mental Health Nursing 6:363–370

Reynolds WJ, Scott B 2000 Do nurses and other professional helpers normally display much empathy? Journal of Advanced Nursing 31(1):226–234

Rogers C 1957 The necessary and sufficient conditions of therapeutic personality change. Journal of Consulting Psychology 21:91–105

Rogers C 1961 On becoming a person. Houghton Mifflin, Boston, MA

Shea SC, Maloney M 1998 Psychiatric interviewing: the art of understanding. Saunders, Philadelphia, PA

Thompson S 1996 Empathy: towards a clearer meaning for nursing. Nursing Praxis in New Zealand 11(1):19–26

Travelbee J 1971 Interpersonal aspects of nursing. FA Davis, Philadelphia, PA

Triplett JL 1969 Empathy is … Nursing Clinics of North America 4:673–681

Walker KM, Alligood MR 2001 Empathy from a nursing perspective: moving beyond borrowed theory. Archives of Psychiatric Nursing 15(3):140–147

Wheeler K, Barrett EAM 1994 Review and synthesis of selected nursing studies on teaching empathy and implication for nursing research and education. Nursing Outlook 42(5):230–236

White SJ 1997 Empathy: a literature review and concept analysis. Journal of Clinical Nursing 6:253–257

Whyte L, Motyka M, Motyka H, Wsolek R, Tune M 1997 Polish and British nurses responses to patient need. Nursing Standard 11(38):34–37

Wiseman T 1996 A concept analysis of empathy. Journal of Advanced Nursing 23:1162–1167

Wispé L 1986 The distinction between sympathy and empathy: to call forth a concept, a word is needed. Journal of Personality and Social Psychology 50:314–421

Yegdich T 1999 On the phenomenology of empathy in nursing: empathy or sympathy. Journal of Advanced Nursing 30:83–93

Zderad LT 1969 Empathic nursing: realisation of a human capacity. Nursing Clinics of North America 4:655–662

CHAPTER 7

Collecting information: exploring

INTRODUCTION

The skills covered in Chapters 5 and 6—attending, listening and understanding— lay the foundation for effective interaction between patient and nurse because their use enables nurses to hear, perceive and reflect back what patients are expressing. Exploration, the subject of this chapter, moves the interaction beyond absorption and reiteration of patients' messages. Exploration opens new areas, focuses on selected areas and delves more deeply into a patient's total experience.

The process of exploration is one of searching, carried out for the purpose of discovery, detection, recognition and identification. Successful exploration results in greater understanding between patient and nurse; it can be directed towards something in particular or it can be open-ended, leading to the discovery of something unexpected, which is the case with interpersonal exploration carried out in the context of patient–nurse relationships. Collecting specific information from patients, the directed type of exploration, is necessary. Is Mr Green allergic to any medications? How long did Ms Geraghty sleep last night? Does Mr Nelson understand his special low-fat diet? Answers to such questions help guide nursing approaches and actions, and nurses need to know how to collect pertinent information from patients.

Nevertheless, effective exploration in the nursing context involves more than merely the collection of specific facts from patients. Open-ended, spontaneous inquiry, the other type of exploration, is also needed because it is the means by which a nurse can come to understand how a patient interprets health and illness. What are Mr Green's expectations about his pending surgery? What is interfering with Ms Geraghty's sleep? How different is Mr Nelson's special diet from his usual one? Exploration into areas such as these is aimed at discovering ideas, thoughts, perceptions, feelings and reactions experienced by patients. It is important that nurses come to understand patients' responses to health and illness, and effective exploration assists in this understanding.

Consider the following story:

Martin Johnson spent his entire life in a rural part of the country. He felt very much at home 'on the land'. He disliked city life and avoided 'the big smoke' at all possible costs. Martin also had another aversion: visiting the doctor. He always put that off as long as he could. However, the obvious problems he was experiencing with his throat made it impossible to ignore his need of medical attention.

When he finally was admitted to a large metropolitan hospital for major surgery, Martin felt very much out of place. However, coping with being in the city seemed minor in comparison to his worry about being ill and in hospital. He did not ask many questions of the surgeons when they came to explain his surgery, which included possible removal of his larynx (voice box). Martin listened as the surgeons explained what they would do, but did not think too much about what it meant. Being a man of few words, he did not ask for clarification.

The night before his surgery, Lucille was the nurse caring for Martin. She felt an instant rapport with him, despite his quiet nature and the paucity of words between them. As she explained to Martin what he could expect following the surgery, she slowly came to the alarming realisation that he did not understand that the surgery would affect his ability to speak. In fact, if the surgeons performed the laryngectomy, he would not speak again. Although he had consented to the surgical procedure, he did not seem to appreciate the potential consequences for his life. Through exploring his understanding and desires, Lucille discovered that Martin preferred a shorter life with the ability to speak rather than a longer life and the inability to speak. As a result of her exploration and understanding, Martin's surgery was cancelled and other treatment options were explored.

This story raises questions as to whether Martin's consent to the surgery was adequately informed and highlights the importance of coming to understand the patient's point of view. And understanding the patient's point of view is contingent on effective exploration of patient perceptions and interpretation.

Chapter overview

This chapter reviews the skills of exploration within the context of patient–nurse interaction. It distinguishes directed exploration, such as a formal interview, from the less formal, spontaneous exploration, which occurs as a result of a trigger or cue from the patient. Both types of exploration rely on the use of the same skills, and these skills are divided into the broad areas of prompting and probing. Prompting techniques include minimal encouragement, one-word/phrase accents, gentle commands, open-ended statements, finishing the sentence and self-disclosure. The section on probing techniques covers open-ended questions and closed questions, and includes a discussion of when to use each type. The next section reviews two processes of exploration: focused exploration and patient-cue exploration. In the final section, there is a review of nurses' control in exploration, with an emphasis on shared control with patients.

Activity 7.1 DEVELOPING EXPLORATORY RESPONSES I

PROCESS

Record how you would respond to each of the following patient's statements. Do not concern yourself with how 'right' or 'wrong' your responses are, but do try to make them helpful to the patient. Assume that all statements are made to you, the nurse caring for the patient making the statement.

1 A hospitalised 65-year-old woman, who has recently undergone a total hip replacement: 'How am I ever going to manage on my own when I return home?'

2 A hospitalised patient speaking to a first-year nursing student: 'Do you know what you are doing? How much experience have you had?'

3 A 20-year-old woman who is undergoing diagnostic tests on an outpatient basis: 'The doctor keeps evading my questions. What is really going on?'

4 A mother of a 5-week-old baby during a routine visit to an early childhood centre: 'I wish I could get a decent night's sleep like I used to.'

5 A long-term resident of a nursing home: 'I can't stand being here. There's nothing to do and no one ever comes to visit me.'

6 A 20-year-old man who is hospitalised with a fractured femur, following a motor vehicle accident: 'Why do these things always have to happen to me? All the bad things like this happen to me.'

7 A hospitalised patient, during medication rounds in hospital: 'I think all of these tablets are really making me sleepy.'

8 A hospitalised patient during morning care: 'I have asked the doctors how long they think I have to live, but they keep avoiding the question. Will you tell me, please?'

9 A hospitalised patient during morning nursing rounds: 'I'm so glad to see you. Those nurses on the night shift just don't help me.'

10 A 70-year-old man in an outpatient clinic, following consultation with the doctor: 'If what the doctor says is true, I don't see the point in going on and suffering ... better to just end it now.'

DISCUSSION

1 Each of the statements presented indicates a situation that requires further exploration by the nurse—more information, clarification and/or elaboration is required. Review your responses and decide which of your responses do explore the patient's statement. Mark these with a tick.

2 Write a new response for those not marked. Try to make this revised response an exploratory one.

(Note: This activity will be further developed in Activity 7.10, 'Developing exploratory responses II'.)

PLANNED VERSUS SPONTANEOUS EXPLORATION

Planned exploration is directive (i.e. the nurse controls the interaction by directing the flow and content of the patient's response). A good example of planned exploration is a formal interview conducted for the purpose of health assessment. Spontaneous exploration is responsive (i.e. the nurse responds to something the patient has said or done). In planned exploration, nurses assume the lead and introduce the topics; in spontaneous exploration, nurses follow patients' leads. The distinction between planned exploration and spontaneous exploration is somewhat artificial because similar skills and techniques are used for both types of exploration. The distinction is drawn to highlight the different contexts in which nurses use exploration skills and techniques.

A common context in which nurses use exploration skills is when they conduct a health assessment. Most often, nurses conduct health assessments when they encounter a patient for the first time (e.g. on admission to hospital). Brown (1995) urges nurses to clarify the purpose of health assessments. If the purpose is to collect data about the patient's health status, then planned interviewing is appropriate. If the purpose is also to explore personal meaning of a patient's health status, then a less formalised, spontaneous exploration is appropriate. In nursing, both purposes are relevant. Nurses need to collect factual data about a patient's health as well as understanding the meaning of the health experience for the patient. As a result, exploration is most effective when it is both planned and spontaneous. Brown refers to this style of exploration as 'conversational interviewing', which closely mirrors the balanced give and take of everyday conversations, as compared to the one-way, controlled structure of a formal interview in which 'questions impose an obligation to answer' (1995 p 340).

Planned exploration

During planned exploration, the nurse directs and leads the search for information regarding pertinent aspects of a patient's 'health story' and current needs for nursing care. Specific data collection is the primary purpose of planned exploration, and topic areas are introduced and explored on the basis of what the nurse needs to know in order to care for the patient. Nurses direct and often control this type of exploration.

Structured, planned exploration occurs in the beginning phase of the patient–nurse relationship, usually upon initial contact between patient and nurse. The manner in which exploration occurs during these initial contacts sets the stage for subsequent interactions and further development of the relationship, by establishing the conditions for trust and openness. A nurse whose approach is authoritarian and rigid may convey a message to the patient that the nurse is in control and obedience in answering the questions is expected. This might happen when the nurse becomes so focused on filling out a nursing history form that patients are left with the impression that completion of the record is more important than them as people. Likewise, an overconcern with the techniques of exploration may interfere with a nurse's ability to fully attend and listen to patients' replies.

Spontaneous exploration

This type of exploration occurs when nurses pick up and follow through in exploring a patient cue. Patients often express their needs to nurses in indirect, disguised ways (Macleod Clark 1984), not because they want to keep the nurse guessing but because patients perceive that an indirect message poses less of a threat to nurses. How nurses respond to these messages, or cues from patients, helps to shape the direction of their continuing relationship. This type of exploration tends to be patient-controlled and patient-led. The nurse follows the patient's lead, instead of the patient following the nurse's lead.

Spontaneous exploration is important to the continuing relationship between patient and nurse, because it affirms that the nurse is attending and listening to the patient. It deepens the relationship and communicates the nurse's continued interest in the patient's welfare, because it is a concrete demonstration of the nurse's ongoing concern for the patient.

The difference between planned and spontaneous exploration

In both types of exploration, information is collected and greater depth of understanding is achieved, but the process is different because the roles of leader and follower are reversed. In the real world of patient care, this distinction in the types of exploration may not be obvious because there is give and take between nurse and patient. The roles of leader and follower are continuously shifting.

Whether leading or following, nurses utilise similar skills and techniques, although the type and frequency of skills used may be different. For example, more questioning techniques are employed in planned exploration than in spontaneous exploration. Planned exploration, such as the formal interview, often follows a prescribed format, even if the sequence is altered; spontaneous exploration has no set format. Planned exploration aims to solicit standard information, while spontaneous exploration is more a search for meaning and for a patient–nurse relationship in which more information and feelings can be shared. The differences are highlighted in Table 7.1.

TABLE 7.1 Planned versus spontaneous exploration

Planned exploration	Spontaneous exploration
Directive	Responsive
Nurse-led	Patient-led
Prescribed format, usually	No prescribed format
Information solicited	Meaning sought
Topic areas determined by the nurse	Topic areas introduced by the patient
More questioning techniques (probes) used	More exploratory statements (prompts) used

Activity 7.2 WAYS OF EXPLORING: QUESTIONS VERSUS STATEMENTS ➡304

PROCESS

1 Form pairs for this activity. The participants in a pair should not be well-known to each other. Designate one person as the interviewer and the other as the interviewee. If the number of participants is uneven, form a group of three, with the third person acting as an observer.

Interview I

2 The interviewer is to find out as much as possible about the interviewee by asking questions only. The interviewer is not to make any statements during the interview. This interview is to last 5 minutes.

3 After the interview, each of the participants records a summary of the information discussed, as well as the reactions and feelings experienced during the interview. Observers (if used) record what type of information (e.g. factual, opinions, feelings) the interviewer actively solicited, as well as general impressions about the comfort level of participants in the interview.

Interview II

4 The interviewer and the interviewee now reverse roles. Conduct a second interview, only this time the ground rule is that no questions are to be asked during the interview. The interviewer is to learn as much as possible about the interviewee by making statements only. This interview is to last 5 minutes. The observer records the specific strategies used by the interviewer during the interaction.

5 After the interview, each of the participants records a summary of the information discussed, as well as reactions and feelings during the interview. Observers (if used) record the type of information that was solicited during the interview, as well as general impressions about the comfort level of participants in the interview.

6 Before proceeding to the discussion section, participant pairs should discuss their reactions to the activity with each other.

DISCUSSION

On a board visible to all participants, record the answers to the following discussion questions, using the grid (Fig 7.1) as a format.

FIGURE 7.1 Grid for Activity 7.2

	Interview I: all questions	Interview II: no questions
Interviewer reactions		
Interviewee reactions		
Type of information		
Strategies used		

Discussion questions for interview I

1 What were the reactions of the interviewer to the first interview?

2 What were the reactions of the interviewee to the first interview?

3 What kind of information was discussed during the interview? How much was learnt about the interviewee during this interview?

4 Observers (if used) report their general impressions of interview I.

Discussion questions for interview II

5 What were the reactions of the interviewee to the second interview?

---

6 What were the reactions of the interviewer to the second interview?

7 What kind of information was discussed during the interview? How much was learnt about the interviewee during the interview?

8 Observers (if used) report their general impressions of interview II.

9 What strategies were used in interview II to promote and sustain the interaction?

The summary of Activity 7.2 will most likely show that the second interview (with no questions used) created more anxiety. The interviewer in these circumstances often feels uncomfortable and sometimes even selfish. Nevertheless, the type of information obtained when no questions are asked often is more personal, focused and meaningful in getting to know the interviewee. Asking no questions usually results in increased reciprocal sharing during the interview and this eventually leads the interviewer to a greater understanding of the interviewee on a personal level. The first interview usually collects a lot of facts about the interviewee, but does not really uncover subjective opinions and ideas. The first interview usually covers more breadth, while the second one covers more depth.

Questions tend to focus on the collection of information and are associated with formal interviews. Exploratory statements tend to focus more on reciprocal sharing of ideas, opinions, beliefs and feelings, and reflect a conversational style of interacting. Each type of exploration yields different types of information: how information is collected affects what information is gleaned.

THE SKILLS OF EXPLORATION

As demonstrated in Activity 7.2, exploration can be accomplished with or without the use of questions. This section divides the skills of exploration into two major categories: prompting and probing. Prompting skills are exploration techniques that are statements; probing skills are exploration techniques that are questions.

Prompting skills

Verbal prompts are a means of instigating further interaction and serve to assist the patient in elaboration and expansion of partially expressed ideas. Prompting skills include:

- minimal encouragement
- one-word/phrase accents
- gentle commands
- open-ended statements
- finishing the sentence, and
- self-disclosure.

Minimal encouragement

Minimal encouragement is expressed by verbal responses such as, 'uh huh', 'mm hum' and 'yes'. Often, they are utterances that are not really classified as words, yet convey messages such as, 'I'm with you', 'I'm following what you are saying' and 'I want to hear more'. They are signals that acknowledge the patient's verbalisation and encourage further elaboration. Visualise a person on the telephone who keeps repeating 'yes' and 'uh huh'. Although you cannot hear the person on the other end of the line, you can ascertain that the person is encouraging the other person to carry on the conversation. A person talking on the telephone uses minimal encouragement extensively because non-verbal messages are limited. In face-to-face communication, minimal encouragement reinforces attentive listening, but is not really a substitute for it. Attentive and active listening (see Ch 5) is, in itself, an effective prompt because it conveys messages similar to those of minimal encouragement.

Sometimes, minimal encouragement is used without conscious awareness, even when active listening is absent. If this is the case, the verbal and non-verbal messages are incongruent. Because of this incongruence, minimal encouragement, without attentive listening, probably would not prompt further interaction. Try it in a conversation. Keep uttering 'uh huh', while not really attending and listening to the other person. Eventually, the person speaking to you either gives up or tells you, 'Hey, you're not listening to me!'.

Minimal encouragement works best when patients are willing and able to continue the interaction. When patients are having difficulty verbalising their experiences, more explicit prompting and probing techniques need to be employed.

One-word/phrase accents

One-word/phrase accents are the repetition of key words or phrases, and are an effective way to both extend and focus the interaction. The choice of which word or phrase to repeat is important because it determines the direction of the exploration; it becomes the focus. It is best to repeat words or phrases that are judged to be the most central or critical. The following example illustrates the uses of accents:

Patient: My son won't be visiting me while I'm here in hospital.
Nurse: *Won't* be visiting?
Patient: Yes, he says he can't stand the sight and smells of the hospital.

Notice how the accent encourages the patient to expand the initial comment. Nurses effectively use the accent to explore what they perceive to be the most significant part of the patient's statement. Had the nurse repeated the words 'your son?', the interaction may have taken a different direction. In this regard, one-word/phrase accents are controlled by the nurse, although they are always in response to what the patient has said. If a patient does not elaborate, a nurse should follow the patient's lead and end the discussion.

Gentle commands

Gentle commands (Shea & Maloney 1988) are explicit requests for information or elaboration. Although specific topics are often introduced with gentle commands, they are open-ended because they allow the patient to determine the direction and flow of the response. Examples of gentle commands include:
- 'Tell me about your family.'
- 'Can you describe that in more detail?'
- 'Tell me more.'
- 'Let's talk about that further.'
- 'Tell me what it's like for you to be in hospital.'
- 'Go on, say what's on your mind.'

In response to the first example, 'Tell me about your family', patients can choose whatever they wish to share about their family. One patient could say how many children they have, while another may focus on relationships with their extended family. The gentle command is directive in one sense, yet allows the patient to control the direction in another sense.

Gentle commands should always be said in a way that allows patients to maintain a sense of control; they should not be demands. Although the idea of commanding patients to tell the nurse something sounds a bit harsh, the qualifier 'gentle' must not be forgotten. 'Gentle' means that the command is stated as an interested request for more information, rather than an order to speak. The qualifying phrase 'Can you?' is often placed before the command for this reason. 'Can you tell me about your family?' sounds less harsh than, 'Tell me about your family'. Technically, the addition of 'Can you' turns the statement into a closed question, and a patient can simply respond 'yes' or 'no' without any further elaboration. In general, this does not happen because the underlying message that the nurse wants to hear more than a simple 'yes' or 'no' is usually understood.

The gentleness of the command is conveyed primarily through non-verbal messages. Practise a few of the examples cited, using a variety of vocal tones and facial expressions, and include the qualifier 'Can you?' at the beginning of the statement. Note that the words can sound harsh if said in a controlling, demanding manner. Nevertheless, if gentleness is put into the tone and facial expression, such commands are quite effective in exploring patients' experiences.

Open-ended statements

Open-ended statements provide a broad introduction to topics for discussion and are sometimes referred to as 'indirect questions' (Benjamin 1969). They indicate to a patient that the nurse would like to hear more about something and provide an open invitation for the patient to speak about a topic. Examples of open-ended statements include:
- 'So, this is the first time you are having surgery.'
- 'I wonder how it is being sick when you've been so healthy all of your life.'
- 'I hear from your family that you are quite the athlete.'
- 'You've been giving yourself insulin injections for a few years now.'

It is clear from these examples that the nurse making the statement is interested in hearing more about the topic that is introduced, and desires the discussion to proceed further. Open-ended statements are invitations to patients to say more, if they choose to accept the invitation. In this way, open-ended statements are similar to gentle commands because they allow the patient to determine the direction and depth of the interaction. Open-ended statements are often a good way to begin an interaction, because they introduce a topic, but still allow the interaction to take various directions. While they introduce a topic, they do not control the direction of the conversation.

Finishing the sentence

This exploration technique is similar to open-ended statements. Instead of completing a sentence the nurse begins it, then trails off with an expectation that the patient will finish the sentence (Carnevali 1983). Examples of finishing the sentence include:
- 'So you're most worried about ...'
- 'And when you are in pain you usually ...'

- 'Today has been …'
- 'What you really would like to know is …'

To be effective, finishing the sentence relies heavily on an inquisitive, anticipatory facial expression, which lets the patient know that the nurse has not had a lapse in memory or become preoccupied with other thoughts or activities. The non-verbal message, conveyed through facial expression and body posture, communicates that the nurse is awaiting completion of the sentence by the patient.

Self-disclosure

Sometimes, the most effective way to encourage patients to explore their experiences with nurses is for nurses to share their own thoughts with a patient. Through self-disclosure, nurses open an area for exploration by stating their own reactions, feelings or thoughts. Self-disclosure must always be honest. There is little point in nurses fabricating information about themselves in an attempt to make patients open up. Self-disclosure is not the same as giving an opinion or a valuative judgment. Examples of self-disclosure as an exploration technique include:

- 'If I were in your place, I'd be angry.'
- 'I don't handle pain all that well.'
- 'I think I'd be wondering, what is wrong with me.'

Self-disclosure lets the patient know that the nurse is not afraid to be open. When used in the context of exploration, it serves as a trigger for the patient to expand and elaborate because it creates a climate of safety.

It works well as an exploration technique with patients who seem reluctant to reveal themselves. While self-disclosure is utilised here as a means of encouraging exploration, a complete discussion of it can be found in Chapter 8.

Probing skills

The techniques of asking questions are probing skills. Carefully worded and well-timed questions frequently provide the backbone of effective exploration and interviewing. Questions come in different varieties, yielding different responses and taking the interaction in different directions, depending on the type used. Both planned and spontaneous exploration combine the various types of questions. There are two major types of probing skills: open-ended questions and closed questions. Closed questions have two subtypes, which are particularly relevant to exploration within the nursing context: focused and multiple-choice questions.

Open-ended questions

Open-ended questions are those that require more than a one-word response, such as 'yes' or 'no', thereby encouraging more elaboration in the answer. Examples of open-ended questions include:

- 'How did you sleep last night?'
- 'What concerns you most about the surgery?'
- 'What types of food do you enjoy eating?'
- 'How was your visit to the outpatient department?'

Open-ended questions begin with interrogative words such as who, what, when, where, why and how. Not all questions beginning with these words are open-ended. For example, 'Where do you live?' is a closed question, while 'Where do you see yourself in 5 years time?' is an open-ended question. Questions that are open-ended often yield more information than closed questions because their replies include more detailed expansion and elaboration. Additionally, open-ended questions allow more flexibility in response than closed questions. In answering open-ended questions, patients can highlight what is most relevant to their experience and therefore retain a sense of control in the interaction. Nevertheless, an open-ended question, no matter how well-stated, can pressure patients to disclose personal matters before they feel trusting enough to share their inner experiences. Because open-ended questions often probe more deeply than closed ones, nurses need to be mindful about the level of trust established before delving too deeply into the patient's experience.

Closed questions

Closed questions are those that are usually answered with a simple 'yes', 'no' or other one-word response. They control the direction of the conversation and limit the amount of information that is shared or obtained. If closed questions are overused, an interaction begins to resemble an interrogation and can result in a patient feeling put on the spot because, short of refusing to answer or lying, the patient often feels obliged to answer direct questions posed by a nurse. Examples of closed questions include:

- 'Have you been in hospital before?'
- 'Do you wear eye glasses?'
- 'Is your wife coming to visit you tonight?'
- 'Do you have any children?'
- 'When did you last have something to eat?'

Focused, closed questions At times, it is necessary for nurses to ask closed questions that are focused and directed at obtaining information about a specific clinical situation. These questions are based on the nurse's clinical knowledge and experience. Without them, important and even vital information may be missed (Shea & Maloney 1998). Examples of focused, closed questions include:

- 'Are you feeling nauseous?' (to a patient recovering from anaesthesia)
- 'Do you ever feel dizzy when you get out of bed quickly?' (to a patient whose blood pressure is low)
- 'Is your mouth dry?' (to a patient taking medication that produces a dry mouth as a side effect)

Each of these examples is a closed, focused question that is appropriate under the circumstances. The trigger for these closed questions is the nurse's awareness and understanding of what is pertinent to explore in a given clinical situation. Patients may not recognise the significance of their clinical symptoms and therefore feel reassured by such questions. An open-ended question may not yield the information needed or reveal progress in a particular direction.

Multiple-choice questions Multiple-choice questions are another form of specific, closed questioning that is based on the nurse's understanding of a particular clinical phenomenon. In multiple-choice questions, the nurse provides options to the patient in an attempt to obtain an answer to the question, 'Which of these is correct?' A good example is when a nurse tries to obtain a complete description of a patient's pain. An open-ended question such as, 'How does the pain feel?' or even 'How would you describe the pain?' is often met with responses such as

Activity 7.3 CONVERTING PROBES INTO PROMPTS → 304

PROCESS

Questions (probes) are often overused as a means of exploration. This activity challenges participants to turn closed questions into exploratory statements (prompts). Table 7.2 demonstrates how this is accomplished.

1 Make a list of closed questions pertinent to the nursing context. Divide a piece of paper into three columns and place the closed questions down the left column.

2 Convert each of these questions into an exploratory statement by first making the closed question into an open-ended one. Place these in the middle column of the page.

3 Now convert the open-ended question into an exploratory statement or a prompt. Place these in the right column of the page.

DISCUSSION

1 Which of your closed questions were easy to convert to exploratory statements? Which were difficult? Were there any that you found impossible to convert?

2 Review each of the exploratory statements and discuss how making a statement instead of asking a question would alter the interaction between nurse and patient.

3 Would you obtain different information from an exploratory statement? If so, is the information obtained more relevant?

4 Which of the exploratory statements seem appropriate to the topic being discussed? Do any seem inappropriate or foolish?

5 Can you imagine yourself using the exploratory statements? Why? Why not?

TABLE 7.2 Converting probes into prompts

Closed question	Open-ended question	Exploratory statement (prompt)
Are you feeling all right?	How are you feeling?	Tell me how you are feeling.
Will it help to make you more comfortable if I rearrange your pillows?	What would help you to be more comfortable in the bed?	Perhaps if I rearrange your pillow, you'll be more comfortable.
Did that medication help to relieve your pain?	How did that medication help in relieving your pain?	You had your pain medication 30 minutes ago, I see.
Do you want your sponge now?	When would you like your sponge?	You can have your sponge now or later.
Would it help if I stayed with you a while?	How would you feel if I stayed with you a while?	Perhaps if I stayed with you a while, it would help.

'It feels like pain, it hurts' or 'I don't know, pain just feels like pain'. A multiple-choice question is helpful under such circumstances. In posing a multiple-choice question, the nurse asks, 'Is the pain burning, grabbing, crushing, pinpoint, dull or sharp?' This type of questioning about pain yields specific information about the nature of the patient's pain. In the example provided, the nurse uses knowledge of the various types of pain to focus and direct the exploration.

Activity 7.4 QUESTIONS AND STATEMENTS FOR CONDUCTING A NURSING HISTORY

PROCESS

Each of the topic areas in step 1 is an aspect of a standard nursing history, completed on admission to hospital. During the gathering of information for a nursing history, the nurse explores specific areas in order to collect data about the patient's functioning and experiences. The manner in which the data are collected depends on the nurse's ability to explore effectively. The wording of the questions and exploratory statements affect not only the type of information collected, but also the amount and quality of that information.

1 For each of the following topic areas, develop and write an open-ended question. The first one is completed to provide an example of how to undertake this activity.

Topic area	Open-ended question
Perception of hospitalisation:	● What do you anticipate will happen while you are in hospital?
	● What are your expectations of this hospital stay?

Understanding of current health status:

Social/living situation:

Activities of daily living:

Nutrition/eating habits:

Sleep and rest patterns:

Elimination patterns:

2 Now develop an exploratory statement for each of the topic areas.

DISCUSSION

1 Which way of exploring—questioning (probing) or making statements (prompting)—seems more effective in collecting information in each of the identified topic areas?

2 Do some topic areas lend themselves more to exploratory statements than others?

Open-ended versus closed questions

As a general rule, open-ended questions are more effective as exploration techniques than closed questions because responses to open questions are more elaborate and encourage expansion of ideas through the addition of subjective opinions and beliefs. They also allow the patient to direct the interaction and therefore the nurse who asks an open-ended question is likely to hear what is most significant to the patient at the time.

Does this mean that closed questions should be avoided? Not necessarily, because closed questions have a legitimate place in the context of patient–nurse interaction. The choice between open-ended and closed questions depends on what information is being sought, who is seeking it, who is being asked, in which context and to what end. In making the decision to use one type or the other, nurses must consider their relationship with the patient as well as the need for specific information. For example, when a nurse wants to know whether a patient can tolerate aspirin, they might begin by asking, 'Have you ever used aspirin?' Then, if the answer is affirmative, questions such as 'How much?', 'How often?', 'For what reason?' and 'What effects were noted?' may follow. Asking open-ended questions such as 'How do you experience aspirin?' or 'What do you think about aspirin?' are nonsensical, and inappropriate to the content being explored and the information required.

On the other hand, a question such as 'How was your first pregnancy?' is appropriate in exploring an experience as personal and unique as pregnancy. Nevertheless, questions such as 'How do you feel about being pregnant?' probe too deeply if patient and nurse have not established a trusting relationship. Questions need to probe at a depth that is appropriate to the level of trust between patient and nurse.

The decision about which type of question to use should be based on an understanding of each type of questioning. Table 7.3 compares the two types of question and provides useful guidelines for the selection.

TABLE 7.3 Comparison of open-ended and closed questions

Open-ended questions	Closed questions
Yield information and facilitate elaboration	Yield information and limit elaboration
Allow patient to determine the direction of the interactions	Focus the patient in one direction
May not be useful when specific information is required	Are useful in obtaining specific information
Probe subjective experiences and may threaten patient if trust is not established	Maintain interpersonal safety by keeping the interaction on a less personal level

If the open-ended type is selected as more suitable, the next choice is which open-ended question is best, given the circumstances. In most instances, questions beginning with 'who', 'what', 'where' and 'when' yield factual, objective data, while questions beginning with 'how' yield more personal, subjective information. For example, 'What surgery did you have in 1988?' will yield a factual answer such as 'I had my appendix removed'. If this is followed by a question such as 'And how was that surgery?', exploration of the patient's subjective experience of the surgery is achieved. This general guideline is not a hard and fast rule. For example, 'What were your feelings about the surgery?' is a question that probes on a personal level. The focus of the question is as important as its type.

The most effective exploration will include a combination of both open and closed questions, as illustrated in the following interaction:

Nurse: Have you ever had surgery before? [Closed]
Patient: Yes, once before.
Nurse: What happened that you needed surgery? [Open]
Patient: I had my appendix removed when I was 10 years old.
Nurse: Were you in hospital? [Closed]
Patient: Yes.
Nurse: How was that hospitalisation? [Open]
Patient: Fine, the nurses were great, my Mum was with me the whole time and I don't remember being in any pain.
Nurse: So, you have good memories of that? [Closed]
Patient: Yes.
Nurse: What do you expect will happen this time in hospital? [Open]
Patient: Well, I am a lot older, so my Mum won't be here the whole time. I am a bit worried about the pain.
Nurse: What worries you most? [Open]
Patient: That nobody will be able to help me with the pain ... I am a bit of a baby.
Nurse: The nurses are here to make sure you are not in pain. You do realise that. [Closed]
Patient: Yes, I guess ... but I don't know what you will do to help.

Notice how, in this interview, the nurse moves between closed and open-ended questioning and each question is appropriate to the content and the purpose of the interview. During the interaction, the nurse gathers objective data (previous experience with surgery) as well as subjective data (the patient's personal experience of the surgery). Open and closed questions are not inherently good or bad, because their 'goodness' or 'badness' depends on what information is being sought, and for what reason.

Pitfalls in the use of probing skills

Despite the fact that questions are neither good nor bad within themselves, there are some common pitfalls in the use of questioning, including some types of question that are best avoided altogether. Common pitfalls include overuse of questions, continuous multiple questions, the 'why' question and the leading question.

Overuse of questions The most common pitfall in probing is the overuse of questions. Asking too many questions during an interaction can interrupt and confuse the patient (Benjamin 1969). Overuse of questions runs the risk of continually shifting the focus of the interaction. Additionally, it has the potential to convey the message that the nurse is in an overbearing position of authority. In order to be effective, questions need to be mixed with exploratory, prompting statements.

Continuous multiple questions Another pitfall in questioning is the use of multiple questions, asked in succession, without allowing time for a reply from the patient. For example, 'How did you sleep last night? Did the sleeping tablet help? Was there too much noise?' While this manner of questioning sounds a bit ridiculous, it does occur in patient–nurse interactions (Macleod Clark 1984). Asking multiple questions in succession is counterproductive to the exploration process. If a question is asked, the nurse needs to ensure that enough time is allowed for the patient to respond before proceeding.

The 'why?' question The 'why?' question is a tricky one because often in the nursing context the answer to why needs to be sought. 'Why does Mr Kendall experience so much pain, even after maximum pain relief is administered?' 'Why is Ms Holmes having so much difficulty breastfeeding her baby?' While it is important to uncover the reasons for such occurrences, asking the question 'why?' directly of patients can have a negative impact, and may not be the most effective way to find the answer. This is partly due to the fact that the question 'why?' often creates anxiety and a defensive reaction. It implies that patients have to justify and explain their actions and feelings, or that something is not right about their actions and feelings.

Imagine you are about to administer a medication to a patient and another nurse approaches you and asks, 'Why are you giving that medication now?' Your internal reaction may range from, 'What's it to you?' to 'Oh no, maybe I've made a mistake!' Perhaps your colleague just wants to know if the patient receiving the medication is still experiencing pain. Somehow, your reaction to the 'why?' question does not acknowledge such a well-intentioned motive on your colleague's part. Instead, you become defensive or anxious.

Activity 7.5 EFFECTS OF 'WHY?' QUESTIONS ➡305

PROCESS

1 Form pairs for this activity. Designate one person as A and the other as B.

2 A discusses an experience that produced a strong feeling reaction.

3 B listens attentively, but keeps asking 'why?' whenever A brings up a feeling. B is to embark 'on a mission' to uncover the reasons behind A's feelings and reactions.

DISCUSSION

1 A reports their response to the interaction by answering the question, 'How did it feel to be constantly asked why?'

2 B reports their response to the interaction by answering the question, 'How did it feel to keep asking why?' What did B notice about A's reactions?

The reaction to 'why?' is often defensive because the question has a way of sounding like a negative evaluation. This may be due to experiences in childhood, such as when Mum asked, 'Why did you spill the milk on the floor?' as she stands there, hands on hips, looking and sounding quite cross. It quickly becomes apparent to the child that Mum is not the least bit interested in why the milk was spilt. (Does she want an explanation about gravitational force?) The message conveyed by the 'why?' question in this instance is, 'Don't do it again; I get cross when milk is spilt.' This possible socialisation as to the interpretation of the 'why?' question, and the potential defensiveness produced by it, are reasons for avoiding its use in patient–nurse interactions.

Frequently, the 'why?' question is asked in an attempt to explore feelings (e.g. 'Why do you feel sad, Kate?'). The use of the 'why' question in this instance assumes that Kate knows why she feels sad, and that these feelings have a rational basis. Patients often do not know why they feel a certain way, but may think they need to justify or rationally explain their feelings when asked 'why?'. Again, the reaction may be a defensive one, a justification of feelings. In general, it is best to avoid the 'why?' question altogether. It is often counterproductive to exploration because of its potential to close off further interaction.

Activity 7.6 ALTERNATIVES TO 'WHY?'

PROCESS

The following patient statements have the potential to elicit a 'why?' question from nurses. Read each and record an alternative to 'why?'.

1 Patient (who has been on renal dialysis for a long time and is awaiting a renal transplant): 'I want to stop dialysis.'

2 Patient (who is awaiting results of diagnostic tests): 'I had a really bad night's sleep because I'm so worried.'

3 Patient (who is a recently arrived resident of a nursing home): 'How would you like being stuck in here? I hate this place and just want to die.'

4 Patient (who has recently undergone coronary artery bypass surgery): 'I really thought I was going to die this morning.'

5 Patient (who has been told she should have a hysterectomy): 'I can't possibly spare the time to have this operation.'

DISCUSSION

1 Did you find you were tempted to ask 'why?' in response to each statement?

2 Review your alternatives to the 'why?' question. Are any of them 'why?' in disguise (e.g. 'How come?' or 'What makes you feel that way?').

3 What type of exploratory response did you develop? Are any of the responses exploratory statements?

4 Compare your responses with those of other participants. How much variety exists between the responses?

5 Try to use some of your responses with other participants playing the role of patient. Ask the person who is playing the role of patient to describe the effects of each response.

The leading question Another type of question to avoid is the 'leading' question. Leading questions are not exploratory but rhetorical, because they have an implied answer and are often designed to confirm what nurses think they already know. Examples of leading questions include:
- 'You're all right, aren't you?'
- 'Why don't you just cooperate with us?'
- 'Are you really going to ring the doctor at this hour of the night?'
- 'Is your anger really justified?'

- 'What's making you so hard to get along with?'
- 'You really don't want any more medication, do you?'

Leading questions are not really questions at all. They are statements in disguise, 'dressed up' to look like questions. Like the 'why' question, they have a tendency to put the other person on the defensive because they usually contain a value judgment. It is far better to make a statement than to pretend to want an

Activity 7.7 RECOGNISING TYPES OF QUESTIONS ➡305

PROCESS

Classify each question according to its type, using the following key:

A closed question

B open-ended question

C leading question

D disguised 'why?' question

1 What makes you feel scared?

2 How are you feeling today?

3 What is your doctor's name?

4 Do you really enjoy drinking heavily?

5 When does your pain get worse?

6 Are you interested in seeing a volunteer from Alcoholics Anonymous?

7 What are your reasons for refusing your medication?

8 What kind of nurse do you think I am?

9 You really don't want any more pain medication, do you?

10 What did the doctor say?

11 Did that medication help with the nausea?

12 How do you like your breakfast tray to be arranged?

13 How did you go with physiotherapy today?

14 What makes you say that?

15 How old are your children?

16 How was the visit with your family last night?

17 Did you sleep well after having the sleeping tablet?

18 When are you going to stop bothering the other patients?

19 Are you worried about having sexual relations after your heart surgery?

20 Don't you think you had better try to stick to your diet this time?

21 How do you usually manage your diabetic diet?

22 Are you still hurting your baby by smoking while you are pregnant?

23 What would help you to be more comfortable?

(Note: The answers to this activity can be found at the end of this chapter.)

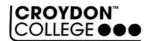

iPoint

You will find useful resources at:

	Silver Zone Science & Technology
610.73 SPO	**Green Zone** History
	Gold Zone – Business Law & Management
	Purple Zone Art & Design
✗	**Blue Zone** Social Sciences
	Yellow Zone Service Industries
	Orange Zone Language & Literature
	Sorry, this item is at the Davidson campus
	Careers
	Study Skills Centre

If you can't find the book(s) on the shelves, or if the item is at the Davidson Campus, please let us know

It may also be useful to look on the following on-line databases:

answer to a question that does not really have one. Review the previous examples of leading questions, turn them into statements and note the difference.

FOCUSED EXPLORATION

The skills of exploration can be employed effectively in the process of focusing an interaction between patient and nurse. The process of focused exploration deepens the nurse's general understanding of the patient's experience by concentrating on a specific aspect. This process of focusing is sometimes referred to as 'funnelling' (Burnard 1989), because of the way in which it continues to narrow the topic being explored. Any of the various exploration skills identified can be employed in the process of focusing. The following interaction, from a postpartum maternity ward, is an illustration of focusing:

Nurse:	How are you today? [Open question]
Patient:	Okay, I guess.
Nurse:	You *guess*? [One-word accent]
Patient:	I didn't sleep very well last night.
Nurse:	Couldn't sleep, huh? [Closed question]
Patient:	No, I kept worrying about my baby.
Nurse:	What, in particular, was worrying you? [Open question]
Patient:	The paediatrician was here last night to examine him and he noticed his high-pitched cry.
Nurse:	And? [Minimal encouragement]
Patient:	Well, the doctor said it was probably nothing to worry about because it was most likely due to some swelling in my son's brain as a result of the labour. I was in second stage for a long time, you know.
Nurse:	Yes, it might clear up in a few days. I have seen babies with that cry before and it was due to temporary swelling that went away after a few days. But, it doesn't really stop the worry, just because you know it might be nothing. [Open-ended statement]
Patient:	What is most worrying is that the doctor said it could be a sign of brain damage.
Nurse:	And that's what has you most worried? [Closed question]
Patient:	Yes. I kept asking the doctor what else besides temporary swelling could be causing the cry. Now I'm sorry I asked. I might have been better off not knowing. There's nothing I can do now but worry and wait.

Notice how the nurse in this interaction begins broadly then keeps focusing and narrowing the conversation. This is accomplished through the use of a variety of exploration skills. The nurse chose to focus on what she perceived to be the most significant aspect of the patient's messages. The focusing process serves to highlight and elaborate on a particular topic.

PATIENT-CUE EXPLORATION

Patients frequently communicate their needs, desires and feelings through indirect messages, indicating what they are experiencing by hints, suggestions and implied questions (Macleod Clark 1984). Indirectly, patients are requesting a response from the nurse by presenting these communication cues.

Cues are small units of information, which are part of a larger, more complex phenomenon (Carnevali 1983). They indicate a need for further exploration into the phenomenon. They signal the need for exploration much like a green light at a traffic intersection signals drivers to proceed. Effective exploration of patient cues, like all exploration, leads to further data collection and greater understanding between patient and nurse. Sadly, nurses frequently either fail to acknowledge patient cues or even actively discourage further exploration of them (Macleod Clark 1984).

Activity 7.8 EXPLORING PATIENT CUES

PROCESS

1 Think of an instance, real or imagined, in which a patient presents a cue, indicating the need for further exploration and/or elaboration (e.g. a facial grimace, possibly indicating pain). Record this patient cue on a slip of paper, providing any information that would be of assistance in understanding the situation (the setting and circumstances).

2 Collect the slips of paper and redistribute them to other participants in the activity.

3 The contents of the slips of paper are then read aloud to all participants. Each participant develops and records an exploratory response, using any type of exploration technique.

4 Form groups of five to six participants and share exploratory responses in this group. Each small group discusses the various exploratory responses and selects the one that is most appropriate as an exploration technique. These are then read aloud to the rest of the participants.

DISCUSSION

Discuss each patient cue and responses selected by the small groups. During the discussion, use the following questions to evaluate the responses bearing in mind that the purpose of the response is to explore the cue presented by the patient.

1 Which exploration technique was used?

2 How effective is the response in exploring the cue?

3 In which context would this response be most appropriate?

4 What purpose does the exploration serve? Is it helpful? How?

5 Could you actually say this to a patient? If not, why not?

Cues and inferences

A cue is a unit of sensory input—a sight, sound, smell, taste or touch that is perceived as important to be noticed. For example, during an interaction, the nurse notices that the patient keeps fidgeting with the bedclothes. By noticing this piece of information, the nurse has perceived a cue.

Almost without awareness, meanings are assigned to perceived cues as a way of making sense of what is experienced. The meanings attached to cues are inferences—conclusions drawn from the cues. Inferences are based on knowledge, previous experience, expectations and needs. For example, fidgeting with the bedclothes may be interpreted as a sign of general anxiety or discomfort with the interaction. Nevertheless, inferences are usually formed on the basis of more than one cue. The combination of fidgeting with the bedclothes, startling easily, pressured speech, non-stop talking and foot tapping are patient cues that may lead to an inference that a patient is anxious.

It is impossible not to make such interpretations about what is perceived; inferences are automatic. What is possible is to differentiate a cue (concrete data) from an inference (the interpretation of the data).

Activity 7.9 CUES AND INFERENCES ➡305

PROCESS

Determine whether each of the following statements is a cue or an inference:

1 Answered interview questions completely.

2 Uninterested in the interview.

3 Changed the topic when asked about her family.

4 An open person.

5 Sleeping quietly.

6 Shallow, rapid respirations.

7 Doesn't understand prescribed medications.

8 Keeps asking questions about diagnostic tests.

9 No eye contact during the interview.

10 Speech is pressured.

11 Puzzled expression on his face when I asked him about the surgery.

12 Doesn't know what to expect.

13 No visible signs of distress.

(Note: The answers to this activity can be found at the end of this chapter.)

DISCUSSION

1 Compare your answers with those of other class participants. Are there any differences in the answers?

2 If differences exist, discuss the item(s) and decide what makes them inferences or what makes them cues.

3 Compare your answers with those provided at the end of this chapter.

Once inferences are recognised by the nurse, they need to be validated with the patient in order to determine if they are correct. In the example of fidgeting with the bedclothes, if the patient admits to feeling anxious, the inference is validated. It is important not to jump too quickly to a conclusion about patient cues. Further exploration is usually the most appropriate initial response to a patient cue.

Communication cues

When nurses prompt and probe during the process of exploration, many verbal and non-verbal cues are elicited because the exploration itself triggers the cues. A straightforward, closed question such as 'Have you ever been in hospital before?' may elicit numerous cues about the patient's experience in hospital. The patient's tone of voice may change, their rate of speech may accelerate, or they may disclose feelings and reactions to previous hospitalisations. In this instance, the exploration triggered the cues and the cue is a trigger for further exploration. This spiralling effect is common in effective exploration.

Patients' questions as cues

Often patient cues come in the form of questions asked of the nurse. Patients' questions that are difficult to answer, yet require a response from the nurse, are examples of cues needing further exploration. For example:

- 'Am I going to die?'
- 'Is Dr Nelson a good surgeon?'
- 'What would you do if you were in my place?'

Questions such as these, which put nurses on the spot, are difficult to answer and are equally difficult to ignore. Perceiving patients' questions as cues for exploration is useful because this enables nurses to respond effectively. Further exploration helps to uncover what is really on the patient's mind. The first example, 'Am I going to die?', can be explored by stating, 'That's difficult for me to answer, but I am curious about the question.' This open-ended statement indicates the nurse's willingness to hear more about what the patient is experiencing. Think 'exploration' whenever patients pose questions that either have no answer or are difficult to answer. It is preferable to do this, rather than ignoring the question or changing the subject, which could happen when nurses feel put on the spot and uncomfortable.

Cue perception

Patient cues must be noticed and perceived if they are to be of use in exploration. Complete attending and active listening keep nurses open and receptive to cue recognition. Observing how a patient reacts and responds to the environment, and the situation at hand, is a skill in itself (see Ch 5).

Often, nurses perceive subtle communication cues from patients on the basis of a 'gut' feeling, hunch or intuition that the patient is trying to tell them something. Cue perception involves not only noticing how the patient is responding, but also trusting a 'gut' reaction about what might be going on. In the following situation, a nursing student relates such a hunch in discussing her observations of a young man, close to her own age, who had recently become a paraplegic:

> He kept joking around all morning about the MRI that was scheduled that day. I was quite comfortable with the banter because I like to joke around a lot too. He kept asking me, in a silly, almost childlike way, if I would be coming with him to 'hold his hand' when he had the procedure. Although I joked back about him being a 'big boy' now and stuff like that, I had the feeling he might have been scared about the test. I wondered how much he really understood about what was going to happen. I guess I am especially sensitive to this because, as I said, I often joke around especially about things that are really upsetting me.

A hunch such as this is often an indication of a need, however well disguised it is by a patient. The nursing student perceived the possibility that this patient was trying to express a need by interpreting the cues that he was presenting. She identified an opportunity for further exploration.

Cue exploration: sharing perceptions

Patient cues can be explored using any of the skills described in this chapter, but one of the most effective ways to explore cues is through open-ended statements in which nurses state their own perceptions. Open-ended statements allow nurses to validate their observations and interpretations of the cue by sharing them with the patient. In the preceding scenario, an effective way for the nursing student to explore her hunch would be to say, 'Hey, all joking aside, I get the feeling you may be a bit uptight about the MRI.' This open-ended statement shares the student's perception with the patient, attempts to validate the perception, and therefore opens the interaction to exploration of the cues. Open-ended exploratory statements, which share the nurse's perceptions, usually begin with:

- 'I notice that …'
- 'I get the feeling that …'
- 'I'm wondering if …'

These sentences are then completed by a concrete description of what the nurse has observed, perceived and/or interpreted from the patient's messages. This is an effective way to validate a cue and explore it further because it acknowledges the patient's message, encourages further discussion of the patient's experience and demonstrates the nurse's willingness to listen.

A word of caution about sharing perceptions

The danger in exploring in this manner is that the nurse may fall into the trap of being a pseudo-psychoanalyst, always looking for hidden meanings and motives. Patients present cues in an attempt to communicate with nurses, so the question nurses must ask themselves is, 'Do I get the feeling this patient is trying to tell me something?', rather than, 'What's really behind this patient's behaviour?'. It is a subtle yet important distinction.

Activity 7.10 DEVELOPING EXPLORATORY RESPONSES II

PROCESS

1 Refer to your responses in Activity 7.1, 'Developing exploratory responses I'. Label each of your responses according to the skills outlined in this chapter. You may have used more than one type of exploratory response.

2 Determine if you have a tendency to use one type of exploratory response in preference to the other types.

3 If you tend to ask closed questions, make these open-ended.

4 Do any of your questions begin with 'why'? If so, find an alternative.

5 Turn your exploratory questions into exploratory statements. What possible effects would these changes have on the interaction with the patient in the situation?

NURSES' CONTROL IN EXPLORATION

Previously in this chapter, planned exploration was differentiated from spontaneous exploration. In planned exploration, the nurse leads and takes charge of the direction and focus of an interaction. In spontaneous exploration, the nurse follows

Activity 7.11 PATIENT INTERVIEW ➡305

PROCESS

1 Each participant is to obtain a blank nursing history form from a healthcare agency. Review the form and determine the most appropriate way to explore each area with a patient.

2 Form groups of three and designate one person as A, another as B and the third as C.

3 A conducts a nursing history interview with B acting in the role of patient. C acts as observer. A informs B about the setting and the circumstances of the patient interview. C records the types of exploratory skills used by A during the interview by keeping a record of the name of each skill used.

4 C now interviews A, who plays the role of patient. B is now the observer. Continue as per instructions in step 3.

5 B now interviews person C, who plays the role of patient. A is now the observer. Continue as per instructions in step 3.

DISCUSSION

1 What types of exploratory skills were used during the interviews? Were some types used more frequently than others?

2 Were there areas of the nursing history that lent themselves to the use of a certain skill more than other areas? If so, what are these areas? Which skills seemed most appropriate for these areas?

3 How did it feel when you were in the role of patient? Did you think you had enough opportunity to tell your story? Did you think the nurse got to know you as a person during the interview?

4 When you were the nurse, what was easy to explore? What was difficult? Were there any areas you thought were not covered adequately? How well did you come to understand the patient during the interview? What would you change in the interview if you had the opportunity?

5 What generalisations can be made from the activity in terms of conducting interviews between patients and nurses?

the patient's lead, usually through clarifying and probing patient cues. The same skills are used in both types of exploration, although not to the same extent. For example, closed questions may be more prevalent when the nurse is leading, and one-word/phrase accents may be more prevalent when the nurse is following.

At the heart of the difference between spontaneous and planned exploration is the notion of who is in control. Control in the context of patient–nurse interaction refers to who dominates in determining the flow of information exchange (Kristjanson & Chalmers 1990). When the patient is in control, they dominate. The reverse is true when the nurse controls the interaction.

Ideally, a balance is achieved when both patient and nurse share control of interactions. Nevertheless, is there any evidence to support the ideal? Answers to this question can be found in research studies in which verbal communication between nurses and patients as they interact in clinical settings is analysed (e.g. Shattell 2004, Hewison 1995, Wilkinson 1991, Macleod Clark 1984). Analyses of patient–nurse interactions in studies such as these reveal that nurses 'block' and 'control' interactions through a variety of strategies. Some of these strategies included focusing on tasks, exerting power over patients, spending little time actually talking to patients and even avoiding interaction with patients. In community-based settings, Kristjanson and Chalmers (1990) found that interactions were either nurse-controlled or jointly controlled by patient and nurse, but no interactions were controlled by patients.

Although the results of these studies suggest that nurses do not pick up patient cues and that they control interactions, other studies suggest that when nurses are expert they are alert to patient cues (Johnson 1993) and offer opportunities for patients to introduce issues that are affecting their lives (Brown 1994).

While the evidence on whether nurses control interactions is inconclusive, some helpful guidelines can be ascertained. These guidelines include the need for nurses to be alert to the cues of patients and to be able to follow that patient lead. Likewise, nurses will at times control the interaction when they are obtaining specific information. Self-aware nurses who reflect on their interactions will notice whether they tend to be controlling in their interactions.

CHAPTER SUMMARY

The process of exploration is one of the most important aspects of patient–nurse interaction because it not only provides the means by which information is obtained, but demonstrates the nurse's active regard for understanding the patient's experience. During planned exploration, nurses focus on what is most significant for them to know about patients. During spontaneous exploration, nurses focus on what is most significant to the patient at the time. Both types of exploration require the use of effective questioning (probes) and exploratory statements (prompts). When used in conjunction with other interpersonal skills, exploration helps to shape effective and facilitative patient–nurse interaction and leads to greater understanding.

Answers to Activities

Activity 7.7 RECOGNISING TYPES OF QUESTIONS

Key:

   A closed question

   B open-ended question

   C leading question

   D a disguised 'why?' question

1   D What makes you feel scared?

2   B How are you feeling today?

3   A What is your doctor's name?

4   C Do you really enjoy drinking heavily?

5   B When does your pain get worse?

6   A Are you interested in seeing a volunteer from Alcoholics Anonymous?

7 D What are your reasons for refusing your medication?

8 C What kind of nurse do you think I am?

9 C You really don't want any more pain medication, do you?

10 B What did the doctor say?

11 A Did that medication help with the nausea?

12 B How do you like your breakfast tray to be arranged?

13 B How did you go with physiotherapy today?

14 D What makes you say that?

15 A How old are your children?

16 B How was the visit with your family last night?

17 A Did you sleep well after having the sleeping tablet?

18 C When are you going to stop bothering the other patients?

19 A Are you worried about having sexual relations after your heart surgery?

20 C Don't you think you had better try to stick to your diet this time?

21 B How do you usually manage your diabetic diet?

22 C Are you still hurting your baby by smoking while you are pregnant?

23 B What would help you to be more comfortable?

Activity 7.9 CUES AND INFERENCES

1 Cue Answered interview questions completely.

2 Inference Uninterested in the interview.

3 Cue Changed the topic when asked about her family.

4 Inference An open person.

5 Cue Sleeping quietly.

6 Cue Shallow, rapid respirations.

7 Inference Doesn't understand prescribed medications.

8 Cue Keeps asking questions about diagnostic tests.

9 Cue No eye contact during the interview.

10 Cue Speech is pressured.

11 Cue Puzzled expression on his face when I asked him about the surgery.

12 Inference Doesn't know what to expect.

13 Cue No visible signs of distress.

REFERENCES

Benjamin A 1969 The helping interview. Houghton Mifflin, Boston, MA

Brown SJ 1994 Communication strategies used by an expert nurse. Clinical Nursing Research 3(1):43–56

Brown SJ 1995 An interviewing style for nursing assessment. Journal of Advanced Nursing 21:340–342

Burnard P 1989 Teaching interpersonal skills: a handbook of experiential learning activities for health professionals. Chapman and Hall, London

Carnevali D 1983 Nursing care planning: diagnosis and management, 3rd edn. JB Lippincott, Philadelphia, PA

Hewison AL 1995 Nurses' power in interactions with patients. Journal of Advanced Nursing 21:75–82

Johnson R 1993 Nurse practitioner–patient discourse: uncovering the voice of nursing in primary care practice. Scholarly Inquiry for Nursing Practice: An International Journal 7:143–163

Kristjanson L, Chalmers K 1990 Nurse–client interactions in community-based practice: creating common ground. Public Health Nursing 7(4):215–223

Macleod Clark J 1984 Verbal communication in nursing. In Faulkner A (ed.) Communication, pp 52–73. Churchill Livingstone, Edinburgh

Shattell M 2004 Nurse–patient interaction: a review of the literature. Journal of Clinical Nursing 13:714–722

Shea SC, Maloney M 1998 Psychiatric interviewing: the art of understanding. Saunders, Philadelphia, PA

Wilkinson S 1991 Factors which influence how nurses communicate with cancer patients. Journal of Advanced Nursing 16:677–688

CHAPTER 8

Intervening: comforting, supporting and enabling

INTRODUCTION

The material in the previous chapters has laid a theoretical foundation and a practical framework for establishing effective patient–nurse relationships. Through knowing self, listening to patients' stories, understanding patients' experiences and exploring patients' personal meanings of health and illness, nurses are able to interact with patients in ways that are helpful. Helpful interactions build relationships that are of assistance to patients and the patient–nurse relationship becomes a vehicle through which nursing actions come to life. The skills of listening, understanding and exploring are fundamental to the development of this relationship and their use must be continuous for the relationship's maintenance and further development.

Thus far, this book has alluded to how nurses take direct action in helping patients, but active intervention has not been fully explained. In fact, moving too quickly into action has been shown to be inappropriate in the absence of a relationship based on understanding. Focusing prematurely on action, intervention and outcome has the potential to stifle the nurse's understanding and appreciation of the patient's current experience.

There is inherent danger in taking action without first understanding the patient's unique orientation to the world. Interventions cannot be applied in a context-free manner, selected from a list of options as one selects a recipe from a cookbook. Such non-specific, potentially hit-and-miss approaches can actually do more harm than good. For example, enabling patients to participate in their care by sharing information is most effective if nurses first determine how much information a patient wants and can use. Some patients want to know every minute detail about their nursing care, while others prefer to know the bare essentials only. It is inappropriate, even potentially harmful, to burden a patient with too much detailed information when the information is not wanted or cannot be put to some use.

This suggestion, to initially curtail direct intervention, may prove frustrating to some nurses, because a felt need to do something often overrides the need to understand the patient's experience from the patient's perspective. Time is a precious commodity in nursing practice, and the time spent in coming to understand patients' experiences may be perceived as a luxury. Nevertheless, the time and effort expended in coming to understand the patient's frame of reference are well spent because actions, which direct and influence patients, are then based on such understandings.

These actions include: comforting patients through interpersonal interaction; supporting patients in the use of resources; and enabling patients to participate in their healthcare by sharing information and encouraging them to reframe their perspective through challenging and self-sharing.

Chapter overview

This chapter presents skills that provide the means for nurses to take action beyond listening, exploring and understanding. These actions are psychosocial in nature—that is, they are interpersonally oriented and enacted through the nurse–patient relationship. Swanson's theory (1993) of nursing as informed caring is presented as a way of situating the skills in this chapter within the context of material in previous chapters. Ways of responding (first introduced in Ch 6) are revisited in order to emphasise when psychosocial actions are appropriate. These psychosocial nursing actions are grouped into three major areas: comforting, supporting and enabling. The primary comforting action is the skill of reassuring patients. Supporting actions, described next, promote patients' use of resources. Enabling focuses on actions that are aimed at encouraging patients to actively participate in their own care. The major enabling action described is that of sharing information and providing explanations to patients. The final skills of challenging and self-disclosure are two further examples of enabling actions.

PSYCHOSOCIAL ACTIONS THAT COMFORT, SUPPORT AND ENABLE

Often nursing actions are aimed at physical care and treatment of a disease (e.g. administration of medication to provide physical relief from pain), and technical competence is perceived by patients as caring (see Ch 2). But nursing actions are also psychosocial in nature. Psychosocial actions are aimed at promoting psychological ease and relief of distress (e.g. through explanations that orient patients to what is happening around them).

Physical actions and psychosocial actions are inextricably linked in nursing practice. For example, hospitalised patients in Cameron's (1993) study indicated that focusing on physical care left them concerned about how they would be able to integrate illness into their lives, while focusing on psychosocial care resulted in worries about their physical care. Despite the artificiality of the separation of physical actions from psychosocial actions, this chapter focuses on psychosocial nursing actions that promote health and healing in patients and are accomplished through the patient–nurse relationship.

Swanson's theory of nursing as 'informed caring' provides a useful model for situating the interpersonal skills necessary for psychosocial actions within the context of the skills outlined in previous chapters. Five processes of caring are explicated in the theory of 'informed caring' (Swanson 1993). The first of these is a philosophical grounding of nursing in an inherent belief in people and a conviction in personal meanings that are attached to health events (such a philosophy is enhanced through self-understanding: see Ch 3). Once 'grounded' in this philosophical stance, nurses 'anchor' their caring through striving to understand the meaning that patients attach to health events. This second process is achieved by 'knowing the patient' (see Ch 2), and is brought to life through the interpersonal skills of understanding and exploring (see Chs 6 and 7). The third process in the theory of informed caring is enacted by nurses when they are fully present and available to patients through attending and listening (Ch 5). Referred to by Swanson (1993) as 'being with' patients, this process was reviewed in Chapter 5 in the form of attending and listening skills.

Once they are 'with' patients, nurses express their caring through actions that pertain to the final two processes in Swanson's theory, termed 'doing for' patients and 'enabling' patients to do for themselves. Although not rigid in the sense that the processes are passed through as stages and phases, there is a sequential aspect to them. For example, 'doing for' requires nurses to understand what must be done (i.e. to understand a patient's frame of reference before attempting to provide psychosocial help).

As seen in Table 8.1, the interpersonal skills for the first three processes of informed caring have been developed in previous chapters. This chapter focuses on the final two processes, 'doing for' and 'enabling'. Although the process of 'doing for' is predominantly expressed through physical care and skilled clinical performance of nursing care, 'doing for' also includes comforting measures that are achieved through interacting with and relating to patients. Comforting measures such as reassurance are discussed in this chapter. Supporting actions are also considered in the process of 'doing for' patients. Swanson's process (1993) of 'enabling' includes having patients participate in their healthcare. Such participation is contingent on patients' knowledge and understanding of their health status and care. The interpersonal skills needed to inform and assist patients in obtaining this knowledge are also reviewed in this chapter.

TABLE 8.1 Processes of informed caring and related interpersonal skills

Processes of informed caring (Swanson 1993)	Interpersonal skills
Maintaining belief in people	Self-understanding
Appreciating personal meanings of health events	Understanding and exploring
Being with patients	Attending and listening
Doing for patients	Comforting and supporting
Enabling patients	Encouraging participation by sharing information and challenging

Indications of the need for psychosocial action

When listening and understanding, nurses are guided by patients. When taking psychosocial action, nurses assume a more active role in guiding patients. This does not mean that a nurse takes charge and control of a patient's life, but rather intervenes in a way that encourages the patient to assume as much control as possible. For example, when an understanding is reached that a patient is facing a decision, the nurse takes action in order to help the patient make the decision, rather than taking over and making the decision for the patient. Actions that are psychosocial in nature are liberating, not restrictive, and they always work from within the patient's experience.

Taking action is based on indications that it is needed. The following list includes examples of patient situations that indicate a need to intervene directly. Psychosocial action may be required when patients are:

- in need of more information
- emotionally distressed (e.g. feeling overwhelmed)
- facing a health-related decision
- learning new skills
- lacking in available resources
- inadequately using existing resources, or
- experiencing difficulties in coping, adjusting and adapting.

Patient outcomes

Psychosocial nursing actions of comforting, supporting and enabling are focused on outcomes and resources. When nurses employ these actions, they do so with the deliberate intention of producing positive changes or reinforcing adaptive ones in patients. While the desired outcome may not always be directly observable and measurable, action is taken for a focused purpose. Some examples of desired outcomes include helping patients to:

- adjust and adapt to changes in living imposed by illness
- maintain self-esteem
- find meaning in illness
- feel secure and in control
- contain and control emotional distress within manageable limits
- make decisions about healthcare, and
- access and use helpful resources.

Outcomes are based on the indication of need for action. For example, the indication that a patient is emotionally distressed calls for an outcome of containing and controlling that distress within manageable limits. Not only is it important for nurses to relate desired outcome to patient need but, more importantly, nurses must work with patients in determining needs and outcomes from the patients' perspective.

Patient resources

Psychosocial nursing actions are most effective when nurses work with patients' natural resources, their capabilities and means for coming to terms with health-related and illness-related issues in their lives. Some actions work with the patients' existing resources, while others focus on the identification, development and use of new or unused resources. It is important for nurses to understand the patient's resources. Examples of resources include: the patient's knowledge, will, desire, strength and courage; their family members and friends; other patients; self-help groups; and health services and providers (Carnevali 1983). Possible resources are endless for some patients and quite limited for others. Essential to the use of patient resources is the recognition and acknowledgment that nurses themselves are but one, usually temporary, resource in helping patients. Nurses must look to longer term patient resources, basing their outlook on the belief that patients are themselves resourceful and capable.

WAYS OF RESPONDING REVISITED

The various ways of responding (presented in Ch 6) include the action-oriented, influencing responses of advising and evaluating, analysing and interpreting, and reassuring and supporting. These responses were rejected as initial responses in favour of understanding responses. The major reason these action-oriented responses were deemed inappropriate early in the course of the relationship between patient and nurse is because the nurse who employs them at this time is exerting too much control and influence on the patient. For example, an interpretation challenges patients to view their situations in a different light—one that is based on the nurse's perceptions rather than the patient's. There is a danger of alienating the patient if a nurse is too directive early in the course of the relationship.

The tendency for nurses to be directive in the face of patient problems was demonstrated in two studies (Motyka et al 1997, Whyte et al 1997). In these studies, nurses were asked to write a verbal response to a patient complaint (tightness in the throat and difficulty swallowing). Of the 150 nurses who participated, the majority responded with directives such as 'Don't worry', 'Don't be upset' or 'I'll tell the doctor and you will be fine'. Only 2% demonstrated an understanding response. When two groups of nurses were compared using the same research methods (Whyte et al 1997), British nurses more frequently responded by collecting information about the patient complaint than did Polish nurses. Nevertheless, the majority of responses of nurses in both studies indicated that they operated from a position of authority and were directive in their responses. That is, the majority of responses indicated that the nurse assumed control, rather than working with the patient to explore the meaning of the complaint further or to respond with understanding of the patient's discomfort.

Each way of responding is appropriate at various levels and stages in the development of the patient–nurse relationship. Nevertheless, the findings of the studies do indicate that nurses may tend to respond in habitual and automatic ways. The skills presented throughout this book, and especially those in this chapter, offer a range of possible alternatives. Nurses are encouraged to reflect and consider which type of response is appropriate at the time and under the circumstances. The importance of timing is highlighted as nurses consider what skills to use when. Early in the relationship, the patient directs the interactions. As the relationship progresses, the nurse can exert more direct influence through direct action.

COMFORTING

Of the five ways of responding (see Ch 6), a response that attempts to comfort and reassure is used most often by people who are trying to be of help (Johnson 2007). Nurses are no different in this respect. In the studies by Motyka et al (1997) and Whyte et al (1997), nurses most often tried to cheer patients with reassurance and consolation. Although participants' intentions were not investigated in these studies, the majority of their responses were most likely meant to comfort patients.

Caring and comforting

Comforting is associated with soothing distress, relieving pain and easing grief. To be comfortable is associated with being relaxed, contented, and free from pain and anxiety. It is understandable that nurses attempt to comfort. In fact, Morse (1992) has urged nurses to reconsider this claim and refocus nursing care on the concept of comfort. She argues that caring focuses on the nurse, while comfort focuses on the patient. Caring is process oriented and is the motivation for nursing actions. Comfort is outcome oriented and is the aim of nursing actions. Caring is *why* nurses act; comforting is *how* they act (Morse 1992).

Morse's argument is compelling in the sense that it offers nurses a focus of care that can be described through practices that comfort patients. Caring is more nebulous in the sense that it offers little in the way of clear guidelines for clinical performance, especially for beginning nurses. Because comfort focuses on outcomes rather than process, it offers a framework for nursing action.

Patients' view of comforting

The meaning of comfort in nursing requires careful consideration, especially in relation to the patients' point of view. The importance of comfort was highlighted in an extensive study into patient's perspectives of care. In this study, patients found interacting with nurses to be comforting and this resulted in their sense of control (Williams & Irurita 2006). This was confirmed in an earlier study exploring patients' views of comfort (Cameron 1993), which indicated that patients are not passive in their view of comfort (i.e. patients did not wait in hope of receiving comfort). Rather, they sought it out by, for example, gathering information about their condition and treatment from caregivers and other patients. These patients also vigilantly monitored nurses' responses to them in an effort to find reassurance that all was well. Patients in this study also delved into themselves as a way of integrating their illness experience into the whole of their lives. These patients' views indicate that comfort is an active process that energises. This view of comfort as enlivening, although part of its original meaning, contrasts to current conceptualisation of comforting as soothing, easing or consoling (Cameron 1993).

In another study of comfort, patients gave an account of an illness in which they experienced agonising pain, trauma or life-threatening conditions. In their analysis of the patients' stories, Morse et al (1994) concluded that comfort measures by nurses included taking control, reassuring, protecting, connecting, distracting (refocusing), acknowledging and supporting. Comfort measures enabled patients to retreat from discomfort and provided the opportunity for patients to regain strength and energy (Morse et al 1994). The enlivening aspects of comfort echo Cameron's findings (1993).

In their analysis of patient biographies of illness, Morse et al (2006) describe a number of actions that promote comfort. These actions include pity (expressing regret), sympathy (conveying sorrow), compassion (sensitively sharing the distress of another), consolation (encouragement that things are not as bad as they could be), commiseration (sharing mutual situations), compassion (sharing feelings) and reflexive reassurance (appearing optimistic in order to counteract negative emotions). Each response has the potential to promote comfort because the response confirms negative emotions (pity), legitimises the patients' response (sympathy), recognises and shares feelings (compassion), reduces patients' distress (consolation), confirms universality of feelings (commiseration) and counteracts anxiety (reflexive reassurance) (Morse et al 2006).

Each of these comforting responses focuses on the patient. More importantly, responses such as consolation and compassion interpersonally engage the patient by confirming their experience. In a similar vein, patients in Drew's (1986) study reported that they felt comforted and confident when they experienced confirming responses that were both cognitive and affective. When nurses' responses were confirming, they expressed a sense of concern for the patient, demonstrated through being unhurried, making eye contact and using a soothing tone of voice. Comfort and confirmation go hand in hand.

Nurses' expression of comforting

The measures described by patients in the studies cited above indicate that spontaneous (reflexive) responses promote engagement and involvement because they express identification with the patient's pain and distress. These responses are natural and naturally human, thus promoting a sense of connection between nurse and patient.

Sometimes, nurses are taught to stifle these spontaneous responses in favour of 'professional' responses that are learnt (Morse et al 2006). Traditionally, nurses are taught to provide comfort by therapeutic empathic responses (see Ch 6). Clinical empathy de-emphasises the emotional involvement of reflexive empathy (Halpern 2003). Emotional empathy, which is developed through experience, enables nurses to implicitly know what to do when patients are distressed (Morse et al 2006). Informative reassurance, which provides explanation and information, is another learnt response. While intended to promote comfort, learnt responses are not as engaging as the spontaneous responses (Morse et al 2006).

Results of studies that explicate comforting strategies (Proctor et al 1996, Bottorff et al 1995) include nursing actions of talking to patients in ways that help them to hold on, especially when they are in pain. Examples of 'holding on' strategies included supporting, praising and affirming the patient. Other comforting behaviours included providing information, explaining what is happening, being informal and friendly, and expressing concern. Offering choices in care is another way that nurses helped patients stay in control and feel comforted.

All the skills in this chapter could be subsumed under the umbrella of the comforting strategies that have been explicated through research; this reinforces the centrality of comforting in nursing. Nevertheless, for the purpose of simplicity and clarity, reassurance is the main skill that is fully developed as a comforting action. Supporting is another comforting action, which is described in a separate section. Other skills, such as informing and challenging, are developed under the umbrella of enabling patients to participate in care.

Reassuring skills

Reassuring the patient is a common nursing activity, often cited as a planned, purposeful intervention in nursing care. But how is reassurance actually offered and provided by nurses? Under what circumstances is it indicated? How can reassurance be engaging and not dismissive of patients? Unless the answers to these questions are clearly thought through and understood, there is a danger that reassurance will be oversimplified as nothing more than a natural human response.

While the responses analysed by Morse et al (2006) as naturally comforting are spontaneous (i.e. they are not learnt), they are culturally conditioned. Sometimes, cultural conditioning will result in a reassuring action that is not focused on the patient, but rather protective of the nurse. This is false reassurance.

False reassurance

In everyday social situations, reassurance is frequently offered in the form of trite, trivial clichés and platitudes, repeated so often that they have lost their meaning. Ready-made comments such as 'Everything will work out', 'Don't worry' and 'It will be all right' are uttered in an almost automatic, stereotypical manner. These types of 'reassuring' response were presented in Chapter 6 as examples of false reassurance. They do little to ease discomfort in the person being offered them. When reassurance is offered in this way, the effect is often opposite to its intention.

In saying to patients 'Everything will be all right', nurses may believe they have been truly reassuring; however, patients often feel dismissed by such an expression. Not only have nurses failed to meet patients in their world, but they have also actually denied its existence or diminished its importance.

False reassurance distances the patient from the nurse and may be used by nurses to distance themselves from unpleasant or difficult aspects of nursing (Faulkner & Maguire 1984 p 135). Telling a patient not to worry may make the nurse feel better but, as a general rule, unless the patient receives concrete reassuring evidence, this alone does little to calm the patient who is concerned and distressed.

Unless they are careful and thoughtful, nurses may inadvertently find themselves slipping into this automatic mode of falsely reassuring patients. Because years of socialisation are difficult to change, it is likely that a platitude or cliché will 'slip out' before a nurse realises it. When this happens, the realisation that such responses are not truly reassuring, and even potentially alienating to patients, may produce a sense of failure in the nurse.

Nevertheless, a nurse who inadvertently utters a trite cliché can recover by following the cliché with a comment that indicates awareness and sensitivity. Here are some examples of how to recover:

- '(Everything will be all right), *but my saying so won't necessarily make it so.*'
- '(Don't worry). *That's easy for me to say, isn't it?*'
- '(Things have a way of working out), *but that thought may not help you to feel any better.*'
- '(Some good will come out of all of this). *That doesn't really help you, though, does it?*'

Recovering comments, such as these, demonstrate the nurse's awareness, and usually result in the interaction proceeding rather than generating feelings of alienation and rejection in the patient. After recovering, the nurse is now free to proceed with a more realistic reassuring response.

Comforting reassurance

If effective reassurance is not about presenting such falsely reassuring responses, then what does it involve? To reassure is to restore confidence and to promote a sense of safety, control, hope and certainty. Reassurance calms the anxious, abates the uneasiness of the worried and decreases concern in the uncertain. Reassurance is concrete and directly related to the patient situation, rather than global and non-specific, as clichés are. Realistic reassurance is novel, imaginative, unique and, most importantly, specific to the patient.

The desired outcome in providing reassurance is a restored sense of confidence and feelings of safety within the patient. To reassure literally means to assure again. In this sense, reassurance is restorative. By supporting their inherent power and ability, effective reassurance enables patients to face situations with equanimity. Reassurance may not 'make everything all right' (sometimes this is not possible), but the patient who is reassured can face experiences with confidence, hope and courage.

Reassurance is often associated with patient coping (Fareed 1994). Like the previous analysis of caring and comforting, reassuring is what the nurse does (i.e. it is nurse-focused), and coping is the desired patient outcome. Nevertheless, the provision of reassurance does not guarantee that the patient will feel more certain and confident, and therefore cope better. This lack of guarantee, however, should not stifle attempts to reassure patients.

Patients' need for reassurance

As with all intervening skills, the recognition of the patient's need for reassurance and an understanding of the patient's experience in relation to this need precede action. Nurses must understand and appreciate the concrete, specific nature of a patient's worry. The following situation serves as an illustration of the importance of assessing a patient's need for reassurance:

James Carroll is scheduled for an above-the-knee amputation of his right leg. He has diabetes, which has been difficult to control and manage. Prior to surgery he expresses concern by making statements such as 'I don't know how this is all going to turn out' and 'It's a bit of a worry'. The nurse caring for him avoids saying, 'Oh, don't worry, everything will be all right', appreciating the futility and potential harm of such a statement. Instead, the nurse explores what, specifically, is worrying Mr Carroll. Perhaps he fears pain postoperatively; he could be worried about how he will manage to get around after the surgery; perhaps he is concerned about loss of income (he is self-employed) during and after hospitalisation; perhaps he fears not being able to return to his usual occupation. Perhaps … perhaps … the list is almost endless.

Unless the nurse responding to him understands what exactly is worrying him, any attempts to reassure him may be misguided. Through the use of exploration and understanding skills, the nurse comes to know that the fear of postoperative pain is worrying him most. Now that the specific focus of his concern is identified, the nurse can reassure Mr Carroll, with specific information, about how much pain he can expect and, more importantly, what will be done to alleviate and control his pain.

In nursing practice, there are common patient situations that indicate the need for reassurance. Awareness of these general situations, however, does not replace the necessity of exploring and understanding each patient's experience in relation to the need for reassurance.

Activity 8.1 SITUATIONS REQUIRING REASSURANCE

PROCESS

1 Working individually, record a patient situation that you have experienced or can imagine that indicates the patient's need for reassurance. Ask yourself, 'What made me think the patient needed reassurance?' Describe the situation as fully as possible.

2 Form groups of five to six participants and distribute the recorded situations randomly among the members.

3 Have each member review the situation and write a key word or phrase from the recorded situation that indicates the need for reassurance. Make a list of patient cues from the recorded situation that expressed the need for reassurance.

4 Record all key words and phrases, including those that are repetitive, on a sheet of paper visible to all participants.

5 On a separate sheet of paper, visible to all participants, record the identified patient cues.

DISCUSSION

1 What themes are expressed in the key words and phrases?

2 How much variation is there in the list of patient cues?

3 What generalisations can be made about patient situations that indicate a need for reassurance?

The need for reassurance arises out of situations in which patients are apprehensive, doubtful, uncertain, worried, anxious, full of misgivings or lacking confidence. In nursing practice, there are myriad circumstances that result in patients experiencing such feelings and perceptions. Some examples include:

• unclear/unknown medical diagnosis
• facing unfamiliar situations
• facing an uncertain outcome/future, and
• painful procedures.

The common theme in situations indicating a need for reassurance is uncertainty (Boyd & Munhall 1989). The need for reassurance arises out of situations that are unfamiliar, unknown, unsettling, threatening and confusing. Patients facing such situations often experience a loss of control, and need to have their confidence restored (Teasdale 1989). They are in need of something on which, or someone on whom, they can rely to decrease their uncertainty. The intention in reassurance is then to decrease uncertainty and restore a sense of control.

Patient cues indicating uncertainty

Because of their uniqueness, patients will express uncertainty in a variety of ways. Return to the list of patient cues indicating a need for reassurance, developed in Activity 8.1. Some examples of patient cues indicating feelings of uncertainty, and therefore the potential need for reassurance, include:

- openly stating fears and anxieties
- asking numerous questions
- continuous activity
- being quiet and withdrawn
- crying, and
- making numerous requests and demands.

The perceptive nurse will notice such cues, place them within the context of the patient's current situation, integrate them with an understanding of this patient's experience, and explore and validate the presence of uncertainty and need for reassurance. A general discussion of how to explore patient cues is found in Chapter 7. Having established the presence of a need for reassurance, nurses now can proceed to provide it in a variety of ways.

Activity 8.2 WAYS NURSES REASSURE PATIENTS

PROCESS

1 Recall a time in your life when you were filled with uncertainty about something that was happening, or about to happen, to you.

2 Reflect on the situation and circumstances surrounding it.

3 What, if anything, would have allayed or did allay your uncertainty? Describe, on a piece of paper, how you were/might have been reassured.

4 Form groups of five to six participants and discuss both the described situations, and the ways of reassuring.

5 List the identified ways of reassuring.

6 Compare each small group's list, developed in step 5.

7 Prepare a list that combines each small group's list.

DISCUSSION

1 Of the identified ways of reassuring, which are appropriate within the nursing context?

2 How might a nurse reassure patients?

3 What hinders nurses in their attempts to reassure patients? What helps?

Nurses reassure patients in a variety of ways, not just through verbal responses. They provide reassurance to patients through their presence and manner, as well as through reassuring actions and verbal responses.

Reassuring presence of the nurse

Patients are reassured by the knowledge that the nurse will be there, as the presence of another human being is reassuring in itself, especially during times of disquiet. Being present involves more than simply a physical presence; it involves the emotional presence of a nurse who is fully attending and listening. Hospitalised patients in Fareed's study (1996) described reassuring presence as 'being with [me]' and 'being there [for me]'. In fact, accessibility of the nurse was the key factor in these patients' sense of feeling reassured. Chapter 5 describes this presence with specific reference to the comforting presence of the nurse whose entire focus is on the patient.

In addition, patients are reassured in knowing that the nurse will remain present and will not abandon them, no matter how difficult, painful or overwhelming circumstances are for them. This vigilant, constant and reliable presence of the nurse promotes confidence within patients, thus providing reassurance.

Reassuring manner of the nurse

When a nurse conveys, primarily through non-verbal means, calmness and confidence, patients are reassured (Fareed 1996). This highlights the need for self-understanding (see Ch 3), because nurses may unconsciously (non-verbal behaviour is largely unconscious) communicate a sense of uneasiness to the patient. A nurse's uneasiness may or may not have reference to the immediate patient, but it will compound the worry of an already worried patient. A nurse who appears unsure or uncertain can contribute to the patient's uneasiness and uncertainty.

The nurse's reassuring presence and manner maintain meaningful human contact between patient and nurse. Other non-verbal forms of communication, including touching, holding hands, massaging and ministering, are examples of physically comforting, reassuring acts (Fareed 1996, Boyd & Munhall 1989). Cultural and age variations in relation to the use of touch are important to understand. These are discussed in Chapters 4 and 10.

Reassuring actions

In addition to the reassuring presence and manner of nurses, there are a number of actions that reassure patients. These include:
- optimistic assertion (Teasdale 1989)
- concrete and specific feedback, and
- explanations and factual information.

These skills are considered facilitative because they encourage patients to reinterpret their situations in light of different or new information. They are especially helpful when a patient's current interpretation of a situation is threatening (e.g. the new mother who believes that her blue feelings after birth are a sign that she is 'losing her mind').

Optimistic assertion

An optimistic assertion is a pledge, promise or guarantee made with the intention of reassuring the patient (Teasdale 1989). Examples of optimistic assertions include:

- 'The pain medication that we will give you routinely after your surgery is quite effective. I think you'll find it really helps.'

- 'This wound is going to heal nicely because you are a fit, healthy person.'
- 'I will visit your family every 2 weeks. Most families find this sufficient, but if you need to contact me in between visits you can reach me on this number.'

Notice how making an optimistic assertion is similar to sharing information (covered later in this chapter). While sharing information is related to optimistic assertion, it is not exactly the same. An optimistic assertion usually contains an interpretation, which the patient is asked to accept without analysis (Teasdale 1989). Information may be added to strengthen an optimistic assertion, but information itself does not provide an interpretation.

Optimistic assertions are similar to false reassurance, although they should not be empty promises or false guarantees. Termed reflexive reassurance by Morse et al (2006), an optimistic assertion is encouragement to maintain an optimistic outlook, even in the face of dire circumstances. Patients in Fareed's study (1996) felt reassured when they were encouraged to remain optimistic, even when nurses used clichés such as 'Don't worry' or 'I'm sure this will get better for you'.

The difference between false reassurance and an optimistic assertion is the nurse's focus. When a cliché or platitude is focused on protecting the nurse and hiding distress, it is not reassuring. When it is focused on the patient, such a comment, genuinely and spontaneously stated, can result in comfort and reassurance.

Concrete and specific feedback

Feedback about how the nurse perceives a situation can be reassuring to patients. In order to be helpful in providing reassurance, feedback needs to be concrete and specific to the patient. Simply saying to a patient, 'I think you are progressing just fine', is not concrete enough to fully reassure the patient. Examples of helpful feedback include:

- 'I can tell that you are getting a little stronger each day because yesterday you could only walk to the edge of the bed. Today you made it to the shower on your own.'
- 'You have been through a lot with your father's illness. It's no wonder you are feeling a bit drained.'
- 'Last month you weren't sure what you were going to do about the tumour. This month, I see a different person.'

Like optimistic assertion, feedback provides the patient with a new interpretation of the situation. This interpretation is based on the nurse's view of the situation, which is usually informed and knowledgeable. It is based on the nurse's view, but helpful feedback is not a judgment, an evaluation or an analysis of the patient's situation.

For feedback to be truly reassuring, it is essential that the nurse establishes first that the patient wants it and can use it. In addition, feedback that focuses on the patient's strengths and resources is more helpful than feedback that highlights weaknesses and shortcomings.

Providing explanations and factual information

Sharing information, especially about what is usual/expected under the circumstances, is reassuring to patients, particularly to those patients whose interpretation is based on faulty or misguided information. For example, a patient who is nil by mouth, and receiving intravenous fluids, may fear that they will literally 'starve to death', due to lack of understanding. Explanations provide patients with an opportunity to re-evaluate their situation, in light of new, more valid information.

Termed informative reassurance (Morse et al 2006), explanations and factual information restore patients' sense of control over situations and reduce their uncertainty. Receiving factual information is a key factor in feeling reassured and gaining control (Fareed 1996). However, because informative reassurance is cognitive, it may not address patients' emotional fears (Morse et al 2006).

Activity 8.3 REASSURING INTERVENTIONS

PROCESS

1 Return to Activity 8.1, 'Situations requiring reassurance', and randomly redistribute the recorded patient situations to each participant.

2 Each participant reviews the patient situation and records how they would provide reassurance under the circumstances.

3 The recorded situations, along with the suggested way to reassure the patient, are once more randomly distributed to all participants.

4 Each situation and suggestion for reassurance is then read aloud by the participants. The types of reassurance suggested are recorded on a tally sheet, under the broad headings provided in the text.

DISCUSSION

1 Which methods of providing reassurance were most preferred? Discuss the possible reasons for this.

2 Which methods of providing reassurance are easy to employ? Which are more difficult? Discuss reasons for this.

SUPPORTING

To support is to provide a means of holding up something to prevent it from falling apart. Foundations support houses. Beams support ceilings. Their enduring presence provides the means to keep a structure intact and prevent its collapse.

In supporting patients, nurses 'stand in the wings' awaiting a call for assistance. Being supportive is an essential quality of nurses and it is needed whenever nurses relate to patients. The foundation skills of listening and understanding are the primary means of conveying a supportive attitude. Their use demonstrates that the nurse is available, accepting and encouraging. Nurses also express their support by upholding an inherent belief in patients' capabilities and resources, and through maintaining a sense of hope. In this regard, support encompasses a variety of skills because it is predominantly an attitude of being with and for the patient. In addition, supporting involves 'knowing the patient' (Skilbeck & Payne 2003).

Types of support

The provision of support occurs within an interpersonal process that involves both emotional support (often expressed as comfort) and instrumental support, which involves the provision of direct assistance and information (Finfgeld-Connett 2005). There are a variety of ways in which nurses provide support to patients. Firstly, there is informational support. Sharing information with patients is supportive because information assists patients in coming to terms with their health status, making decisions about healthcare and understanding what is usual and expected for a given situation. Another type of support comes in the form of direct aid and assistance. This type of support is the concrete, often observable, 'lending a helping hand'. Helping a hospitalised patient out of bed is a clear example of this type of support. Another type of support is the provision of positive affirmation and encouragement to patients. This type of support is emotional in nature, and an example of it is the proverbial 'pat on the back'. It involves standing by and offering encouragement to the patient. The last type is the most common usage of the term 'support'.

Wortman (1984) provides a useful schema in defining support. Support is conveyed to patients through:

- expressions of positive regard and esteem
- encouragement to express and acknowledgment of feelings and points of view
- access to information
- practical and tangible assistance, and
- a sense of belonging.

Most of what hospitalised patients describe as supportive is captured in this description of support (Edgman-Levitan 1993). The most important aspects of support for the patients in Edgman-Levitan's study were expressions of concern, acceptance, understanding and hope. In addition, patients felt supported when they were offered useful information and realistic expectations.

From the preceding description of the types of support, it is apparent that nurses provide support to patients in a variety of ways. An effective relationship with a patient provides support. Most of the actions patients find supportive are discussed in the previous chapters of this book (e.g. listening with understanding). The previous section of this chapter on comforting, and the following section on sharing information, are both examples of supportive nursing actions.

Nevertheless, nurses must also bear in mind that they are but one, often temporary, source of support for patients. Too much emphasis on nurses as providers of support can result in them feeling overwhelmed by patients' needs.

Mobilising patient resources

Another way for nurses to provide support for patients is through direct intervention to mobilise 'other' sources of support. This section focuses on such mobilisation. The following example is an illustration of how nurses mobilise support for patients:

> Barbara Frenzell is in hospital following the stillbirth of a baby girl at full term. The pregnancy, her first, was planned and both she and her husband eagerly anticipated the birth. The loss and disappointment following the stillbirth were devastating

for Barbara. As expected under the circumstances, she was extremely sad, upset and distraught. The nurses found her to be remote, non-communicative and inaccessible, although her emotional pain was visible to them. They understood Barbara's sadness, but were especially concerned by her lack of responsiveness when interacting. Although every effort was made to interact with Barbara, the nurses began to feel helpless because they could not 'connect' with her. They recognised that their concern was greater than usual, and assessed the need for active intervention.

Of all the nurses caring for Barbara, Sue had established the most meaningful relationship with her. Although mostly unresponsive, Barbara spoke more with Sue than any of the other nurses. Through exploration, Sue learnt that Barbara's husband, John, had refused to discuss the death of their daughter with her. John's attitude and approach was one of a 'stiff upper lip' style. He saw no reason to 'cry over spilt milk' and dwell on the negative; he just wanted their lives to return to normal as soon as possible. Sue noticed that, when Barbara discussed John's reaction, she became a bit more communicative and animated. More than anything, Barbara wanted to talk to John about her feelings of despair and sadness. In this situation, one of Barbara's supports, John, was not available to her. What she needed, more than anything, was to be able to talk to John about what had happened. Sue decided to intervene to mobilise this support for Barbara.

The next time John came to visit, Sue made the effort to spend time with them both. Up to this point, the nurses had left the two of them alone during visiting time, out of respect for their need for privacy. During the interaction with Barbara and John, Sue encouraged John to discuss his reactions to what had happened. When he stated that there was no reason to cry and feel sorry for himself, Sue suggested that, although he himself may not wish to cry, perhaps his approach was preventing Barbara from expressing how she felt. At this point, Barbara began to cry. John appeared a bit surprised, but made an effort to console her. Sue left the room, with Barbara and John in an embrace. The next day Barbara's general appearance and demeanour had changed. Although still quite sad, she was more talkative and open. Clearly, she felt better as a result of receiving support from her husband John.

This story illustrates, quite clearly, the importance of nurses perceiving support as more than something they supply directly. Through mobilising support for Barbara, rather than focusing exclusively on the patient–nurse relationship, Sue provided intervention that was helpful and effective.

ENABLING PATIENTS TO PARTICIPATE IN CARE

Patient participation has become a popular concept in nursing (Jonsdottir et al 2004, Gallant et al 2002, McQueeen 2000, Cahill 1996) because it moves away from the notion of the patient as a passive recipient of care to the patient as an active agent in care. It shifts the role of nurse from provider of care to partner in care. Patient participation is concordant with a modern view of the patient as a collaborator in care.

Patient participation varies from involving patients in care by considering their viewpoints to having patients acting as equal partners in decisions about care. Partnership implies a working association between two people, which is usually based on a contract (Cahill 1996). As such, both partners are knowledgeable about the work of the partnership. Involving patients in care, on the other hand, is more one-way, with the nurses being more knowledgeable, yet taking into consideration the patient's point of view. Whether at the level of partnership or involvement, there must be a relationship between patient and nurse in order for patient participation to occur (Cahill 1996).

Partnership must be negotiated between patient and nurse (Bidmead & Cowley 2005), and this negotiation process is essential as patients vary in their desire and capacity to participate (Sahlsten et al 2007, Florin et al 2006). Not all patients either want to or are able to participate in their own healthcare, and the extent to which they do depends on congruence between their desire to participate and the extent to which nurses allow such participation (Schoot et al 2005). Nurses are not always aware of the extent to which patients want to participate and can overestimate their desire to do so (Florin et al 2006).

Having patients participate in their healthcare is both an ethical ideal and a practical reality. From an ethical point of view, all patients should have a say in their care (i.e. having a legitimate voice in care is a recognised patient right). From a practical standpoint, patients who participate in their healthcare are more likely to commit to that care because the care takes into account their particular circumstances. In this regard, health outcomes are more likely to be successful when patients have input into that care.

But having patients participate in their own care is not simply a matter of believing in an ideal or acknowledging a reality. Although healthcare practitioners acknowledge the value of patient participation, they prefer patients to be passive and are challenged to determine whether and to what extent patients want to participate (Clover et al 2004, Cahill 1998, Guadagnoli & Ward 1998).

Do patients want to be involved in their care? Research indicates that the answer to this question is both complex and variable. In most of the research on the topic, patient participation has been viewed as patient involvement in decision making about healthcare. That is, participation is viewed as the extent to which patients are involved in healthcare treatment decisions. Reviews of these studies reveal that patients want to participate to variable degrees *if* options exist and *when* they feel well informed (Schoot et al 2005, Cahill 1998, Guadagnoli & Ward 1998).

Studies have consistently demonstrated that patients want to participate in care if they feel well enough to do so, know enough and are permitted to participate (Eldh et al 2006, Biley 1992). Other studies reveal that patients are more likely to 'toe the line' and fit in with the nurses than exercise their right to participate in healthcare (Shattell 2005, Waterworth & Luker 1990). Another study that reveals insight into patient participation involved patients who were chronically ill and not hospitalised (Thorne & Robinson 1989). These patients involved themselves as 'team players' when they felt competent in managing their illness and when they trusted the healthcare professionals. In the absence of trust and the presence of personal competence, these patients used their knowledge to manipulate the system to obtain necessary services, but did not engage with professionals.

The major theme in the literature on patient participation is the amount of information that patients have to participate. In the absence of information, patients do not feel capable of participating. Therefore, having patients participate in their care is contingent on them having knowledge about that care. Herein lies one of the major challenges to participation. Sharing information with patients is an important skill in meeting this challenge.

Sharing information

The skill of sharing information encompasses a range of actions—from providing explanations, to giving instructions, to imparting knowledge, to formal teaching. When explaining to a patient the reasons for an extended delay in a scheduled procedure, the nurse is sharing information. When engaged in informing patients what they can expect to happen postoperatively, the nurse is sharing information. When teaching a patient how to care for a colostomy, the nurse is sharing information.

What nurses perceive as ordinary and everyday in the routine of healthcare delivery can seem foreign to patients. Patients may have little previous knowledge and experience to draw on in trying to understand this sometimes strange, often frightening, world of healthcare. Clearly, nurses are in a prime position to help patients make sense of the environment and their experiences in it through the sharing of information.

Nurses play a key role in keeping patients informed, not only because of their sustained, continual presence, but also because of their close proximity to the patient's specific experience. When sharing information, a nurse operates from within a patient's experience. It is the nurse who comes to know how much adjustment Mr Jones must make in order to follow a prescribed therapeutic diet. It is the nurse who appreciates the demands being placed on a new mother who has recently arrived in the country and is isolated from her usual support systems. Empathy and understanding of the patient's experience enable nurses to share information that is subjective to the patient, and to appreciate what the patient wants to know in relation to health status and care.

Sharing information is more than merely providing information, or imparting knowledge. In sharing, there is concern with how the information is received, understood and used. It is a two-way process. Providing information involves merely supplying information to patients and is a one-way process. In this sense, books, pamphlets and videos provide information to patients. Sharing information, on the other hand, is interactive: it connects the patient's experience with the need for information; it concerns itself with how the information is received; and it views the patient as an active participant, not as a passive recipient.

As with all the skills of intervening, sharing information is grounded in the nurse's understanding of the patient. To some patients, remaining fully informed, down to the level of minute detail of their care, is extremely important to their sense of wellbeing. Other patients prefer not to know every detail and feel best when told only the bare essentials. Nevertheless, some information (e.g. orienting information about the routine of the clinical setting) is necessary, regardless of the patient's frame of reference and expressed desire to know.

Effects of sharing information

Having meaningful information about their health status and care helps patients gain a sense of control over sometimes uncontrollable, confusing or disturbing events. Frequently, information is shared when a patient is prepared for an anticipated health event. For example, knowing what can be expected following abdominal surgery assists patients in coming to terms with the usual postoperative course of events. Accurate information can do much to alleviate unnecessary anxiety stemming from false beliefs, misconceptions and even fantasies. Patients facing decisions in relation to healthcare are able to determine the best course of action when they are fully informed. Explanations alleviate the anxiety of guessing what will happen next.

The skill of sharing information has been mentioned elsewhere in this chapter in the sections on reassuring and supporting. In the case of reassuring, information is shared so that patients remain aware of what is usual and expected in relation to their health status. In this regard, reassurance through sharing information is similar to informational support, a type of support mentioned in the section on supporting. In the next section of this chapter, sharing information is considered as a challenging skill, because of its potential to trigger patients in reappraising their situations. This section contains a general overview and discussion of how best to employ the skill of sharing information.

A nursing perspective on sharing information

Nurses sometimes are reluctant to embark on sharing information with patients, because the information to be shared is perceived as exclusively medical in nature. While it is inappropriate for nurses to assume the role of doctor in presenting initial information about a medical diagnosis, nurses frequently serve as the interpreters of such information. Patients frequently ask nurses questions that are medical in nature. Simply referring them to the appropriate doctor is often not enough. Nurses can assist patients to obtain relevant medical information by helping them to develop questions to ask of the doctor and suggesting appropriate questions to ask. In this sense, nurses act as guides for patients.

Nevertheless, there is more to sharing information than helping patients to obtain and understand input that is medical in nature. Patients also need assistance in understanding how their health status, including their medical diagnosis (when present and known), will affect their day-to-day living. They need to learn how to adjust and adapt to the demands that are placed on them by alterations in health status. When nurses share information about these aspects of health, they are functioning within a nursing perspective. By focusing on these aspects, nurses concern themselves more with patients' responses to their health status, rather than just their health status per se.

Examples of a nursing perspective on sharing information include helping patients to:
- make sense of what is happening to them
- learn new skills in caring for self, and
- make adjustments and adaptations in relation to the demands placed on them by alterations in health status.

In short, nurses are in a position to share information about patients' daily living in relation to health status (Carnevali 1983).

Sharing information versus giving advice

It is easy to confuse giving advice with sharing information (this was mentioned briefly in Ch 6). In sharing information, nurses offer a range of alternatives to patients. In giving advice, nurses present solutions to patients. There are times when patients expect advice and place nurses in the role of knowledgeable expert. Before assuming this role, however, nurses need to be clear that certain risks are inherent in advising.

When functioning within the nursing perspective, nurses share information in an attempt to help patients adjust and adapt to their daily living. By advising patients about what is 'best' to do, nurses assume they are experts about each patient's life. Clearly, patients are the most qualified experts when it comes to managing their lives. The risks of playing the expert when it involves another person's life are apparent—the advice can be unsuitable, unacceptable, inappropriate or even dangerous.

It is better to present alternatives, through sharing information, and enable the patient to determine which course of action might be best. The following scenario highlights the process of presenting alternatives versus giving solutions:

June Ford has been visiting the local early childhood centre on a regular basis since her first son, Ted, was born 11 months ago. During a recent visit she related that she is becoming increasingly distressed because Ted is still waking during the night to breastfeed. Although Ted feeds quickly during the night and settles back to sleep quite easily, June is distressed by her continual nights of broken sleep.

Eleanor, the registered nurse in the centre, has been working with mothers and babies for 12 years. June asks Eleanor for advice about what to do, because she is becoming desperate for an unbroken night's sleep. Eleanor begins by explaining that Ted is of sufficient weight and age to go through the night without a feed. She then proceeds to explain that June has various options. She could let Ted cry until he returns to sleep; she could use the 'controlled crying method' to get him back to sleep without a feed; June's husband could tend to Ted in the middle of the night; or she could continue to feed him, knowing that some day waking during the night will cease. Eleanor then continues, explaining how other mothers she knows have dealt with similar circumstances. Finally, she shares her own experiences learned through caring for her three children.

After presenting the options, Eleanor explains to June that only she can decide what is best for herself, Ted and the family. She finishes by stating that there are numerous theories about how to care for babies, and a variety of possible approaches, but it really comes down to what June can live with. She then explores each of the options with June, to determine what June would like to try.

Obviously, Eleanor could have advised June about what she should do, rather than share information and let June decide. In doing so, however, she would have run the risk of suggesting a solution that is unacceptable or unworkable for June. Even if the advice is acceptable, it may not work, so June would be left with no other options. Under these circumstances, June probably would not ask Eleanor again, and may even blame her for the failure of her recommendation. Most importantly, by giving advice, Eleanor becomes responsible for the outcome. June could be left with feelings of inadequacy as a result. These are the risks of presenting solutions, rather than alternatives.

Giving advice is not the same as presenting factual, clinical information to patients, or explaining the potential consequences of certain health-related behaviours. Advice offers solutions when patients are facing situations that they can potentially manage. Instructing a patient to cough and breathe deeply following surgery, in order to help prevent pulmonary complications, is an example of presenting information and instructions, although this could be construed as advice. There are times when nurses effectively offer advice to patients, but this should be undertaken with full awareness of the risks involved.

Approaches to sharing information

Sharing information begins with the nurse's recognition of the patient's need for it. While it could be said that all patients need certain information in order to cope with changes in health status, the specific need within each patient may be variable. Recognition and appreciation of the patient's unique requirements for information stem from the nurse's understanding.

While the patient's unique experiences provide a useful starting point for the use of any intervening skill, there are some general situations that indicate a specific need for information. These include:
- facing new and unfamiliar situations
- coping with demands of altered health status
- developing new skills
- being misinformed
- requesting information and explanations, and
- expressing the need for reassurance and informational support.

Readiness to learn

Timing is crucial when sharing information, and this is best expressed as capturing the patient's readiness to learn (Benner 1984 p 79). If information is shared before a patient is ready, it may fall on deaf ears or, worse, create undue anxiety in the patient. When it occurs too late, sharing information fails to achieve its desired outcome.

Capturing a patient's readiness to learn is a sophisticated process, which is described as an aspect of expert nursing practice (Benner 1984). The degree of sensitivity to patient cues that is required for this level of practice is developed through experience and involvement with numerous patient experiences. To beginning nurses, the concept of the 'right time' to share information may seem vague and elusive. Nevertheless, an acceptance and recognition that there is a right time to 'strike while the iron is hot' enables beginning nurses to make the effort to observe and notice patient cues that indicate readiness.

A good example occurs in the teaching of patients to care for a colostomy—a complex, sometimes overwhelming, task for most patients. Because patients must first come to terms with the reality of a colostomy, they will not be ready to learn the details of caring for it and themselves until this happens. Cues indicating readiness include looking at the colostomy in more than just a fleeting manner, not reacting with disgust when looking at it, and asking questions of the nurse who is changing the colostomy bag. This is but one example of the importance of noticing when the patient seems ready to learn.

Obviously, capturing the patient's readiness means that nurses must be flexible enough to change their immediate plans in order to accommodate this readiness.

Beginning to share information

Once the need for information is established, and the readiness to receive the information is noted, it is best to begin sharing information by establishing what the patient wants to know. Often patients will ask questions without prompting or probing, but it may be necessary for the nurse to use exploration skills (see Ch 7) to establish what the patient wants to know first. Questions that are useful include:

- 'What questions are on your mind?'
- 'What would you like to know?'
- 'Where would you like me to begin explaining this?'

Through exploring what patients want to know, the nurse is requesting and encouraging the patient to ask the questions. It is important that these questions are answered at the depth and level at which they are asked. A simple question need not be met with a complicated, involved answer. Likewise, a complex question should not be brushed aside with a superficial answer. It is often a good idea to paraphrase (see Ch 6) the patient's question prior to attempting to answer it.

After answering a patient's question, the nurse needs to check that the response satisfied the question. This is accomplished by following the response with another question, such as 'Does that answer your question?'. The nurse may be surprised when the patient answers 'No'. Under this circumstance, it is obvious that the nurse needs to develop another response, or have the patient pose the question again, using different words.

From this point, the nurse now can move into further, more focused exploration of what the patient already understands. A person who has experienced repeated hospitalisations may understand a great deal about ward routine. This exploration provides a good opportunity to correct any misinformation or misperceptions. The nurse can also use the patient's current level of understanding as a springboard for expansion and elaboration of further information. Notice how beginning in this manner encourages the patient to direct the flow of information. It also provides an opportunity for the nurse to further assess the patient's readiness to receive information.

Limiting the amount of information shared

When nurses are expanding into sharing new information, they need to appreciate that there are limits to how much information can be absorbed at one time. Too much information presented at one time can overload the patient's information-processing capacity. Presenting detailed, complex information all at once can create more confusion within the patient. For this reason, the general guideline of presenting no more than three new items at one time is recommended (Cormier et al 1986).

Using appropriate language

Another important facet of sharing information is to use language that matches the patient's age, experience and cultural background. Nurses sometimes become so accustomed to the jargon of healthcare that they fail to appreciate that patients do not understand some of the language used. Terms such as 'IVs', 'nil by mouth', 'obs' and even 'bedrest' can create confusion in patients. For example, some patients think 'bedrest' literally means to have a rest in bed and liken it to an afternoon nap, thinking this is sufficient to maintain bedrest. Not only should standard medical and nursing terms and jargon be fully explained to patients, but also their use should be kept to a minimum, if not avoided altogether.

Tailoring information to the patient

Of even greater importance when sharing information is the need to tailor explanations to the individual patient. Obviously, age (see Ch 10) and cultural variations (see Ch 4) need to be taken into account. But it is equally important to work from the patient's background and experience. For example, an engineer can easily relate the functioning of the heart to already acquired knowledge of closed systems that work on pressure, pumps, one-way valves and electrical conduction. Knowing a patient's background is necessary for this guideline to be enacted.

The need for reinforcement

It is often helpful to reinforce explanations and information verbally shared with prepared pamphlets, diagrams, models and spontaneously written notes. Using an alternative means of expression such as one or more of these provides helpful reinforcement for patients. Summarising (see Ch 6) the shared information is another helpful means of reinforcing. Often patients' anxiety levels interfere with their ability to absorb information, and reinforcing will aid in the retention of presented information.

Additionally, there may be a need to reiterate information. Repetition provides reinforcement, although the need to repeat information may prove frustrating to the nurse. The patient may need to hear it more than once in order to incorporate the information, and put it to some use.

Checking the patient's understanding

Sharing information is more than imparting knowledge, so the nurse sharing the information needs to periodically check that the patient understands the information. It is better to check frequently throughout an information-sharing interaction than to wait until it draws to a close. The skills of exploration (see Ch 7) are employed for this purpose.

Expressing understanding when sharing information

When nurses are sharing information, they need to be sensitive to the impact of the information on the patient. For the patient, there may be surprises and challenges contained in the information received. Observing patient cues, which indicate their reactions, reflecting observed feelings and expressing empathy are all helpful skills to employ for this purpose. In the absence of patient cues, it may be necessary for nurses to explore patients' reactions to the information that is shared.

A final word on sharing information

Before embarking on sharing information, nurses must be reasonably confident with their own level of knowledge related to the patient situation. This is not to say that nurses should 'know everything' there is to know about all patient situations, but there is little point in trying to share information when the basics of the situation are not understood. If this is the case, a cursory assessment of the patient's need for information could be undertaken, but there are limits (e.g. a patient's misunderstanding might not be immediately corrected if the nurse lacks knowledge).

There are likely to be situations in which a patient's request for information is beyond what a nurse currently understands and knows. There is no real harm in nurses admitting that they do not know, as long as they are willing to find out for the patient or refer the patient to an appropriate resource. When referral to another person (e.g. the patient's doctor) is the most appropriate course of action, nurses can assist patients in framing questions to ask of this person.

Activity 8.4 SHARING INFORMATION ➡305

PROCESS

1 Working in groups of five to six participants, develop a list of patient situations that indicate that the patient needs more information.

2 Each group member now writes a brief scenario, based on one of the situations from the developed list. Include patient cues indicating a need for information.

3 Distribute the scenarios to each of the group members. Members are to take the scenario away from the session and gather the information required to fully inform the patient described in the scenario.

4 At the next class gathering, participants form groups of three. Identify one member of the group as the patient, one as the nurse who will share information and the third person as an observer.

5 For each scenario, have the 'nurse' share information with the 'patient'. The observer uses the 'Guide for sharing information' (see the appendix, page 306).

DISCUSSION

1 What was easy about sharing information? What was hard?

2 What were some of the difficulties experienced in sharing information? Refer to questions on the observer guides that were answered 'no'.

3 How did the 'nurses' assess the 'patient's' current level of knowledge?

4 How did the 'nurses' determine the 'patient's' comprehension of the information?

5 What kind of wording and language was used in sharing the information?

Challenging

When challenging, nurses urge patients to reconsider their current perspectives and assist them in the development of new perspectives. A challenge encourages patients to evaluate their views, feelings and interpretations of a situation. This can be achieved by directly presenting a different interpretation, or by exploring alternative perspectives with the patient. Either way, a successful challenge enables patients to reframe their experiences in a new light and therefore participate in care with this new view.

Challenging is a skill that is high in terms of influencing patients. This is because the nurse is asking patients to call into question their experiences and to develop new perspectives on their experience. Challenging often forces patients to call on new or unused resources.

The challenging aspects of other skills

The section on reassuring skills makes reference to responses that encourage patients to reinterpret their experience. When enacted in this way, reassurance has a challenging edge to it. Sharing information can also be challenging because the presentation of new information often results in the formation of new perspectives. Even exploration and empathy expression can be challenging. When nurses express empathy, reflect feelings and engage in exploration, the result may be that patients begin to challenge their own perspectives.

The nature of challenging

Effective challenging is beneficial because it encourages patients to look at their situations in new and different ways. This reframing and reinterpretation may prove unsettling at first, and patients may experience anxiety as a result. For this reason, nurses are often uncomfortable with the notion of challenging a patient, because it seems unsupportive to cast doubt on the patient's current perspective. Perhaps this is due to a lack of understanding of the nature and helpfulness of a challenge.

Challenging is not the same as disagreeing with or rejecting the patient's perspective, although it does rely on the nurse's judgment that another perspective may be more productive. For example, a patient may believe that having a myocardial infarction results automatically in permanent disability and dramatic alteration to previous functioning. An interpretation such as this can lead to feelings of depression and even despair. Such a patient is at risk of becoming a 'cardiac cripple'. By challenging this perspective, the nurse enables the patient to develop a more realistic view of the situation post-infarction.

The conditions needed for effective challenging

As with all the psychosocial action skills, challenging is preceded by an understanding acknowledgment of the reality of the patient's current experience (see Ch 6). Nurses 'earn the right' (Egan 2007) to challenge patients by first demonstrating understanding of their viewpoints and experiences. In this sense, understanding is a prerequisite to challenging.

Before embarking on challenging skills, a nurse must also consider the strength of the relationship with the patient. If little rapport, trust and understanding is developed, it is likely that a challenge will be ineffective. In fact, without trust, challenging may be counterproductive to the further development of the relationship. Patients will accept a challenge from a nurse who has demonstrated interest, accessibility, reliability and understanding. Challenging is more likely to be effective in longer term rather than shorter term relationships.

Other aspects to consider before embarking on a challenge relate to the vulnerability and fragility of the patient. Nurses must be reasonably certain that the patient being challenged has the strength, resilience and resources to develop and accept a new perspective. Minimally, the patient needs to be able to acknowledge that alternative views are possible.

The need to challenge

The need to challenge stems from the existence of patient perspectives that are unproductive, unsatisfying, poorly informed, unacceptable, and/or unnecessarily painful or distressing to the patient. The importance of that final phrase, *to the patient*, cannot be stressed enough. It is important that challenges are not presented as negative judgments that give the impression that patients 'should not' think or feel the way they do. Although nurses rely on a judgment that a new perspective may be needed, they must operate from within the patient's value system in order to be most effective. A nurse cannot decide, without consultation, that the patient's perspective needs to be altered.

Tentativeness of the challenge

Challenges are best presented in a tentative manner, but not so tentative that nurses lack assertiveness in the process. A nurse wishing to challenge a patient can begin by suggesting that there may be another way of looking at the situation. This is an effective way to determine the patient's readiness to accept alternative perspectives.

Approaches to challenging

When patients indicate, often through subtle cues, that their current view is unproductive or difficult to maintain and acknowledge the possibility of alternative perspectives, nurses can proceed by:

* exploring alternative perspectives
* presenting their own interpretation and perspective, and
* sharing factual information.

The first approach relies on the use of exploring skills (see Ch 7). The second approach uses the skill of feedback, covered in the section on reassuring in this chapter. The third approach is also covered in this chapter, under the heading of 'Sharing information'.

Exploring consequences

Another way to begin the challenge is to explore the consequences of the patient's present perspective. While this approach relies on the effective use of exploring skills (see Ch 7), it is a focused exploration into the possible effects of the patient's current perspective, and delves into the potential risks and benefits of that perspective.

A nurse may be tempted to take the idea of consequences one step further and actually point them out to patients. This approach should be used sparingly (Ivey & Ivey 1998), because of its potential to degenerate into a judgmental, coercive activity, which preaches warnings and punishment. Nurses need to be cautious about admonishing patients because this can translate to 'blaming the victim'. If this happens, patients may form the impression that the nurse does not care to understand.

Assertiveness in challenging

The ability to be assertive (see Chs 3 and 10) is necessary when challenging. Some examples of assertive challenging responses include:

* 'I see your situation in a different light from you.'
* 'I'm concerned that if you continue along these lines, you will just wither away.'
* 'You say you are doing everything to help yourself, but I can see some more things that you could do.'

When challenging, it is important to focus on the patient's strengths and resources, not just weaknesses and failures. In this regard, challenging is employed with an attitude of respect for the patient's inherent capabilities.

Reframing through self-disclosure

Self-disclosing is a skill whereby nurses share their own thoughts, feelings, perceptions, interpretations and experiences in the interest of helping the patient. Self-disclosure is both a form of commiseration, which is a way of comforting patients (Morse et al 2006), and a way of helping patients reframe their situations.

Reference to the use of this skill is made elsewhere in this book. In Chapter 7 it is presented as a means of opening areas for exploration. Using self-disclosure to prompt patients and encourage them to express themselves is one of the most common forms of this skill. Self-disclosure is also discussed in Chapter 6 as a way to clarify what patients have expressed. The skill of self-disclosure is included in this chapter because it can also be used to directly influence patients.

Sharing own experiences

One of the most frequent ways that self-disclosure is effective occurs when a nurse has experienced a situation that is similar to the patient's. For example, a nurse who has had the experience of a family member with cancer may share this experience with the family of a patient who is diagnosed with cancer. Under circumstances such as these, nurses share their experiences (commiseration) not only to demonstrate to the patient a personal understanding of the situation, but also to present an alternative perspective (reframing).

Self-disclosure also serves as a way to reassure patients that nurses are real people, with real lives. Being open enough to share their own stories with patients demonstrates that nurses trust patients as much as they want patients to trust them. The genuineness and personal involvement that is demonstrated by self-disclosure has the potential to draw the nurse and patient closer together. But it also may frighten some patients who do not desire this degree of intimacy, or who prefer nurses to remain distant.

How much of the self should be shared?

This notion of sharing one's self with patients does challenge some notions of 'professionalism'. At times, professionalism is equated with distance, detachment and non-involvement with patients. This notion of professionalism is explored fully in Chapter 2. Self-disclosure raises questions about how much information about themselves nurses should share with patients.

In deciding how much of one's self to share with patients, there will almost certainly be differences that are based on the personality of each nurse. Like all people, some nurses are more willing to share personal experiences than others. Irrespective of personality, a general rule of thumb can be applied in deciding how much of self to share. The general rule stems from the nature of the relationship between patient and nurse. Although this relationship involves give and take and, at times, is quite intimate, the nurse must remain oriented towards the patient. When self-disclosure is used to benefit the nurse, the orientation has shifted onto the nurse.

Activity 8.5 SELF-DISCLOSURE

PROCESS

1 Discuss the following:

   a How much personal information about themselves should nurses share with patients?

   b Is there anything of a personal nature that nurses should not share with patients? If so, what?

   c Discuss the reasons for the answers to each of these questions.

DISCUSSION

1 How much disagreement was there between participants in answering questions 1a–c?

2 Were there areas of agreement about what should and should not be shared with patients? What are they?

3 How do you account for the agreement and disagreement in the questions posed?

Pitfalls of self-disclosure

Self-disclosure does not mean that nurses should ask patients to bear some of the burden of their own personal difficulties and problems. This is one of the potential pitfalls of self-disclosure. Self-disclosing has the potential to shift the focus from the patient to the nurse and, as a result, the nurse dominates the interaction with discussions about self. In this case, the self-disclosure runs the risk of burdening the patient with the nurse's personal story. Obviously, if this happens, questions are raised about how helpful this might be for the patient. It takes awareness to recognise when this is happening and an aware nurse will shift the focus back onto the patient, perhaps by employing an exploration skill.

When sharing their own experiences with patients, nurses need to be careful not to use the self-disclosure as a subtle way of rejecting a patient's experience in favour of the nurse's. Nor should self-disclosure be used in a competitive manner of 'let's see who has the best/worst story to tell'. Before disclosing themselves to patients, nurses should pass the disclosure through the following proverbial gate: 'Am I sharing this in order to benefit the patient or our relationship?' If the answer is 'yes', the gate opens for self-disclosure.

Patient requests for personal information

The discussion about self-disclosure also raises the question of how nurses should respond when patients request information that is personal in nature. In this regard, the patient prompts the self-disclosure. Clearly, the decision about how much nurses share of themselves is a personal one, but there are also professional reasons to disclose or not to disclose. Firstly, the context must be considered. In an inpatient mental health setting, for example, there may be sound reasons for nurses to avoid too much disclosure of personal

details about their lives. Other aspects of the context that should be considered include:
- the possible reasons the patient requests the information
- the degree of personal depth in the request, and
- the potential consequences of answering or not answering the question.

Nurses are encouraged to reflect and explore how much or how little information about themselves they are willing to share with patients.

CHAPTER SUMMARY

The skills presented in this chapter focus on psychosocial actions of comfort, supporting and enabling. Nurses employ the skills of comforting in order to reassure patients. Effective reassurance releases patient anxiety so that energy can be used for dealing with the health event at hand. Effective support offers assistance and aid, again freeing the patient's energy to cope. Enabling patients to participate in care by sharing information and challenging helps them to reframe their perspectives on their situation. All of these skills involve taking direct action to positively influence patients and, more importantly, free energy to cope with health events.

The power necessary for nurses to influence patients in these ways is not automatic; the nurse who has taken the time to fully understand the patient earns it. Taking action is most effective when it works from within the patient's experience; therefore, the continual need to listen, explore and understand has been emphasised throughout the chapter. Nurses are most effective when they use psychosocial actions with the view that patients are capable and resourceful. With this view, the skills in this chapter are used to mobilise, utilise and reinforce patients' capabilities and resources.

REFERENCES

Benner P 1984 From novice to expert: excellence and power in clinical nursing practice. Addison-Wesley, Menlo Park, CA

Bidmead C, Cowley S 2005 A concept analysis of partnerships with clients. Community Practitioner 78(6):203–208

Biley FC 1992 Some determinants that effect patient participation in decision-making about nursing care. Journal of Advanced Nursing 17:414–421

Bottorff JL, Gogag M, Engelberg-Lotzkar M 1995 Comforting: exploring the work of cancer nurses. Journal of Advanced Nursing 22:1077–1084

Boyd CO, Munhall PL 1989 A qualitative investigation of reassurance. Holistic Nursing Practice 4(1):61–69

Cahill J 1996 Patient participation: a concept analysis. Journal of Advanced Nursing 24:561–571

Cahill J 1998 Patient participation: a review of the literature. Journal of Clinical Nursing 7: 119–128

Cameron BL 1993 The nature of comfort to hospitalized medical surgical patients. Journal of Advanced Nursing 18:424–436

Carnevali D 1983 Nursing care planning: diagnosis and management, 3rd edn. Lippincott, Philadelphia, PA

Clover A, Browne J, McErlain P, Vandenberg B 2004 Patient approaches to clinical conversations in the palliative care setting. Journal of Advanced Nursing 48:331–341

Cormier LS, Cormier WH, Weisser RJ 1986 Interviewing and helping skills for health professionals. Jones and Bartlett, Boston MA

Drew N 1986 Exclusion and confirmation: a phenomenology of patients' experiences with caregivers. Image: Journal of Nursing Scholarship 18(2):39–43

Edgman-Levitan S 1993 Providing effective emotional support. In: Gerteis M, Edgman-Levitan S, Daley J, Delbanco TL (eds), Through the patients' eyes: understanding and promoting patient-centered care, pp. 154–177. Jossey-Bass, San Francisco, CA

Egan G 2007 The skilled helper, 8th edn. Brooks Cole/Thomas Learning, Boston, MA

Eldh AC, Ekman I, Ehnfors M 2006 Conditions for patient participation and non-participation in health care. Nursing Ethics 13(5):503–514

Fareed A 1994 A philosophical analysis of the concept of reassurance and its effect on coping. Journal of Advanced Nursing 20:870–873

Fareed A 1996 The experience of reassurance: patients' perspectives. Journal of Advanced Nursing 23:272–279

Faulkner A, Maguire P 1984 Teaching assessment skills. In: Faulkner A (ed.),Communication, pp. 130–144. Churchill Livingstone, Edinburgh

Finfgeld-Connett D 2005 Clarification of social support. Journal of Nursing Scholarship 37(1):4–9

Florin J, Ehrenberg A, Ehnfors M 2006 Patient participation in clinical decision-making in nursing: a comparative study of nurses' and patients' perceptions. Journal of Clinical Nursing 15:1498–1508

Gallant MH, Beaulieu MC, Carnevale FA 2002 Partnership: an analysis of the concept within the nurse–client relationship. Journal of Advanced Nursing 40:149–157

Guadagnoli E, Ward P 1998 Patient participation in decision-making. Social Science and Medicine 47:329–339

Halpern J 2003 What is clinical empathy? Journal of General Internal Medicine 18:670–674

Ivey AE, Ivey M 1998 Intentional interviewing and counseling: facilitating client development, 4th edn. Brooks/Cole, Pacific Grove, CA

Johnson DW 2007 Reaching out: interpersonal effectiveness and self actualization, 10th edn. Allyn and Bacon/Merrill, Boston, MA

Jonsdottir H, Litchfield M, Dexheimer M 2004 The relational course of nursing practice as partnership. Journal of Advanced Nursing 47:241–250

McQueen A 2000 Nurse–patient relationships and partnership in hospital care. Journal of Clinical Nursing 9:723–731

Morse JM 1992 Comfort: the refocusing of nursing care. Clinical Nursing Research 1(1):91–106

Morse JM, Bottoroff J, Anderson G, O'Brien B, Solberg S 2006 (originally 1992) Beyond empathy: expanding expressions of caring. Journal of Advanced Nursing 53(1) :75–90

Morse JM, Bottoroff JL, Hutchinson S 1994 The phenomenology of comfort. Journal of Advanced Nursing 20:189–195

Motyka M, Motyka H, Wsolek R 1997 Elements of psychological support in nursing care. Journal of Advanced Nursing 26:909–912

Proctor A, Morse JM, Khonsari ES 1996 Sounds of comfort in the trauma center: how nurses talk to patients in pain. Social Science and Medicine 42:1669–1680

Sahlsten MJM, Larsson IE, Sjöström B, Lindencrona CSC, Plos KAE 2007 Patient participation in nursing care: towards a concept clarification from a nurse perspective. Journal of Clinical Nursing 16:630–637

Schoot T, Proot I, Ter Meulen R, De Witte L 2005 Actual interaction and client centeredness in home care. Clinical Nursing Research 14(4):370–393

Shattell M 2005 Nurse bait: strategies hospitalized patients use to entice nurses within the context of the interpersonal relationship. Issues in Mental Health Nursing 26:205–223

Skilbeck J, Payne J 2003 Emotional support and the role of clinical nurse specialists in palliative care. Journal of Advanced Nursing 43:521–530

Swanson KM 1993 Nursing as informed caring for the well-being of others. Image: Journal of Nursing Scholarship 25(4):352–357

Teasdale K 1989 The concept of reassurance in nursing. Journal of Advanced Nursing 14: 444–450

Thorne SE, Robinson CA 1989 Guarded alliance: health care relationships in chronic illness. Journal of Advanced Nursing 21:153–157

Waterworth S, Luker KS 1990 Reluctant collaborators: do patients want to be involved in decisions concerning care? Journal of Advanced Nursing 15:971–976

Whyte L, Motyka M, Motyka H, Wsolek R, Tune M 1997 Polish and British nurses' responses to patient need. Nursing Standard 11(38):34–37

Williams AM, Irurita VF 2006 Emotional comfort: the patient's perspective of a therapeutic context. International Journal of Nursing Studies 43:405–415

Wortman CB 1984 Social support and the cancer patient. Cancer 53(supplement):2339–2362

Part III
Skills in context

In Part II various skills and concepts of interacting with patients were presented without direct reference to situational variables that affect the use of these skills. The skills of interacting were placed in the context of the relationship that develops between nurse and patient. While the various patients' stories in these chapters have served as illustrations in the use of the skills, no attempt has been made so far to place the skills into specific nursing-care contexts.

Part III places interpersonal skills in context by addressing transitions through health and illness and how people cope with these transitions in order to successfully navigate through them (Chapter 9). In addition, there is information regarding how nurses can assist in these transitions. Chapter 10 includes a discussion of difficult encounters that may challenge nurses in their therapeutic endeavours, and includes a discussion of conflict and the need for assertiveness in its resolution. This chapter also includes a discussion of the importance of age and inclusion of family members in the care of patients. The final chapter explores stress in nursing and describes the ways in which nurses can cope with this stress by building a supportive workplace and using interpersonal skills to enhance relationships with nursing colleagues.

CHAPTER 9

Transitions through health and illness

INTRODUCTION

Nurses relate to people in a variety of contexts, and for the most part these people will be in the throes of significant life events such as transition from health to illness. These transitions, whether major or minor, often create interruptions and disruptions in the lives of the people experiencing them. Understanding the particular ways in which people experience illness enables nurses to help people navigate their transition, because nurses can use this understanding to individualise their care for each person. Individualising care involves recognition of personal responses to illness and the patient's own particular journey in healthcare transitions.

People experiencing transition often feel uncertain and vulnerable, especially as they meet the demands and cope with the changes that often occur as a consequence of transition. Nurses are in a prime position to ease the path of transition by decreasing uncertainty and vulnerability, and by assisting people to cope with changes brought about by illness.

A clear understanding of coping and illness enables nurses to appreciate the variety of ways that people may respond. Nurses can adapt their interpersonal approach to how a particular patient is responding in order to assist that person through their transition. However, the emphasis is not simply to understand how patients are coping, but rather to use this understanding in making interpersonal connections. Forming helpful relationships remains at the heart of nursing care.

Chapter overview

This chapter begins with a discussion of the process of transition through health and illness, focusing on how people cope with the consequent stress of transition. The transitions that most concern nurses involve changes from health to illness and from illness to health, and how people make efforts to cope with such changes is important for nurses to understand. An overview of coping efforts is included for this reason. Coping resources such as resilience, a sense of coherence and social support bolster understanding of how people handle transitions.

Coping efforts often reflect how patients conceptualise illness and change. Referred to as illness representation, this conceptualisation of an illness refers to how people think about their situation, and, more importantly, how they feel about it. The relationship of coping efforts and illness representation is included in this chapter for this reason.

Common themes in the experience of illness are highlighted in the final section and these include uncertainty, vulnerability, distress, loss and grief, and hope.

TRANSITIONS AND COPING

The people who are cared for by nurses often are experiencing life transitions. They may be adults moving from being independent to being permanently or temporarily dependent on others for their survival. It may be a family coming to grips with a catastrophic illness or a terminal diagnosis of one of its members. Others may be awaiting a medical diagnosis after experiencing symptoms of illness. For others, it will be dealing with the challenges of chronic illness, often exacerbated by bouts of acute illness and the continual need for readjustment. All of these circumstances involve transition—a movement from one way of being to another. The process of transition is important for nurses to understand, not only because of its pervasiveness in healthcare, but also because nurses are in a position to help facilitate a transition (e.g. by assisting patients to learn new skills in their healthcare).

In its simplest definition, transition is a passage from one place to another. In this regard, transition refers to relocation; in healthcare settings such passages are often far reaching. Transitions through health and illness are often transformative in the sense that lives are altered. A health transition is 'a process of convoluted passage during which people redefine their sense of self and redevelop self-agency in response to disruptive life events' (van Loon & Kralik 2005, cited in Kralik et al 2006 p 321). Distress, anxiety, loss and grief may also mark health transitions, as people cope with life alterations such as being unwell, getting well again, becoming disabled and approaching death.

In the process of facilitating transition with patients, nurses' efforts are aimed at understanding the patient's experience of illness. Understanding the illness requires knowledge of the patient's physical condition, medical diagnosis and treatment; this is 'case knowledge', described in Chapter 1. Nevertheless, understanding illness is more than simply knowing about diseases; it entails knowing something about the person who experiences illness. This is knowledge of how the person is responding to the disease, also discussed in Chapter 1, as 'patient and person knowledge'.

In nursing practice, the focus is on the relationship between illness and disease (Benner 1984)—that is, the personal, subjective experiences of patients. Disease is a medical diagnosis that explains symptoms of an illness. Illness is the experience of disease—that is, how disease affects a person's life. Illness is also the whole personal experience of a disease—the 'story' of the patient. 'Illness is the human experience of loss or dysfunction whereas disease is the manifestation of aberration at a cellular, tissue, or organ level' (Benner & Wrubel 1989 p 8).

Illness is the human response to disease; however, there can be illness in the absence of disease. Similarly, a person can have a disease, yet not experience illness.

The experience of illness is not inherently negative in nature. Transitions, even one from health to chronic illness, are neither positive nor negative; often they are both. This is because transitions bring with them opportunity for positive growth (Meleis et al 2000). Consider the following story:

When Ted Johnston had a myocardial infarction (heart attack) at the age of 52, he was not surprised. Many years earlier he had witnessed his father suffer numerous myocardial infarctions that eventually left him debilitated and ultimately resulted in his death. Ted knew that there was a strong possibility that he also might experience a fate similar to his father. Because of his family history, Ted had quit smoking and reduced both his cholesterol intake and his weight, 10 years prior to his infarction. Ted received early warning signals in the form of angina 3 years prior to his infarction and the diagnosis of coronary artery disease was confirmed at that time. When Ted had the diagnosis confirmed, he began an exercise program and visited a cardiologist regularly. None of these measures prevented his ultimate heart attack; however, Ted knew that his efforts had helped to decrease both the severity and the effects of the infarction.

One aspect of Ted's life had not been altered in his efforts to reduce his risk of progressive coronary artery disease. It was his job. His work as an information technology expert in a large multinational company was stressful, and recent events in the industry had placed more demands than ever on Ted. When he had the heart attack, Ted realised that it was time to consider altering his current work activities. Just how he would or could do so was not immediately apparent, but the recognition that something had to be done to either reduce his work-related stress or cope with it in different ways became clear in Ted's mind as he lay in that hospital bed inside the coronary care unit.

Ted underwent coronary artery bypass surgery within weeks of his infarction. His recovery from a medical and surgical viewpoint was uneventful, but the experience dramatically altered Ted's life. When he returned to work 6 weeks after the surgery, he did so on a part-time basis. No longer would he spend endless hours at work. Ted also altered his attitude towards work. No longer would he react with anger and frustration at what he perceived to be improper decision making at upper management levels. He successfully changed both his attitude and reactions to work-related demands. While still functioning effectively on the job, he successfully altered his perception of his work environment and his response to it.

After 2 more years as an information technology manager, Ted was offered and accepted a newly created position in his company. This position was more relaxed and enabled him to have more flexibility and control over his work environment. After 3 years in this position, Ted decided to take a lucrative early retirement package when it was offered.

Prior to his illness, the idea of retirement had frightened Ted, because he could not imagine what he would do with his time if he was not at work. His illness changed all that. He took up more leisure activities in an effort to relax and keep physically fit. When his final days at work approached, Ted was ready and able to leave it all behind, eagerly anticipating his new life as a retired worker. Many years later, he remains content in his retirement, relaxed and able to enjoy the slower pace of life that it brings. Ted sometimes reflects back to his illness and wonders what might have happened had he not seized the opportunity to slow down and enjoy life. He remains grateful that his heart attack caused him to reconsider his lifestyle and take action to alter what had become unhealthy work practices.

The story illustrates how a transition to illness can serve as a catalyst for learning and change. Ted met the challenges presented by his illness by seizing the opportunity in a positive manner as he achieved a sense of wellbeing with a life now redefined. Transition is not simply change, but rather the process that people go through to incorporate the change or disruption into their lives (Kralik et al 2006). Success in transition is considered to occur when feelings of distress are relieved and the person feels a sense of mastery of the event that brought about changes in their life (Schumacher & Meleis 1994).

In facilitating successful transitions, it is important that nurses have a basic understanding of how people make sense of life changes and make efforts to cope. Coping is concerned with efforts to manage demands for adjustment and adaptation, and the emotions that they generate (Lazarus 2006).

Coping efforts

The link between coping and transitions is premised on the notion that transitions mean change and this engenders demands for adjustment. When helping to facilitate a smooth transition, nurses need to understand how the patient is attempting to cope with such demands. Coping is defined as 'constantly changing cognitive and behavioral efforts to manage specific external and/or internal demands that are appraised as taxing or exceeding the resources of the person' (Lazarus & Folkman 1984 p 141). Coping efforts include all attempts that are made in response to these demands. Attempts to cope range from denying the significance of an event to mastering new skills in order to meet the demands of the situation. Coping efforts may be focused on reducing the anxiety, mastering the situation, minimising its significance or simply tolerating it.

People make efforts to cope in two identifiable ways. They can attempt to change the situation and meet its challenges by developing capabilities such as self-care, so that it does not continue to be so stressful; or they can attempt to change the way the stressful situation affects them, thus altering their response to it. The first of these attempts is known as 'problem-focused' or active coping, as they address problems directly. The second is known as 'emotion-focused' or passive coping, as they regulate emotional responses. Active coping focuses on the problem at hand, by solving the problem and developing new skills. Passive coping focuses on the emotional response to the problem at hand (e.g. by pushing the problem to one side and thinking about something else) (Lazarus & Folkman 1984).

Active coping efforts are related to meeting the demands of the situation through direct actions. Such efforts include problem solving, seeking further information in preparation for an event, talking it over with a trusted person, finding alternative ways to meet needs and goals that are thwarted by the event, learning new skills, and altering goals or expectations. These efforts directly confront the situation at hand.

Passive coping efforts are aimed at keeping uncomfortable feelings within manageable limits and thinking about the situation in a different way. Examples of these types of effort include avoiding the situation, minimising the significance of the event, distancing techniques, focusing on the bright side, maintaining an optimistic outlook, deriving positive value from negative events, meditating, turning to religion, laughing it off, and using physical exercise to decrease tension. These efforts are aimed at attempts to avoid the situation and are often considered to be a form of denial.

Denial

Denial is frequently used as a means of emotion-focused coping and is effective in containing anxiety within manageable limits. Denial can take many forms, ranging from denial of feelings about an illness to denial of the existence of a disease even when it has been diagnosed and explained to a patient. It is an effective way for patients to manage the perceived consequences of an illness. Denial is often used whenever these consequences are dire for the patient (e.g. when life goals are under threat).

There is often an automatic tendency by nurses to confront and challenge denial, because nurses often perceive denial as an ineffective way of handling an illness. Before challenging denial, nurses need to understand and appreciate the benefits of it.

Denial serves as a buffer for a disturbing and disruptive reality, by allowing a temporary respite from this reality. Because patients will let reality (*their* reality) seep into their awareness at a rate that is manageable for them, the degree of denial is in keeping with this rate. This rate may be different from the nurse's desired rate. Whenever nurses are tempted to challenge a patient's denial, it is essential that the patient's readiness to accept the challenge be assessed. The nurse wishing to challenge denial must ask, 'Is this for the *patient*, or for *me*?'

Cognitive appraisal

The way an event is perceived in terms of its relevance affects how it is handled. In order to cope effectively, people must be able to construct an interpretation of an event so that meaningful action can be taken. The perception of the event, referred to as 'cognitive appraisal' (Lazarus & Folkman 1984), affects coping efforts that are made. Cognitive appraisal relates to how an event is evaluated in terms of its perceived outcome in relation to personal life goals and values, and an assessment of coping skills to achieve this outcome. The appraisal influences the person's coping response.

Coping efforts that are aimed at keeping anxiety under control (passive or emotion-focused coping) are effective in situations that are perceived as futile (i.e. when there is considered to be a lack of control over the outcome). These types of coping efforts usually are focused on maintaining emotional control. When the outcome is perceived as overwhelming or disruptive to major life goals, and there is little that can be done to alter the outcome, then temporary denial or avoidance may be the most effective alternative.

When people believe that they can influence the outcome of an event through some effort, they are likely to take active measures to meet the challenges and demands of the event (active or problem-focused coping). Most people use a combination of both types of coping efforts. People must be able to keep emotional responses within manageable limits through the use of avoidance mechanisms (emotion-focused coping), while simultaneously altering, adjusting and adapting to the demands placed on them by stressful events (problem-focused coping) (Lazarus & Folkman 1984).

People need to be able to employ both types of coping effort. Passive coping efforts assist in maintaining emotional equilibrium by diffusing emotional responses and keeping anxiety under control. Active coping efforts enable people to change and grow through stressful experiences. Although it is a somewhat paradoxical concept, people simultaneously maintain equilibrium and grow throughout life and its transitions. According the Lazarus (2006), there are dangers in treating the two types of coping as separate and competing, as they often complement each other and combine to form the complete coping process.

Lazarus (2006) has warned that an emphasis on the two types of coping, while necessary, may be inadequate as the types refer to only part of the coping process—the cognitive or thought processes. He urges an equal emphasis on the personal meaning of events, especially in relation to the emotions that are engendered when facing life stresses. For nurses to appreciate how a patient is coping, they must also understand meanings that the patient attaches to illness (i.e. their own perception of the event and their feelings about it).

Coping effectiveness

Like transitions, coping methods are not inherently good or bad, and nurses need to view patients' coping efforts within the overall context of the situation (e.g. the effects of coping on significant people in the patient's life). An evaluation of the effectiveness of coping efforts relies on the use of a variety of criteria, expressed in the following questions:

- Does the coping effort help to keep anxiety and distress within control?
- What are the long-term effects of the coping efforts?
- Does the coping effort help to maintain a sense of self-esteem?
- Is the coping effort helping to maintain interpersonal connections?
- Is there flexibility in the thinking about and the approach to the situation?

Effective coping is a sophisticated juggling act, which simultaneously maintains self-esteem and internal equilibrium, sustains interpersonal relationships, assists in securing adequate and relevant information, and promotes autonomy and freedom and flexibility of approach. These factors are important to take into account when nurses are considering the effectiveness of coping efforts.

Some people have a characteristic style of coping that is not effective for the health situation at hand. For example, when symptoms are experienced yet no definitive diagnosis can be made, or is delayed through extensive testing, patients with the tendency to attack situations head on may not cope effectively because they are essentially trying to come to grips with an unknown. As long as there is effort made to determine the cause of symptoms, patients in this situation may be better off temporarily forgetting or denying the possibilities. Focusing on 'what-if' scenarios could lead to increased distress and anxiety.

Consider the following story:

Leanne was 43 years old when she was diagnosed as having a brain tumour. Her symptoms during the 3 years prior to diagnosis had been annoying, puzzling and, at times, alarming to her. But, despite these symptoms, she did not see herself as ill. It was her gradual loss of hearing in her left ear and the subsequent referral to a neurologist that finally resulted in tests that confirmed the presence of the tumour. Initially, she was shocked and frightened, but somewhat relieved when a biopsy showed that the tumour was benign.

Nevertheless, she was informed that she would need to undergo a lengthy and complicated surgical procedure for the removal of the tumour. She began to prepare herself for this. She was accustomed to leading an active and involved life, filled with a job she enjoyed, friends and family, and extensive travel. From what the surgeon explained, Leanne realised that her life would change dramatically in the immediate months following the surgery. Although the long-term prospects for full recovery were hopeful, Leanne realised that there were no guarantees. She understood the implications of her surgery and knew her future was filled with uncertainty.

Leanne's friends and family were amazed by the way she was facing the situation. Naturally, she had periods of distress, anxiety, sadness and even anger. But most of the time she thought about and discussed her impending surgery with an informed awareness of what it would entail. She understood and accepted that her recovery would take time and require effort to relearn some daily functions that she previously took for granted.

In the weeks leading up to the surgery, however, Leanne found that she focused less and less on what was about to happen. Instead, she busied herself by sewing fancy nightgowns so she would at least 'look nice' while in hospital. There was really no more for her to do but wait and try not to dwell on her worries.

Leanne's story illustrates how a combination of efforts is used to cope with an illness. Initially, she focused on 'attacking' the problem by having all the necessary tests and gathering information that would help her to understand the surgery. Once plans for surgery were under way, she coped with the waiting period by focusing her energies elsewhere. Worrying seemed of little value to Leanne at this time, so she coped by 'not thinking too much about' the surgery.

Experienced nurses who are involved with people dealing with major life transitions that are disruptive and sometimes shattering can't help but be struck by the strength of the human capacity to cope. Some people seem to have limitless capacity to psychologically weather the storm of serious illness, while others become overwhelmed and incapacitated by minor inconveniences. The difference is not necessarily related to the seriousness and extent of an illness, but rather to how the person perceives the situation and uses resources in the dynamic process of coping.

Coping resources

Coping resources are personal assets that increase the likelihood of effectiveness as people adjust and adapt to health transitions; as such, they provide protection against distress. Three such resources are of particular relevance in relation to the process of coping with illness. Those selected for review here are resilience, a sense of coherence and social support. Not only can nurses learn to recognise these particular resources, but also they can use an understanding of them when facilitating the process of transition through health and illness. Much like the process of enabling (see Ch 8), nurses can assist people to mobilise and strengthen these resources.

Resilience

People who are resilient have the ability to 'bounce back' in the face of adversity and remain optimistic in the face of threats to their wellbeing (Earvolino-Ramirez 2007, Tugade & Fredrickson 2004, Jacelon 1997). Resilient people are capable of being injured and they do bend under stress, but they are equally capable of subsequent rebound and recovery (Garmezy 1993). They demonstrate minor or transient disruptions in their functioning whenever they are under stress (Bonanno 2004).

Resilience is characterised by a strong sense of self-esteem and self-determination, high flexibility and adaptability, an optimistic outlook that includes a sense of humour about oneself and life in general, which is accompanied by positive, caring, strong social connections and support (Earvolino-Ramirez 2007). Resilient people possess a strong sense of self and they are able to find meaning and purpose in life (Waaktaar et al 2004).

Once considered a personality characteristic that moderates the negative effects of stress (Jacelon 1997, Wagnild & Young 1993), resilience is now recognised as a dynamic process that is learnt and therefore modifiable (Earvolino-Ramirez 2007).

As a process, resilience is a response to stress in which a person directs energy to minimise the impact of stressful events through novel approaches to problem solving and reframing their perception. When faced with negative circumstances, resilient people use positive emotions and are likely to construct positive meaning in negative events (Tugade & Fredrickson 2004). They are able to manage adversity through positive adaptation and maintain functioning at an optimal level (Earvolino-Ramirez 2007).

Resilience is the direct opposite to the concept of vulnerability (Jacelon 1997). When people feel vulnerable, they feel inadequate to meet the demands of a situation. Resilient people feel adequate and are resourceful. Consider the following story:

> Sue Campdon wouldn't rest until she had an answer that made sense to her about what she felt in her breasts. Dissatisfied with what the doctors were telling her about her symptoms, she persisted in seeing more medical specialists. She did not believe that there 'was nothing wrong'. She told herself and her friends, 'Just because the tests have come back negative doesn't mean I am fine. I know there is something wrong and I am not going to settle until somebody does something.' Sue knew she could not afford to take any chances. Her family, especially her three children, needed her.
>
> She was not at all surprised by the diagnosis of cancer when finally a specialist agreed to do a breast biopsy. While the diagnosis and subsequent mastectomy were extremely distressing, at least some action was being taken. She felt strong because she knew what she was fighting. And fight she did. Through every course of radiotherapy and chemotherapy, Sue remained incredibly optimistic. She reassured her friends and family members when they expressed worry or fear. In fact, Sue's fortitude was an inspiration to everybody. When secondary sites of the cancer were found, she was a bit disheartened, but not discouraged. She courageously endured 3 years of cancer therapy and never lost the beaming smile on her face. Her major frustration was a low level of energy and the need to curtail her usual activities. Sleeping during the day was not her style, but she did adjust to the change of pace

in her life. Her friends and family members stepped in to assist with her daily responsibilities of caring for her children.

Despite ongoing treatment, the cancer gradually invaded all of Sue's body. When it became clear that no more active treatment was indicated, some of her friends and family members fell apart. Nevertheless, Sue did not. She remained an inspiration to all. Her cheerfulness was unending. Even though her 'fight' with the cancer was over, she did not feel or act defeated. She enjoyed every day that she had with her family. Sue was thankful for and cherished every moment until the end of her life. When she died peacefully and in comfort in her home, her friends and family members were grief-stricken. But they also knew that Sue and her phenomenal strength and human spirit had enriched their lives.

Sue showed remarkable resilience throughout her illness. Her ability to remain optimistic in the face of adversity, along with her equanimity and responsiveness to others, are demonstrations of the characteristics of resilience.

Sense of coherence

Aaron Antonovsky (1987) developed a theory about how people stay healthy in order to counteract the tendency in healthcare to focus on why people get sick. In doing so, he emphasised the resources that people use to successfully cope with the stresses of life. These resources combine and converge to form what Antonovsky (1987) refers to as a sense of coherence, an orientation towards life's challenges that averts tension and assists in managing life stress and transitions. Such a disposition also contributes to perceptions of being healthy (Souminen et al 2001) and results in a resistance to stress (Hart et al 2006).

A sense of coherence (Antonovsky 1996, Antonovsky 1987) is marked by three attributes: an ability to understand and make sense of situations that happen in life (*comprehensibility*), an abiding trust that things will work out because there are resources available to meet the demands of life's various situations (*manageability*), and the motivation to invest time and effort in life's challenges (*meaningfulness*).

People who have a strong sense of coherence perceive life's challenges as having some structure and clarity as opposed to the perception that life is a series of random events. This is what is meant by comprehensibility. Manageability, the second attribute, is the extent to which a person perceives that resources to cope successfully are available and adequate. The final characteristic, meaningfulness, is the extent to which a person believes it is worth putting time and effort into coping with life stresses (Hart et al 2006, Amirkhan & Greaves 2003, Wolff & Ratner 1999, Antonovsky 1987).

Comprehensibility is the cognitive or thinking aspect of coherence, manageability is the behavioural or action aspect, and meaningfulness is the motivational or feeling aspect. All three—thoughts, behaviours and feelings—come together to form a sense of coherence.

A strong sense of coherence is likely to diffuse the negative effects of stressful situations and promote health in two ways (Amirkhan & Greaves 2003). First, a sense of coherence diffuses negative effects of stress through a perceptual process of accenting the positive. This is referred to colloquially as 'seeing the world through rose-coloured glasses'. In addition to its effect on perception, a sense of coherence results in coping that involves problem solving (active coping), rather than avoidance (often associated with emotion-focused coping). Not only does the disposition towards coherence result in effective coping, it also positively influences health status in general (Hart et al 2006).

Antonovsky's theory has received attention in the nursing and healthcare literature. Studies indicate that a sense of coherence is related to alleviating the development of distress in cancer (Gustavsson-Lilius et al 2007), lowering levels of depression and anxiety in illness (Schnyder et al 2000), remaining healthy and socially connected (Wolff & Ratner 1999), maintaining hope in the face of a diagnosis of cancer (Post-White et al 1996), and returning to work following a liver transplant (Newton 1999). A sense of coherence is associated with quality of life in illness, regardless of other factors such as self-esteem, social support and illness outcome (Dantas et al 2002).

While initially considered by Antonovsky as stable by the age of 30 years, a sense of coherence can be promoted by assisting people to 'restructure' the meaning of illness, framing it in a positive light (Baarnhielm 2004). In this manner, the disposition of coherence could be enhanced through helpful interventions such as finding meaning in illness, or assisting in the development of useful coping methods. That is, it is not a static disposition, but rather a dynamic process that is open to change through life experiences and interactions with others.

Promoting the positive aspects of coping, such as the enhancement of a sense of coherence, rather than focusing on problems, such as medical diagnoses, is concordant with a nursing perspective of healthcare (McAllister 2003). With an emphasis on health, nurses assist patients in dealing with the whole of a health event, not simply managing a disease. They do so as people who are skilled in the practice of comforting, supporting and enabling (see Ch 8).

Social support

Both resilience and a sense of coherence have a common thread—that of the presence of a social network that provides support to the person. Social support involves connection with and mutual obligation to other people; people who experience social support feel cared for, loved and esteemed (Cobb 1976). Social support is based on the assumption that people need to have supportive relationships with other people in order to manage the demands of daily living and cope with life transitions (Norbeck 1988). These relationships serve to fulfil social needs for affection, approval, belonging, security and identity (Thoits 1982).

In Chapter 8, the concept of nurses as providers of support was explored, but emphasis was placed on the importance of nursing care that mobilises other sources of support for patients. In this chapter, social support is referring to these other sources that come from close associates such as family and friends. When these usual sources cannot provide needed support, people look to others (e.g. healthcare professionals) (Finfgeld-Connett 2005).

Support from other people in the form of aid, assistance, personal affirmation and information is necessary when stressful events such as transitions in health and illness are experienced. While support from other people does not necessarily alter the demands of a situation, it does lessen its consequences. Support aids in the response to the situation, provides further capability for meeting the demands, and counteracts feelings of helplessness and hopelessness.

Social support helps people to evaluate their situation realistically, to challenge and alter their existing perspectives, to maintain their self-esteem by reinforcing a belief that they are able to manage and to establish emotional balance by absorbing the impact of strong feelings. Other people's involvement can also serve as a temporary distraction from distress. Cultural and religious rituals, beliefs and practices, largely social in nature, can also provide support during stressful events.

As a result of supportive social networks, people experience a sense of competence, empowerment and wellbeing (Finfgeld-Connett 2005). There is a positive correlation between being strongly connected through a social network and health (Griffiths et al 2007, Östberg & Lennartsson 2007, Ell 1996). That is, people who have a strong, supportive social network remain healthier than people who are socially isolated and lacking in a social network. In addition, social support is positively related to health and recovery from illness (Tomaka et al 2006, Luttik et al 2005, Ell 1996), as well as self-care in chronic illness (Sayers et al 2008, Gallant 2003) and adherence to medical treatment (DiMatteo 2004). That is, family and friends offer needed assistance and emotional support in illness, thus helping in recovery.

Apart from the provision of tangible aid (e.g. physical assistance with getting around), just how does support from other people assist with coping? There are two main hypotheses (Keeling et al 1996). The first is having people around who are caring and concerned boosts a person's self-esteem and sense of security. In addition, other people may provide tangible and practical aid, such as providing transport to medical appointments or encouraging shared, regular exercise. Another way that other people provide support is by helping with the perception and appraisal of a situation (i.e. looking at the world with different eyes). Whether by providing information or offering a different perspective, other people often help with seeing a situation in a new and different light. All of these instances of social support have a positive effect on coping and being healthy.

To be effective in stressful situations, support from other people must be available, usable and suitable to the context. A hospitalised patient's relative who cannot cope with the sights and sounds of a hospital will be of little value in the situation. In this sense, the effectiveness of the support needs to be evaluated in light of the current context. Supportive people must be suitable to the context and available in the situation. A supportive person who lives in another state or country may not be able to provide support, regardless of how helpful this person may be. That is, social support must always be considered specifically within a context (Finfgeld-Connett 2005, Williams et al 2004). And in the case of a person without a network, nurses can become an integral feature of support.

The concept of social support is sometimes presented as all positive, expressed through catch phrases such as 'your friends are your best medicine'. Nevertheless, this is a simplistic notion of social connections because people in a social network can place demands on each other as well as offer assistance. Friends and family can create stress as well as alleviate it. Also, support that is offered must match what is needed (Hupcey 1998). There is no use in a friend offering help that actually hinders (e.g. offering advice that is neither wanted nor useful).

Therefore, social support is a complex, multidimensional concept, which means there are many aspects to it. One aspect is that social support encompasses an acknowledgment of the importance of social relationships. Other aspects include descriptions of social networks and the interrelationships between the people in that network (e.g. an extended family). In addition, there are functional aspects of social relationships, the perceived availability of support and actual support that is received (Keeling et al 1996). Because of its complexity, social support has many definitions (Finfgeld-Connett 2005, Hupcey 1998, Keeling et al 1996). At their most basic level, social connections between people are part of a healthy life.

FACILITATING TRANSITIONS IN ILLNESS

In coping with an illness, patients call upon needed resources. Nurses are potential resources if they are involved, interested and concerned. But nurses can only be resources when they have taken time to understand the situation from the patient's perspective.

Nurses help patients cope with illness by assisting them in many ways; they can help patients to contain uncomfortable feelings, generate a sense of hope and redefine the situation in solvable terms. Perhaps most significant is the way in which nurses assist patients in maintaining or regaining their self-esteem.

Throughout an illness, patients must be able to maintain a sense of self-esteem and their capability for meeting the demands of the situation. Illness often threatens this sense, for example, when there is loss of physical functioning or an alteration in body image. Acknowledging and understanding patients' experiences is one of the most effective ways that nurses can help maintain patients' self-esteem.

Whenever patients become ill, there is a personal assessment of the meaning of the illness. Benner and Wrubel (1989 p 9) express this by stating that, 'Every illness has a story—plans are threatened, relationships are disturbed and symptoms become laden with meaning depending on what else is happening in the person's life'. 'When illness strikes, the illness and possible ways to cope with it are understood in light of personal background meanings, the situation and ongoing concerns in the patient's life' (Benner & Wrubel 1989 p 88).

While it might be easier for nurses to consider a patient's responses in light of what they know about the clinical condition of the patient, they also need to understand how the patient perceives and interprets the meaning of the illness in relation to its impact on their life. The impact and meaning of an event will influence whether or not the event will create anxiety and distress. Some patients view admission to hospital for routine surgery as a minor inconvenience. But a mother of small children who is unable to arrange adequate childcare in her absence may view the same event as a major inconvenience and disruption to her daily life.

Often there is a perception of threat or danger in illness, especially when it begins or exacerbates—threat that the person's life may no longer be the same; threat that there may be an inability to proceed with life as anticipated and planned; and threat in the sense that the body once relied on to perform and work effectively is no longer able to do so. This sense of threat is often accompanied by anxiety and fear, and if these feelings become too strong or pose too much of a disruption, they are met with efforts to keep them under control.

Of primary importance in coping with illness is the ability to maintain emotional balance. Patients must be able to keep distressing feelings within manageable limits in order to cope with other demands of illness. If feelings of anxiety and fear become overwhelming, patients become disorganised or almost paralysed. Passive coping efforts such as minimising, denying, rationalising and ignoring are all examples of how feelings of anxiety are kept in check.

In Chapters 6 and 7 there are references to the importance of recognising when patients are trying to control their emotions and appreciating the importance of not focusing on feelings during these times. The reasons for this are reinforced in this section, and nurses who understand the importance of timing their responses will be able to refrain from discussing feelings with patients who are coping by containing and controlling their emotional responses.

Illness representation

How patients perceive an illness (i.e. how they make sense of it) involves a complex cognitive and emotional process that results in the creation of a mental representation of the illness (Leventhal et al 1980). Referred to as the lay view, or commonsense model of illness, this representation is based on the sources of information that are available to people in order to make sense of and manage an illness event (Hagger & Orbell 2003). The sources include: previous experiences and cultural understandings, information from other people including authoritative sources such as healthcare professionals, and current perception of and previous experience with the illness (Hagger & Orbell 2003).

The illness representation includes five cognitive dimensions: cause, consequences, identity (of the symptoms), timeline and cure/controllability. The dimension of *cause* refers to biological factors such as a virus, as well as psychological ones such as overwork or mental attitude. In this regard, causes can be seen as internal and/or external to the person. The next dimension, *consequences*, relates to the impact of the illness on the person in relation to overall quality of life as well as functional capacity. *Identity* refers to the recognition and experience of the symptoms of illness, and *timeline* involves beliefs about the course of an illness (e.g. whether it is perceived as short-term or chronic). The *cure/controllability* dimension includes the perception of the effectiveness of coping behaviours (e.g. the belief that taking medication, as an active coping effort, will cure an illness).

The original work on illness representation included these five dimensions that are cognitive in nature. More recently, the role of emotional representation (i.e. how a person feels about the illness) has been recognised as equally important (Hagger & Orbell 2003). Illness representation is not only what people think, but also how they feel about what is happening to their health. For example, the diagnosis of an 'incurable' cancer may have different emotional meaning to a 96-year-old person who feels satisfied that they have lived a good life than it would to a 26-year-old person who is the mother of small children. The emotional stakes and impact are different in each of these situations.

Each of the dimensions of illness representation affects how people cope with a health event. In a comprehensive analysis of the research into how illness representation related to coping, Hagger and Orbell (2003) reported there is evidence that there are predictable relations between illness cognition, coping and outcomes. For example, they reported that a strong illness identity (i.e. the recognition and experience of symptoms) was correlated to the use of avoidance-coping methods and lack of emotional expression. Perceived controllability was associated with problem-focused coping, expressing emotions and cognitive 'reappraisal' (e.g. belief in coping capabilities). A chronic timeline and serious consequences of an illness were correlated with emotion-focused coping. Perceptions of controllability and curability were positively related to wellbeing and social functioning, and negatively related to distress.

Consider the following story:

The discovery of a lump on her breast during a routine visit to her GP took Angela by complete surprise. At the age of 39 she felt fit, well and quite happy with her life. Her two sons, aged 8 and 10, were doing well with school and friendships. She was happily married to a loving man and enjoyed an active social and community life. She adored her part-time work as an interior designer, a job in which she not only found enormous professional satisfaction, but also one that had brought her public accolades and honours from peers. Having just learnt that she had been nominated for an international industry award for innovative design, the news of the lump in her breast that same day brought her right down to the ground.

When a biopsy revealed that the lump was cancerous, Angela faced the resultant surgical removal of the lump and radiotherapy with the optimistic and cheerful outlook that pervaded the rest of her life. She did not dwell on thoughts of 'why me?' and accepted the illness as happenstance for her; she did not 'blame herself' for the illness, nor did she dwell on what she might have done to contribute to it. She was mindful of the frequency with which she heard of more and more women experiencing breast cancer and considered that she was just one of the unlucky many.

This did not stop her from taking every action she could to restore her health and wellbeing. She altered her diet dramatically based on advice of a naturopath; she began the regular practice of yoga in an effort to learn to more effectively relax and meditate. Her close and supportive network of friends, family and work colleagues were involved and included in all of her efforts. Because of her outgoing nature, she met many women who had experienced breast cancer and was eager to hear of their experiences, whether good or bad.

In addition to her changes in lifestyle, Angela remained diligent in her regular health checks and yearly mammograms. After 5 years, a mammogram revealed 'suspicious' changes in the breast that initially had the cancer, and Angela was once again confronted with the fear of ongoing cancer and the need to have further treatment. Complete removal of her breast was indicated and she faced the surgery with her usual level of optimism, albeit with an ongoing, nagging fear of cancer spreading throughout her body.

The results of the biopsy of the removed breast and further exhaustive testing revealed that there was no need for ongoing concern. Her surgeon was most reassuring that the cancer had been removed from her body. However, he did recommend referral to a doctor who specialised in cancer treatment, an oncologist. Until this point in time, the medical practitioners caring for her shared Angela's optimism about her future health. While she willingly accepted the advice of her surgeon to see an oncologist, she was filled with anxiety because doing so somehow made her a 'real' cancer patient.

She easily formed a good working relationship with the oncologist, as she had with her other doctors. She was willing to heed any advice that she was offered.

However, the oncologist was not as directive as her GP and surgeon had been. Instead, she presented Angela with a set of statistics and options: she offered little in the way of advice. The oncologist assured Angela that there were no signs of cancer in her body at present, but did inform her that there was a 5% chance that her cancer would recur as there could be 'rogue' cancer cells present in her body even in the absence of any current medical evidence to indicate this was so. The oncologist informed Angela that chemotherapy was an option to eliminate the shadow of doubt, based on the 5% probability. However, she stressed that the decision to undergo chemotherapy was entirely Angela's decision and would not offer advice either way.

Suddenly, what seemed fairly straightforward in relation to treatment became murky and ambiguous. Chemotherapy had numerous side effects that Angela found distasteful, especially the loss of her hair. Her family and friends were reluctant to say what they thought she should do, and she did not place them in the position of doing so as she did not ask. She knew that she alone would have to make the decision.

After a few weeks of serious contemplation and much soul-searching, Angela decided to undergo the chemotherapy. She based her decision on the fact that she had a young family to raise and that she was still young herself. More importantly, she reconciled that living with even a small chance of cancer recurrence could become too burdensome mentally and she preferred to relieve her anxieties by undergoing the treatment. She came to terms with the hair loss and purchased a stylish wig to get her through what seemed to be the most troublesome aspect of the therapy.

She underwent the chemotherapy with a positive attitude, secure in the knowledge that it would relieve a large degree of her worries. It was temporary pain for long-term gain. She was extra cautious in her self-care, taking even more time for herself and her health than was her usual nature.

One year following the chemotherapy, Angela was feeling herself again. Her body had been through much and would never be the same in appearance. She mentally accepted that she would always be considered a 'cancer patient'. Yet she was able to move forward with her life. Receiving the international design award had helped to boost her spirits, but she realised that what mattered most in life was her health and the love of her family and friends. She was proud of her achievement and at ease with her body. She experienced a renewed sense of her life values.

Angela's story reveals how an illness representation affects a person's response to a transition in health. She perceived that the cause was external to her and just a matter of happenstance. Nonetheless, she did take measures to control its consequences through changes in her lifestyle that improved her overall quality of life. Prior to her illness, she was more likely to place the needs of others in priority to her own. As a result of the illness, she was able to match concern about her own wellbeing with her concern for others. While she accepted that she would continue to be a 'cancer patient', she did not perceive her illness as chronic. The measures she took to seek and accept medical treatment were based on her belief that the cancer could be contained, if not controlled. Her abiding belief in the treatment that she chose enabled her to progress with her life in a reassured manner. In summary, her representation of her illness affected how she coped with it.

Themes in illness

Nurses come into contact with patients who are facing a variety of situations. For example:

- a disease is suspected yet unknown or unclear, and the patient feels unwell and is ill but no identifiable cause is known
- the patient's condition is one in which full recovery is anticipated, although the patient may be ill and incapacitated for a period of time
- although recovery is likely, the patient experiences complications that delay recovery and create the possibility of a long-term illness
- an acute condition is present for which the patient will need to make dramatic adjustments and alterations to daily living and lifestyle
- the patient's condition is one that is likely to proceed on a progressive downhill course, leaving the patient increasingly incapacitated and ill
- the patient develops a chronic condition that is usually characterised by periods of illness and periods of wellness
- there is a life-threatening condition that brings uncertainty both immediately and in the future, and
- the patient's condition is one in which death is likely to occur in the near future.

Each of these situations represents a different set of circumstances, and each patient facing the situation will experience it differently. Nevertheless, there are commonalities that specifically relate to how nurses approach patients who are experiencing these situations. These commonalities are uncertainty, vulnerability, distress, loss and grief, and hope.

Uncertainty

Whenever there is an alteration to patients' health status, they are dealing with uncertainty. What is wrong? Will recovery occur? What type of medical intervention will be required? Can the demands of such intervention be met? Will there be a permanent alteration to lifestyle? Will there be pain and suffering? Uncertainty in illness is the inability to assign meaning and to predict the outcomes of a health-related event (Neville 2003, McCormick 2002, Penrod 2001).

Uncertainty is experienced as fear of the unknown, confusion and ambiguity, and is often accompanied by lack of information (Neville 2003), and is the opposite of feeling confident of the way forward and in control. A high level of uncertainty results in emotional distress and anxiety (Neville 2003, McCormick 2002), and is considered to be the greatest single psychological stress when adults experience an acute illness (Mishel 1997). There is substantial evidence that uncertainty influences the psychosocial outcomes in serious illness (Neville 2003).

In understanding the experience of illness, nurses are often sensitive to the uncertainty that is part of the experience. There may be clinical uncertainty in establishing a diagnosis of an illness, or there may be functional uncertainty in understanding what will happen after a diagnosis occurs (Neville 2003). Perhaps the widespread existence of uncertainty in the illness experience is the reason that nurses so frequently offer false reassurance by directing patients not to worry (see Ch 6).

Factors thought to contribute to and influence the level of uncertainty in illness include: severity of illness, specificity of diagnosis, cognitive capacity of the patient, resources to aid in the interpretation, degree of social support, and trust and confidence in healthcare providers (Neville 2003, Mast 1995). Of these possible contributors to uncertainty in illness, the lack of useful and relevant information (e.g. a specific diagnosis) is associated with increasing uncertainty. Therefore, the provision of relevant information by healthcare professionals has been shown to decrease uncertainty. Nurses are seen by patients as credible authorities in health and illness, and therefore patients will turn to them for information to reduce uncertainty (Ch 8).

Furthermore, support from family and friends eases the anxiety that accompanies uncertainty (Neville 2003, Mishel 1997). These people assist in the production of meaning of an illness event in relation to a person's life. This makes the mobilisation of social support (Ch 8) particularly relevant in reducing uncertainty.

Like other aspects of transitions in illness, uncertainty can be perceived as both threat and opportunity (McCormick et al 2006). Patients who perceive uncertainty as a threat are likely to use emotion-focused coping (passive); those who see uncertainty as an opportunity will use problem-focused coping (Mishel 1997). Passive coping efforts, such as not thinking too much about the possibilities of illness especially when a diagnosis is unknown or ambiguous, are effective in reducing anxiety and distress. Active measures such as seeking further information or reevaluating life goals address the uncertainty directly. Nurses need to appreciate and support both types of efforts, as both are effective means of coping.

Vulnerability

Vulnerability is a term that is used in epidemiology to describe groups of people who are 'at risk' of certain health problems (Spiers 2000). For example, Type II diabetes is associated with risk factors such as obesity and a sedentary lifestyle. While useful as an objective measure in population studies that identify 'at risk' groups of people, vulnerability as it is discussed in the context of this chapter refers to the subjective state of vulnerability as individual people experience it.

In this sense, vulnerability refers to the subjective experience in which people make the interpretation that the demands of a situation exceed their personal capabilities for meeting these demands (Spiers 2000). Most people will experience a sense of vulnerability, as it is considered to be part of the human condition (Sellman 2005). However, the vulnerability experienced by people who are ill and in need of healthcare exceeds this fundamental level of vulnerability (Summer 2001). In serious or critical illness, the sense of vulnerability may be great as patients in these circumstances are highly dependent on healthcare providers and therefore unable to meet their own basic needs for survival (McKinley et al 2002).

Coming into contact with nurses can compound patients' vulnerability. The very fact that they perceive their situation as one that requires the use of healthcare resources (e.g. nurses) indicates that they evaluate their own capabilities for dealing with the situation as inadequate. The potential dependence resulting from the need for healthcare may further increase feelings of vulnerability. On the other hand, the fact that patients have mobilised healthcare resources may indicate a sense of competence and resilience. They may still perceive themselves as capable of handling the situation, but recognise the need for professional assistance.

Professional healthcare practices may actually increase a patient's sense of vulnerability (Scanlon & Lee 2007, Rydeman & Törnkvist 2006). For example, when patients are not involved in decisions that affect them, they are denied choice and influence, thus increasing their sense of vulnerability. Providing information and explanations reduces a patient's sense of vulnerability (McKinley et al 2002) and enables them to be involved in decisions that directly affect them (see Ch 8).

Distress

Perceptions of uncertainty and vulnerability can lead to feelings of psychological distress. Distress is characterised by uncomfortable emotions of anxiety, depression, sadness, irritability and even aggression. It occurs when people sense high demand or their needs are unmet; they sense a loss of control and perceive that they are unable to cope with the demands of a situation (Ridner 2004). When an illness makes little sense to a patient (i.e. they lack a coherent 'illness representation', and they feel out of control), distress is likely to be experienced (Fortune et al 2005, Rabin et al 2004).

Attempts to alleviate a patient's distress occur in the context of a trusting relationship (Ridner 2004). The presence of a nurse who listens (Ch 5) provides an atmosphere for the discussion of feelings and the relief of distress (Cossette et al 2002). In addition, praising patients for their efforts to cope, encouraging them by pointing out their strengths and inner resources, and identifying positive aspects of their situation are supportive interventions that help to reduce distress (Cossette et al 2002).

However, listening, encouragement and reassurance alone may not help in the relief of distress. Patients also need information that helps them to understand their illness and to structure its meaning, as these interventions provide the strongest research evidence in relieving distress (Hermele et al 2007, Mishel 1997).

Loss and grief

Losses are often experienced during illness. There may be loss of ability to function, loss of ability to achieve life goals, loss of hope, loss of contact and connection with significant people, or loss of flexibility and freedom to determine life goals. Coping with loss is a process of letting go of what was lost, often accompanied by feelings of sadness, anxiety and sometimes guilt. Patients who are facing or experiencing loss are frequently consumed by this process and therefore are unable to focus their thoughts.

Most often, there is emotional pain as patients come to grips with a loss. There is a tendency to focus on the deprivation created by the loss. Patients whose loss is acute often feel immersed in the experience. When this natural process of healing is allowed to happen, what often follows is a new sense of gain in meeting the demands of the illness.

Grief is a natural reaction to loss. It, too, is a process of letting go, mourning, reflecting, reliving memories, and eventually summoning resources to proceed with life, despite the fact that it may never be the same. Through the experience of grief, people learn to 'let go' and adjust, and eventually adapt to changed life conditions. Grief is a process of closing a chapter of life and gathering energy to begin the next chapter. While there may be energy to begin new phases of life, unveiling the closed chapter is still possible. But this is done as a way of recollecting how it was, of choosing to remember, rather than remaining in the acute pain of loss and grief.

A nurse who understands and appreciates that grieving is a natural process of healing is able to facilitate its spontaneous progression. Through understanding, nurses are able to accept patients' expression of feelings, their reliving and reflecting, as an expected and usual progression towards healing. The process of reflection is often associated with a search for meaning.

It is better for nurses to come to grips, on a personal and professional level, with the reality of the pain of loss. Accepting that loss is an aspect of nursing that cannot be denied or avoided minimises the risk of treating it as something that can be intellectually 'problem solved'. In dealing with patients who are experiencing or facing loss, nurses must be able to assist them with reviving memories of what has been lost. Nurses must be comfortable in allowing patients' feelings to emerge and be expressed. When the experience of loss is shared with and understood by nurses, patients feel consoled and nurtured.

Hope

Throughout interactions with patients in transition, it is also important that nurses maintain a sense of hope that the successful passage through the illness can occur. Hope is an emotion considered to be a vital resource in coping and counteracts feelings of despair (Lazarus 1999). Hope is characterised by a sense of possibility and creates the anticipation of a positive outcome, even when life goals have been altered and there is a redefined future (Fitzgerald Miller 2007). Hope is engendered through a sense of belonging and affiliation with other people (i.e. it is a relational process). It is promoted through the presence of other people who demonstrate acceptance, tolerance and understanding.

During an illness, no matter how serious or minor, a sense of hope must be promoted and maintained. Nurses who demonstrate confidence in patients' capabilities to cope with and manage the situation promote hope. In addition, helping people to find meaning in illness promotes a sense of hope (Fitzgerald Miller 2007).

In the absence of hope, patients often give up, perceiving that their efforts to cope are in vain. This frequently occurs for brief periods during recuperation from a long-term illness or when illness is chronic. If it becomes pervasive, patients may fail to put any effort into recovering or adjusting.

While it is important that nurses maintain a sense of hope, this should not take the form of presenting false reassurance, minimising the significance of patients' distress, or promoting a false sense of wellbeing through deception. At times, nurses may think that deceiving patients is in the patient's best interest. Conversely, deceit signals a lack of respect for the patient's abilities to cope and undermines any trust the patient may be feeling in the nurse. While it may be tempting to offer false hope, such actions are usually counterproductive to the establishment of an effective relationship and successful transition.

Successful transition

Despite the vulnerability, uncertainty and distress that accompanies illness, people are often able to make a smooth transition. Consider the following story:

Sally was returning home from work one rainy evening when she was involved in a low-speed, head-on collision close to her home. Awaiting her arrival at home were her five children, ranging in age from 3 to 12 years, and her husband. The accident left Sally's legs severely damaged and mangled. There was a chance that one of her legs would need to be amputated. Her family, friends and neighbours were shocked and devastated by the news of Sally's condition.

But Sally's outlook was positive right from the beginning of what was to become a long journey back to functioning. She was grateful to be alive, and thankful that she had not sustained injuries to her brain or other internal organs. Although her physical pain was great, especially in the early days after the accident, she remained pleasant and cheerful. Even during the time when amputation of her leg was being considered, Sally maintained that if it eventuated she could find 'other ways of getting around', despite the fact that she may do so 'with only one leg'.

Friends who visited her in hospital in the early days found her attitude uplifting and remarked that they left her bedside feeling better because Sally herself was in such good spirits. Some thought that it was only a matter of time before Sally would plunge into despair, sadness and anxiety about what was happening to her. But this was not to happen, for Sally's outlook remained positive throughout the immediate and long-term recovery periods.

As soon as she was able, she contacted the driver of the other vehicle involved in the collision. She expressed her concern and reassured this young man, who was not physically injured in the accident, that it was just an unfortunate incident for which no one could be blamed. Sally's family and friends rallied around and took care of her family's household needs while she was in hospital. The day she was able to get out of bed and into a wheelchair, Sally began visiting the other patients who were on the hospital ward. She spent the remaining 6 weeks of her acute hospitalisation visiting other patients, bringing encouragement and showing genuine interest in each of them.

Sally's hardiness and the way she approached her situation impressed the nurses who cared for her. She remained optimistic, pleasant and understanding, even when she was suffering excruciating pain. Fortunately, Sally's leg did not require amputation, but she did undergo a long period of rehabilitation during which time she learnt to walk again. Throughout the entire recovery period, Sally demonstrated an ability to cope, had available resources for her assistance, and was able to maintain a realistic and positive view of the situation.

Contrast the following story:

Joanne and Harold had been married 50 years when Harold suffered a heart attack. The heart attack was minor from a medical viewpoint and physical recovery was expected. Harold's hospitalisation and convalescence were following the usual pattern of recuperation, without complications. The nurses in the coronary care unit recognised that although Harold was progressing towards recovery, Joanne remained extremely anxious. Each time she visited Harold, she asked the same questions over and over again. Her questions centred around the theme of Harold's recovery and she expressed fears that he was not going to be 'all right'. She kept focusing on a fear that Harold might die.

No matter how many times the nurses attempted to reassure Joanne, through offering factual, encouraging information about Harold's continued improvement, she remained visibly anxious. In fact, her anxiety seemed to be escalating as Harold recovered. With each visit she appeared more distraught. One day as she was leaving the hospital, Joanne's anxiety mounted to near panic. She began to cry uncontrollably and reached a state where her behaviour became disorganised. She was making random attempts to cope with the situation and her verbalisation reflected that she was having difficulty keeping her thoughts on one track. Joanne needed immediate attention.

Victor, one of the nurses caring for Harold, took Joanne to a quiet area of the ward. He listened to Joanne in an effort to understand what was happening. It took some time to piece together the story that Joanne relayed. Victor learnt that Joanne and Harold had both been survivors of a train crash that occurred many years ago when they were young. They lived through the ordeal, but lost family and friends in the accident. The event brought them close together, bonding them in a common experience that would remain significant for the rest of their lives.

Joanne's major worry now was that Harold would die. She believed the nurses were just telling her everything was all right because they did not want to worry her. She had not been sleeping or eating since Harold was in hospital because 'they always did these things together'. Harold and Joanne's only son was out of town on a business trip that had been delayed because of Harold's illness, but could not be postponed any longer. Many of Joanne and Harold's friends had either died or moved away after retirement.

Joanne's perception of the situation was that Harold would die, despite what she was hearing from the nursing and medical staff. Her major way of coping previously was to talk things over with Harold, an avenue that was not available to her under the circumstances. Joanne's son, a potential source of support, was unavailable to her at the moment. Her representation of illness as fatal, her lack of adequate and usable coping skills, and the absence of available social supports disrupted her ability to make a smooth transition in Harold's illness.

CHAPTER SUMMARY

Whether it is temporary or long term, an illness places coping demands and challenges on people, requiring the use of physical, personal and social resources. Through their interactions and relationships, nurses assist patients in meeting the challenges and demands of illness. Appreciating and understanding the nature of the illness experience—the narrative in the person's life—enables nurses to provide such assistance. Understanding such narratives is considered to be a central aspect of nursing care (Fredriksson & Eriksson 2003).

When forming relationships with patients, nurses must consider how the health status of the patient affects the relationship and their interactions. This chapter has explored patients' health status from the viewpoint of transitions and themes in illness. The many considerations that illness brings to the relationships between patients and nurses create a context for these relationships.

While these considerations may seem to complicate the process of learning how to interact effectively with patients, they also add richness to the experience. While nurses are interacting with patients, they come to appreciate and know the complexity and abundance of human experiences of illness.

REFERENCES

Amirkhan JH, Greaves H 2003 Sense of coherence and stress: the mechanics of a healthy disposition. Psychology and Health 18(1):31–62

Antonovsky A 1987 Unraveling the mystery of health: how people manage stress and stay well. Jossey-Bass, San Francisco, CA

Antonovsky A 1996 The sense of coherence: an historical and future perspective. Israel Journal of Medical Sciences 32:170–178

Baarnhielm S 2004 Restructuring illness meaning through the clinical encounter: a process of disruption and coherence. Culture, Medicine and Psychiatry 28(1):41–65

Benner P 1984 From novice to expert: excellence and power in clinical nursing practice. Addison-Wesley, Menlo Park, CA

Benner P, Wrubel J 1989 The primacy of caring: stress and coping in health and illness. Addison-Wesley, Menlo Park, CA

Bonanno GA 2004 Loss, trauma, and human resilience; have we underestimated the human capacity to thrive after extremely aversive events? American Psychologist 59(1):20–29

Cobb S 1976 Social support as a moderator of life stress. Psychosomatic Medicine 38:300–313

Cossette S, Frasure-Smith N, Lespéance F 2002 Nursing approaches to reducing psychological distress in men and women recovering from myocardial infarction. International Journal of Nursing Studies 39:479–494

Dantas RAS, Motzer SA, Ciol MA 2002 The relationship between quality of life, sense of coherence and self-esteem in persons after coronary artery bypass graft surgery. International Journal of Nursing Studies 39(7):745–755

DiMatteo MR 2004 Social support and patient adherence to medical treatment: a meta-analysis. Health Psychology 23(2):207–218

Earvolino-Ramirez M 2007 Resilience: a concept analysis. Nursing Forum 42(2):73–82

Ell K 1996 Social networks, social support and coping with serious illness: the family connection. Social Science and Medicine 42:173–183

Finfgeld-Connett D 2005 Clarification of social support. Journal of Nursing Scholarship 37(1):4–9

Fitzgerald Miller J 2007 Hope: a construct central to nursing. Nursing Forum 42(1):12–19

Fortune DG, Varden J, Parker S, Harper L, Richards HL, Shaffer JL 2005 Illness beliefs of patients on home parenteral nutrition (HPN) and their relation to emotional distress. Clinical Nutrition 24(6):896–903

Fredriksson L, Eriksson K 2003 The ethics of the caring conversation. Nursing Ethics 10(2):138–148

Gallant MP 2003 The influence of social support on chronic illness self-management: a review and directions for research. Health Education and Behavior 30(2):170–195

Garmezy N 1993 Children in poverty: resilience despite risk. Psychiatry 56:127–136

Griffiths R, Horsfall J, Moore M, Lane D, Kroon V, Langdon R 2007 Assessment of health, well-being and social connections: a survey of women living in Western Sydney. International Journal of Nursing Practice 13:3–13

Gustavsson-Lilius M, Julkunen J, Keskivaara P, Hietanen P 2007 Sense of coherence and distress in cancer patients and their partners. Psycho-oncology 16(2):1100–1110

Hagger MS, Orbell S 2003 A meta-analytic review of the common-sense model of illness representations. Psychology and Health 18(2):141–184

Hart K, Wilson TI, Hittner JB 2006 A psychosocial resilience model to account for medical well-being in relation to sense of coherence. Journal of Health Psychology 11(6):857–862

Hermele S, Olivo EL, Hamerow P, Oz MC 2007 Illness representations and psychological distress in patients undergoing coronary artery bypass graft surgery. Psychology, Health and Medicine 12(5):580–591

Hupcey JE 1998 Clarifying the social support theory–research linkages. Journal of Advanced Nursing 27:1231–1241

Jacelon CS 1997 The trait and process of resilience. Journal of Advanced Nursing 25:123–129

Keeling DI, Price PE, Jones E, Harding KG 1996 Social support: some pragmatic implications for health care professionals. Journal of Advanced Nursing 23:76–81

Kralik D, Visentin K, van Loon A 2006 Transition: a literature review. Journal of Advanced Nursing 55:320–329

Lazarus RS 1999 Hope: an emotion and a vital coping resource against despair. Social Research 66(2):653–678

Lazarus RS 2006 Emotions and interpersonal relationships: toward a person-centered conceptualization of emotions and coping. Journal of Personality 74(1):9–46

Lazarus RS, Folkman S 1984 Stress, appraisal and coping. Springer Verlag, New York

Leventhal H, Meyer D, Nerenz D 1980 The common sense model of illness danger. In: Rachman S (ed.), Medical psychology, Vol. 2, pp 7–30. Pergamon, New York

Luttik ML, Jaarsma T, Moser D, Sanderman R, van Veldhuisen DJ 2005 The importance and impact of social support on outcomes in patients with heart failure: an overview of the literature. Journal of Cardiovascular Nursing 20(3):162–169

Mast ME 1995 Adult uncertainty in illness: a critical review of research. Scholarly Inquiry for Nursing Practice: An International Journal 9:3–24

McAllister M 2003 Doing practice differently: solution-focused nursing. Journal of Advanced Nursing 41(6):528–535

McCormick KM 2002 A concept analysis of uncertainty in illness. Journal of Nursing Scholarship 34(2):127–131

McCormick KM, Naimark BJ, Tate RB 2006 Uncertainty, symptom distress, anxiety, and functional status in patients awaiting coronary artery bypass surgery. Heart and Lung 35(1):34–45

McKinley S, Nagy S, Stein-Parbury J, Bramwell M, Hudson J 2002 Vulnerability and security in seriously ill patients in intensive care. Intensive and Critical Care Nursing 18(1):27–36

Meleis AI, Sawyer LM, Im E-O, Hilfinger Messias DK, Schumacher K 2000 Experiencing transitions: an emerging middle-range theory. Advances in Nursing Science 23(1):12–28

Mishel MH 1997 Uncertainty in acute illness. Annual Review of Nursing Research 15:57–80

Neville KL 2003 Uncertainty in illness: an integrative review. Orthopaedic Nursing 22(3):206–214

Newton SE 1999 Relationship of hardiness and a sense of coherence to post-liver transplant return to work. Holistic Nursing Practice 13(3):71–79

Norbeck JS 1988 Social support. Annual Review of Nursing Research 6:85–109

Östberg V, Lennartsson C 2007 Getting by with a little help: the importance of various types of social support for health problems. Scandinavian Journal of Public Health 35:197–204

Penrod J 2001 Refinement of the concept of uncertainty. Journal of Advanced Nursing 34(2):238–245

Post-White J, Ceronsky C, Kreitzer MJ, Nickelson K, Drew D, Mackey KW, Koopmeiners L, Gutknecht S 1996 Hope, spirituality, sense of coherence, and quality of life in patients with cancer. Oncology Nursing Forum 23:1571–1579

Rabin C, Leventhal H, Goodin S 2004 Conceptualization of disease timeline predicts posttreatment distress in breast cancer patients. Health Psychology 23(4):407–412

Ridner SH 2004 Psychological distress: concept analysis. Journal of Advanced Nursing 45(5):536–545

Rydeman I, Törnkvist L 2006 The patient's vulnerability, dependence and exposed situation in the discharge process: experiences of district nurses, geriatric nurses and social workers. Journal of Clinical Nursing 15:1299–1307

Sayers SL, Riegel B, Pawlowski S, Coyne JC, Samaha FF 2008 Social support and self-care of patients with heart failure. Annals of Behavioural Medicine 35:70–79

Scanlon A, Lee GA 2007 The use of the term vulnerability in acute care: why does it differ and what does it mean? Australian Journal of Advanced Nursing 24(3):54–59

Schnyder U, Morglei H, Nigg C, Klaghofer R, Renser N, Trentz O, Buddegerg C 2000 Early psychological reactions to life threatening injuries. Critical Care Medicine 28(1):86–92

Schumacher K, Meleis A 1994 Transitions: a central concept in nursing. Image: The Journal of Nursing Scholarship 26(2):119–127

Sellman D 2005 Towards an understanding of nursing as a response to human vulnerability. Nursing Philosophy 6:2–10

Souminen S, Helenius H, Blomberg H, Uutela A, Koskenvuo M 2001 Sense of coherence as a predictor of subjective state of health; results of 4 years of follow-up of adults. Journal of Psychosomatic Research 50(2):77–86

Spiers J 2000 New perspectives on vulnerability using emic and etic perspectives. Journal of Advanced Nursing 31(3):715–721

Summer J 2001 Caring in nursing: a different interpretation. Journal of Advanced Nursing 35(6):926–932

Thoits PA 1982 Conceptual, methodological and theoretical problems in studying social support as a buffer against life stress. Journal of Health and Social Behavior 23:145–259

Tomaka J, Thompson S, Palacios R 2006 The relation of social isolation, loneliness, and social support to disease outcomes among the elderly. Journal of Aging and Health 18(3):359–384

Tugade MM, Fredrickson BL 2004 Resilient people use positive emotions to bounce back from negative emotional experiences. Journal of Personality and Social Psychology 86(2):320–334

Waaktaar T, Christie HJ, Borge AIH, Togersen S 2004 How can young people's resilience be enhanced? Experiences from a clinical intervention project. Clinical Child Psychology and Psychiatry 9:167–184

Wagnild G, Young HM 1993 Development and psychometric evaluation of the resilience scale. Journal of Nursing Measurement 1:165–178

Williams P, Barclay L, Schmied V 2004 Defining social support in context: a necessary step in improving research, intervention, and practice. Qualitative Health Research 14(7):942–960

Wolff AC, Ratner PA 1999 Stress, social support and sense of coherence. Western Journal of Nursing Research 21(2):182–197

CHAPTER 10

Challenging interpersonal encounters with patients

INTRODUCTION

There are times when therapeutic relationships may prove difficult to establish, thus challenging nurses in their interpersonal efforts to relate in a helpful manner. There are fundamental skills, such as those reviewed in previous chapters, which assist nurses in meeting the challenges of difficult encounters with patients. But some encounters require the use of more advanced skills. For example, all nurses should be able to respond to patient anger in a helpful manner; they need basic skills of successful conflict negotiation, such as the ability to be assertive. However, dealing with patients whose anger has escalated to physical aggression and even violence requires advanced skills and training. The initial focus of this chapter is on those skills that are most basic to meeting difficult and challenging encounters with patients.

Another area that may prove challenging to nurses is the need to adjust communication with patients in relation to their age and stage of life development. Interacting with a toddler of 2 years requires specialised skills based on the developmental level of the child. Likewise, elderly adults bring a wealth of life experience to an interaction and the central aspects of ageing must also be taken into account by nurses. In addition, family involvement in relation to the care of children and older adults is paramount, as it is often family members who will be communicating with nurses.

Chapter overview

There are times when the challenges of illness and the need for healthcare will create enormous anxiety and distress in patients, and they may act out in anger towards nurses and other healthcare workers. There may be conflict associated with the anger and this can escalate into physical aggression. This chapter reviews how nurses can approach conflict in ways that preserve the nature of the relationship through the use of assertive communication skills. These skills are useful in the successful resolution of the conflict and maintenance of the helping relationship.

The next section of the chapter includes information specific to age-related matters. Included is a discussion of interacting with children and older adults. In the former, emphasis is placed on understanding a child's developmental age. The latter includes information about healthy ageing, as well as problems related to sensory loss or cognitive impairment. Both include discussion of family needs when caring for children and older adults, as family involvement is central to nursing care with these populations.

CHALLENGING SITUATIONS

While nurses are in a prime position to make interpersonal connections that assist people with successful transitions through health and illness, some circumstances make such connections challenging. These circumstances often involve the expression of strong emotions, for example, when patients become angry or demanding. During these times, nurses often feel frustrated in their attempts to help and this can lead to nurses themselves feeling angry because their efforts are impeded by the situation. As a result, there may be difficulties in the development and maintenance of the patient–nurse relationship; and nurses may perceive the difficulty as residing within the patient rather than in the social context of the relationship. That is, the patient is perceived to be 'difficult'.

'Difficult' patients

The behaviours of patients who are considered to be 'difficult' are consistently reported and described in the nursing literature. These behaviours include acting helpless and overly dependent, not cooperating with requests, demanding special treatment, expressing anger towards nurses, making insulting remarks, and threatening, even assaulting, nurses (Wolf & Robinson-Smith 2007). In addition, 'difficult patients' are perceived by nurses to be emotionally unstable, highly anxious, depressed, hostile, aggressive, impatient, unappreciative and non-conforming (Santamaria 2000).

Although documented as 'difficult patients' in the nursing literature, and used by nurses in clinical practice, this term has the potential to stigmatise patients with a label that implies deviance. The term reflects a general acceptance that the problem or difficulty is located within the patient (Macdonald 2007). Such labelling of patients leads to inadequate care because nurses are inclined to distance themselves, blame the patient and withdraw from interactions (MacDonald 2007, Wolf & Robinson-Smith 2007, Olsen 1997). In addition to withdrawing, nurses may respond to difficult patients by enforcing control over them. Patients who are labelled difficult receive the least supportive care and are generally dissatisfied with that care (Macdonald 2007).

Not only is good nursing care challenged by labelling the patient as 'difficult', but also the nurse's wellbeing may be affected. For example, uncooperative patients who thwart nurses' efforts to help can lead to feelings of distress in the nurse. Therefore, both patient and nurse are dissatisfied when the patient is labelled 'difficult' (Macdonald 2007).

Rather than thinking that the patient is 'difficult', it is more productive for nurses to interpret situations that are challenging as difficult interpersonal encounters. The difficulty should be recognised as residing within the relationship rather than within individual patients. When viewed as relationship-based, there is acknowledgment of the social context of the patient's behaviour (Russell et al 2003, Johnson & Webb 1995).

In an effort to understand this social context, Macdonald (2007) explored nurses' perceptions of difficult encounters, rather than having them describe which patients were perceived as 'difficult'. 'Time constraints' were found to be the most important factor in difficult encounters because nurses reported that such constraints prevented them from 'knowing the patient' (Ch 1). Thus, they were challenged in personalising patient care. In addition, nurses in this study recognised that often they resorted to controlling patients, rather than engaging them in care, under conditions of tight time constraints.

During difficult encounters, patients and nurses experience interpersonal conflict (Wolf & Robinson-Smith 2007). Interpersonal conflicts occur when people have goals, needs, wants and desires that are at odds with each other. Difficult encounters between nurses and patients involve conflict because the goals of nursing care seem incompatible with the patients' response. Patients may be in conflict with nurses when they are not cooperative with nursing care. Nurses may experience conflict in relation to being unable to achieve a level of care that they deem professionally desirable.

In order to be successful in managing conflict, nurses must first come to appreciate the nature of conflicts that occur between people.

Interpersonal conflict

Interpersonal conflicts arise when there is lack of congruence between what people in a relationship want and need. A want is a desire for something, while needs include love, belonging, and things necessary for survival (e.g. water and food). Wants and needs give rise to goals and interests. Conflicts of interests exist when the actions of one person attempting to reach their goals prevent, block or interfere with the actions of another person attempting to reach their goals (Deutch 1973, cited in Johnson 2005 p 253). Although conflicts are a natural part of life, they are especially likely when they involve goals that matter and relationships that are valued.

Interpersonal conflicts have their origins in relationships among people and are especially likely when these people are working together to achieve shared goals and assume complementary roles that involve interdependence (Johnson 2005). How each person behaves in the relationship influences the other (see mutuality and reciprocity in Ch 2), although each person will have different perceptions, desires and needs. The combination of interdependence and differing perspectives makes it impossible for a relationship to be free from conflict (Johnson 2009).

From the context described by Johnson, it is easy to ascertain that a patient–nurse relationship has characteristics that are associated with conflict. First, good nursing care is best achieved when patients and nurses have a mutual understanding of the aims of care (shared goals). Second, patients need help and nurses are there to help them (complementary roles that are interdependent). Finally, patients and nurses hold different perspectives by virtue of their individuality as people. Thus, in the context of the patient–nurse relationship, conflicts are likely to occur.

The outcomes of conflict situations can be destructive or constructive. When constructive, conflicts result in greater understanding between people, as each person better appreciates the viewpoint of the other, no matter how different. Constructive resolution of conflict leaves each person feeling satisfied with the outcome and helps to build a better working relationship between them. Destructive outcomes are those in which differences are not appreciated, anger ensues, and the interpersonal relationship between the people involved is harmed if not destroyed.

Conflict in the patient–nurse relationship

From the above description, it is clear how conflicts of interest can occur within the nursing context. Patients may want and even demand more of the nurses' time than they have to offer due to a heavy workload. Nurses may want patients to become independent in their healthcare when patients prefer to remain dependent and want nurses to do everything for them. Patients may want to decide the course of their care, while nurses want them to just 'do as they are told'. When patients are controlled in this manner, the difficulties often get worse instead of better.

Nurses often try to avoid further contact with patients who are seen as difficult, thus attempting to resolve the conflict in ways that are destructive to care. While avoidance is one way of coping (i.e. emotion-focused) with the distress experienced when encountering 'difficult patients', Santamaria (2000) found that avoidance was associated with increased stress in nurses. The results of this study were confirmed by Chang et al (2007) who found that nurses who used problem-focused (i.e. directive) coping experienced less stress associated with nursing work (see Ch 9 for a discussion of coping responses). Therefore, avoiding the 'difficult' patients not only compromises good nursing care, but can actually result in greater distress for nurses.

While it is desirable for patients to negotiate conflict successfully, it is the nurse who is professionally accountable for managing conflict situations. The nurse must assume responsibility for learning the successful conflict negotiation skills. This requires a basic understanding of the nature of interpersonal conflict and negotiation of conflict resolution through effective problem-solving strategies.

A recent study of nurses considered as skilled in dealing with difficult patient encounters found a number of strategies were used (Wolf & Robinson-Smith 2007). The strategies included: demonstrating respect for the patient; focusing on the issue at hand; moving towards solutions rather than focusing on the problem; avoiding becoming emotionally immersed in the situation; and keeping own feelings such as anxiety in check. These are all related to successful strategies in the resolution of conflict, a key characteristic of difficult encounters between nurses and patients.

Strategies to resolve conflict

There are two major considerations in resolving conflict: achieving goals and maintaining a relationship with the other person (Johnson 2009). These characteristics of conflict resolution are synonymous with the basic aspects of communication competence discussed in Chapter 3. Nurses who are competent communicators are able to meet goals of patient care while maintaining good working (i.e. therapeutic) relationships with patients. Achieving these goals requires skills of assertion and maintaining relationships requires responsiveness to the needs and feelings of others. Responsive skills are covered fully in Chapter 6 and termed 'understanding'. This chapter focuses on the skills of assertion.

Each nurse will enter the profession with customary or usual strategies for handling conflict. Directly related to the skills of assertion (meeting goals) and responsiveness (maintaining relationships), these conflict-handling strategies have been classified by Johnson (2009) in the following manner:

- **Withdrawing**. People who use this strategy neither meet their goals nor maintain their relationships with other people. Quite simply, they try to 'bury their heads in the sand' whenever conflicts arise. In relation to communication competence, this style is considered incompetent (see Ch 3).
- **Forcing**. People who use this strategy will meet their goals at all costs, including their relationships with others. They demand that other people cooperate with their goals and are quite authoritarian in their approach. In relation to communication competence, this style is considered overly domineering and aggressive (see Ch 3).
- **Smoothing**. People who use this strategy will ignore achieving their own goals in an effort to maintain the relationship. They relinquish what they want in order to 'keep the peace'. In relation to communication competence, this style is considered to be overly accommodating (see Ch 3).
- **Compromising**. People who use this strategy are willing to give up part of their goals and sacrifice part of the relationship in order to reach an agreement. In relation to communication competence, this style is considered competent (see Ch 3); however, a compromise may leave both parties in the conflict unsatisfied, and not be constructive to either goals or the relationship.
- **Problem solving/collaboration**. People who use this strategy initiate negotiations in order that both people in the conflict meet their goals and maintain a good working relationship. With this strategy, agreements are achieved that benefit each person, and negative feelings engendered by the conflict are dissipated. In relation to communication competence, this style is characteristic of competent communicators, as goals are met and relationships maintained in a mutually beneficial manner (see Ch 3).

People who are successful in resolving conflicts are able to use all five strategies, as each can be effective depending on context. While 'forcing' may be effective when buying a used car, it is not recommended in encounters with people with whom there is an ongoing relationship. If the goals are not important, yet the relationship is valued, then smoothing over the conflict by letting the other person have their way may be effective. However, if personal goals are sacrificed just to 'keep the peace', then smoothing may not effectively resolve the conflict. When the relationship is of moderate importance and the goals of each person cannot be met, or when time is short, compromising may be the best solution to a conflict (Johnson 2005).

Nonetheless, problem solving through negotiation is the strategy that produces the best resolution to conflicts, as this approach reaches goals and maintains relationships (Jordan & Troth 2007). It is the work of true collaboration. This strategy takes the most time and requires skills of both assertiveness and responsiveness. In addition, success in collaboration has been linked to emotional intelligence (Jordan & Troth 2007), as it involves emotional regulation of oneself as well as the ability to understand the feelings of others (see Ch 3). Emotional intelligence is particularly relevant because conflicts often involve the expression of intense feelings such as anger, anxiety and depression.

Each nurse will enter the profession with preferred and sometimes ritualised ways of addressing conflicts in their interpersonal interactions with others. Most people tend to use one strategy most of the time and usually have a 'fall back' strategy when this is not effective (Johnson 2009). The strategies used often reflect the interpersonal skills of the person using them. A high degree of self-awareness and reflection (Ch 3) on how conflict is managed enables nurses to understand their preferred strategies. This enables them to work on developing skills in the use of other, less preferred, strategies.

Studies that explore the strategies used by nurses have demonstrated that they most often use the techniques of forcing, accommodating (i.e. smoothing) and compromising (Skjorshammer 2001, Valentine 2001). These findings suggest that nurses do not employ the skills of collaborating, which is considered to be more effective in conflict management.

Process of negotiation

The process of negotiation is necessary to successful collaboration. There are identifiable steps that, when followed, will result in successful negotiation. Johnson (2009) has described them as follows:

1 **Describe what you want**, by using 'I' statements. For example, 'Sam, I want you to stop shouting at me', 'I would prefer if we could work together in your care', and 'I want you to try and do this for yourself'. In describing what you want, it is important to be specific in your communication.

2 **Describe how you feel**, again by using 'I' statements. For example, 'I am afraid when you shout at me', 'I am much happier when I am able to work with patients', and 'I am more pleased when patients can do things for themselves'. Quite often, feelings are hidden in a conflict situation, so bringing them out helps with its resolution.

3 **Exchange reason for positions**, by explaining what you want rather than assuming an unwavering stance. For example, 'It is difficult for me to help you when you shout at me' (rather than 'I do not tolerate shouting from anybody'), 'Working together will help you get better faster' (rather than 'The Lord helps those who help themselves', and 'Doing this for yourself will aid in your recovery' (rather than 'With an attitude like that, you will never get well').

4 **Understand the other person's perspective**, by listening with understanding and encouraging the other person to express their ideas (see Chs 5, 6 and 7).

5 **Initiate options for mutual gain**, by suggesting how to resolve the conflict. For example, 'We can discuss this further in a quiet way', 'Let's discuss what you want from your recovery', and 'Perhaps if I explained what I want you to do, you can tell me the difficulties you are experiencing'.

6 **Reach a constructive agreement**, by being flexible and adaptable in finding a mutually agreeable solution.

Like communication competence (Ch 3), the process of negotiation involves both the ability to express one's ideas and opinions, as well as to listen and understand the ideas and opinions of others. The former requires skills of assertion and is task or goal focused, while the latter requires skills of responsiveness and is relation focused (see Ch 6). The skills of assertion are reviewed in this chapter.

The skills of assertion

The skills of assertion are those in which a person expresses their needs and wants without denying the rights of others to express their needs and wants. Acting assertively is sometimes confused with being aggressive (i.e. a 'forcing' strategy of conflict management). Aggressive behaviour tramples on the feelings of others and ignores their right to be heard.

Assertiveness is in contrast to being passive (i.e. avoiding or withdrawing) and smoothing strategies of conflict management. Passive people do not express their ideas, but rather allow others to dominate in their opinions. The person does not stand up for their own rights to be heard and respected.

The 'I' messages outlined in steps 1 and 2 of the negotiation process are the backbone of assertive communication, as these focus on the issue at hand and the facts of the situation. An 'I' message does not impart blame on the other person, but rather assumes responsibility for actions and responses. In contrast, a 'you' message, such as, 'You are being unreasonable', 'You are just plain uncooperative' or 'You are just not that interested in helping yourself' blames the other person and will probably fuel the conflict further.

In addition to 'I' messages, there are two other useful assertive techniques that can be employed in the process of negotiation. First is the use of the 'broken record' (i.e. to keep repeating what you want and how you feel). The use of repetition can be effective when feelings are strongly expressed. Next, it is important to keep focused on the issue at hand through the use of 'fogging over', as this prevents getting sidetracked by other issues. For example, if a patient states that 'You are just one of those nurses who doesn't care', rather than engaging in a conversation to the contrary (e.g. 'Yes I do'), it is more useful to simply fog over by saying, 'That may be the case, but I still want you to try to get out of bed by yourself'. In this example, it is irrelevant whether the patient thinks that the nurse cares, and engaging in a conversation about this does not progress the resolution of the conflict.

Sometimes, it is difficult for nurses to be assertive in their workplace. A study by Timmins and McCabe (2005) revealed that nurses were more likely to be passive, rather than assertive, in their workplace interactions. They conclude that conformity to the image of nurses as 'nice people' resulted in nurses behaving in a manner that was accommodating of others. In another study, McCartan and Hargie (2004) found that caring behaviour did not necessarily relate to assertive behaviour, suggesting that a caring, concerned attitude does not preclude nurses from being assertive.

CONSIDERING AGE

Age-related factors also require nurses to adjust their communication and this may prove challenging. For example, when interacting with children, nurses must consider the child's developmental age. The cognitively determined limits this brings to understanding present nurses with challenges of a different kind.

The most obvious adjustments that may be made include altering the level and sophistication of the language and concepts used. Just as nurses must adjust the dosage of medication on the basis of a child's weight, so must communication be altered to adjust for the child's developmental age.

Likewise, relating to older adults can pose challenges to nurses, especially when there is a perceived 'generation gap' between them. Older adults bring a wealth of experience and wisdom to their interactions with nurses.

Relating to children

Relating to children is inherently different from relating to adults for a number of reasons, including the limited amount of experience most children have had in healthcare situations, the negative preconceptions children commonly have of healthcare and healthcare workers, the power differences that exist within adult–child interactions, and the implications of age-related cognitive structures for children's capacity to assimilate and accommodate new experiences and material. It should be remembered, however, that the influence of these factors decreases as infants grow out of childhood and into adolescence. For example, the more powerful position of the adult in the interaction diminishes as children develop a stronger sense of their own identity.

A basic understanding of major theories of child development provides a useful framework for interacting effectively with children and enhances understanding of the major issues involved. In the following sections, a brief discussion is presented of Piaget's theory of cognitive development and Erikson's theory of psychosocial development (Bee & Boyd 2006, Santrock 2004).

Cognitive development

Theories of cognitive development in children are commonly used to track the level of reasoning children demonstrate at different ages. One such theory is that of Piaget, who describes how children's thinking develops from concrete to abstract. Models or explanations based on Piagetian theory have been developed that may assist nurses in understanding how children of different ages tend to perceive and come to terms with different health-related situations.

Methods of explaining health-related events have been developed on the basis of how children come to understand such events. At a certain stage, children's thinking is not developed beyond a concrete level of understanding, which means they are unable to think in the abstract. Children at this stage of development who are diagnosed with cancer will experience difficulty in understanding both their illness and why chemotherapy and other treatments are necessary. How can their illness and treatment be explained adequately when they have a disease that often cannot be seen (they may even be feeling well), and needs to be treated with 'medicine' that makes them feel sicker than they have ever felt in their lives? On a concrete-thinking level, this doesn't make sense.

The work of Bibace and Walsh (1981) provides insight into some of the major issues surrounding children's explanations for the causes of their illness. This model includes two substages within each of Piaget's preoperational, concrete operational and formal operational stages. According to Bibace and Walsh, children within the *preoperational*, or first, stage focus on the physical environment, with cause–effect relationships ascribed to events or factors that are spatially or temporally familiar. Magical thinking and self-centredness are characteristics of thinking within this stage. Bibace and Walsh describe the substages of *phenomenism* (e.g. 'You just get it ... from the bad man, by magic I think') and *contagion* (e.g. 'The wind blows around and around you and you get sick') at the preoperational level.

The second stage within the model, the *concrete operational* stage, contains the substages of *contamination* (e.g. 'You get it when other kids have it and they put it on your face') and *internalisation* (e.g. 'The germs go in your mouth and it feels awful'). In this stage, children are said to move from a position where they attribute the cause of illness to external objects, events or activities (contamination) to viewing the cause as the taking into the body of a harmful external agent (internalisation).

The third stage, *formal operational*, contains the substages of *physiological* (e.g. 'Your lungs get filled up with mucus and stop doing their job') and *psychophysiological* (e.g. 'When you're all stressed out, your immune system does not work properly'). Children in this stage move from a position where illness is viewed as a breakdown in the functioning of internal structures or physiology triggered by external events, to one where the potential role of thoughts and feelings in the production of some illnesses is acknowledged.

Returning to the problem of children who have cancer and are not capable of abstract thinking, discussions concerning the cause of the illness need to focus on external manifestations of their disease. Internal structures and functions of their bodies are outside their understanding. In addition, because children in this group have been found to view illness as punishment for their own misbehaviour (Burback & Peterson 1986), nurses may need to work at dispelling this belief. The need for particular treatments should include a focus on any external or obvious symptoms of the particular cancer, and related to the child's physical environment and priorities. For example, if the child is being given a blood transfusion, a possible explanation would be: 'The new blood will make you pink and strong enough to play with the other children.' The use of 'magical' properties of the treatments ('This is a magic medicine that will make the pain go away') may be used to replace intricate explanations of complex treatments. It would be of no use, for instance, to try and explain links between intravenous therapy, the circulatory system and movement of the medicine to the affected part.

While cognitive developmental level is often closely related to age (sensorimotor 0–2 years, preoperational 3–6 years, concrete operational 7–11 years, and formal operational after 12 years), individual differences in cognitive performance exist within age groups. No recipe-like directions, therefore, are available (nor appropriate) to be used with children of particular ages. Probable cognitive developmental level, and the significance of this for the level of understanding a child *should* display, may be used as a guide only. Applying stereotypes that relate to children of certain ages, gender or temperament is as risky as any other stereotype. Taking the time to talk to children about their major concerns, understandings, expectations and fears is central to meeting the needs of individual children.

Activity 10.1 DEVELOPMENTAL LEVEL

PROCESS

The focus of the activity is the psychological preparation of children of different ages for the procedure of insertion of an intravenous cannula. (Participants who are not familiar with this procedure can either become so prior to the activity or select a potentially painful procedure that is familiar and understood.)

1 Form into groups of four to six participants. Each group discusses preparation of the procedure for one of the following age groups: 1 year, 4 years, 9 years and 14 years.

2 Develop the means of explaining to each child the need for the procedure.
 a How would you describe what is involved?
 b What would you say if the child asked how much it was going to hurt?
 c How would you determine the best means of comforting and supporting the child throughout the procedure?
 d What would be the best measure of the effectiveness of your preparation?

DISCUSSION

1 The spokesperson shares the findings of the group with all the participants in a plenary session.

2 Discuss the commonalities and differences in the explanations that exist across the four age groups.

3 Relate the explanations to the theories of cognitive growth and development.

Previous illness experience

Children who have had previous hospitalisations will probably be better equipped to understand language associated with particular activities (e.g. needle = injection = medication). This experience has ramifications that extend beyond simple links across common terms children will encounter. As children's experiences with aspects of health-related areas (e.g. illness) increase, they may develop a relatively precocious ability to deal with difficult cognitive concepts and require relatively advanced explanations and information.

On the other hand, children of the same age, and for whom acute illness requiring hospitalisation is a novel experience, may encounter a great deal of difficulty maintaining their 'usual' level of cognitive sophistication. In fact, children faced with new and stressful situations may even regress to an earlier stage of development. For example, an 8-year-old child who usually performs at a concrete operational level of reasoning in most areas may regress to a preoperational level when faced with such a situation.

Psychosocial development

It can be seen that children's cognitive developmental stages have a significant impact on their ability to absorb and process new material. Another factor with crucial implications for interaction is the child's stage of psychosocial development. For example, prior to attaining the ability to grasp that their caregiver exists whether or not they are in sight (object permanence), infants are basically content to accept anyone who is available to provide them with the things they require—food, warmth, company and so forth. Once object permanence is obtained, however, and children become attached to their primary caregiver, interactions with others become severely affected. When they encounter strangers or when their primary caregiver disappears out of sight, they become upset and often begin to cry. It is best that nurses, relative strangers, who try to relate to children do so through the child's primary caregiver, and a primary goal in caring for these children involves developing a supportive relationship that facilitates this process.

At the other end of the childhood developmental spectrum are adolescents, primarily focused on developing a strong sense of self and their own identity. Any attempts to develop meaningful relationships with adolescents are doomed to failure if nurses ignore this very real preoccupation. Working through their parents or caregivers would be a misguided approach. Major concerns of adolescents include their peer relationships and body image and, if a pimple can disrupt the life of an average adolescent, imagine the potential impact of a major body change such as the formation of an ileostomy. No matter how necessary the procedure is seen to be by healthcare professionals and the adolescent's family, convincing the adolescent of its worth will involve understanding of the situation from the perspective of the adolescent.

Communication strategies

Table 10.1 outlines specific strategies that can be used when adapting communication to specific age groups.

TABLE 10.1 Developmental aspects of communication
Communicating with infants
Use firm touch and gentle physical contact such as cuddling, patting or rocking
Hold the infant so they can see the parents
Talk softly to the infant
Communicating with toddlers and preschoolers
Interact with parents before communicating with the child
Assume a position that is at the child's eye level
Allow children to touch and examine objects that will come in contact with them
Offer a choice only if one exists
Focus communication on the child, not on the experience of others
Don't use analogies—small children are very literal, direct and concrete
Use simple words and short sentences
Keep unfamiliar equipment out of view until it is needed
Keep facial expression appropriate to activity (don't smile while doing something painful)
Communicate through transition objects such as dolls, puppets or stuffed animals before questioning a young child directly
Communicating with children
Allow time for the child to feel comfortable
Avoid sudden or rapid advances, broad smiles, staring, or other threatening gestures

➡

➡

Talk to the parent if the child is initially shy

Give older children the opportunity to talk without the parents present

Speak in a quiet, unhurried and confident voice

Use correct scientific/medical terminology

Give the correct reason for why something is done or how equipment works

State directions and suggestions specifically and positively

Be honest and let the child know what to expect and how to participate

Allow the child to express concerns and fears; allow time for questions

Use a variety of communication techniques such as drawing or play

Communicating with adolescents

Give undivided attention

Listen, listen, listen

Be courteous, calm and open-minded

Try not to overreact; if you do, take a break

Avoid judging or criticising

Avoid the 'third degree' of continuous questioning

Choose important issues when taking a stand

Make expectations clear

Respect their privacy and views

Praise good points and tolerate differences

Encourage expression of ideas and feelings

Source: Used with permission from Crisp J, Taylor C 2009 *Potter & Perry's Fundamentals of Nursing*, 3rd edn, Elsevier Australia, Sydney (modified from Hockenberry MJ et al 2006, *Wong's Nursing Care of Infants and Children*, 8th edn, Mosby, St Louis).

Communicating with parents and carers

When caring for children, nurses must also be skilled at interacting and forming relationships with parents and carers. In fact, their relationships with children will almost certainly include a relationship with an adult who knows and cares for the child. All of the skills that have been explained in Chapters 5–8 are applicable when interacting with parents. For example, listening for understanding, expressing empathy, comforting and enabling are all relevant when caring for parents and carers.

Of particular importance is the involvement of parents in the care of their children. Nurses must listen and understand the level at which parents want to be involved and participate in the care of their children. Parents do want to be with their children and at least want to participate in care by performing their usual childcare duties, such as bathing and feeding (Power & Franck 2008, Corlett & Twycross 2006). They want their knowledge of the child to be recognised and respected by nurses. Parents are able to participate in care of their children when nurses invite them to do so, discuss the parents' expectations, and provide them with necessary information, especially for the provision of technical care.

Nurses need to assess parental willingness and ability to participate in care beyond the level of basic care. This requires that they be able to negotiate the level to which parents want to be involved (Corlett & Twycross 2006). If willing, then nurses need to offer information, instruction and guidance in order that parents will be able to provide care (see Ch 8). In addition, parents who do participate actively in their child's care need to know that the nurses will take over the care in order to provide parental relief, and when the child becomes very ill (Power & Franck 2008).

Relating to adults

Human growth and development does not end with the identity tasks of childhood and adolescence. Physical, psychological and spiritual growth occurs throughout the whole of the human life span; adulthood is no different. Results of an extensive study of adult development, conducted for more than half a century, reveal that psychological and spiritual growth occur long after the physical body peaks in the early 20s. Referred to as the Harvard study (Vaillant 1977), participants were surveyed from late adolescence to old age (Vaillant 2002).

Healthy ageing is associated with the capacity to meet the developmental tasks of generativity (Erikson 1963)—that is, the capacity to pass the 'baton' to the next generation. People who meet the task of generativity take pleasure and pride in the wisdom that comes with ageing. They willingly share this knowledge with the next generation, and achieve a sense of integrity and peace in their final years. Generativity seems to be the key (Vaillant 2002).

Older people who have a strong sense of coherence (see Ch 9) manage their life well, cope with everyday living and find meaning in life (Neikrug 2003). While most people are capable of healthy ageing, societies that revere youth and longevity may stereotype older people as useless. Such a view is culturally dependent, with some social groups holding their older members in great reverence.

Young adult nurses may be challenged in their interactions with older adults whose life experience has been different from their own. Adults who are a lot older than the nurse may have worldviews that have been developed by experiences that for the nurse are nothing more than a page in a history book. Young adults are likely to be looking forward to a life yet unknown, yet eagerly anticipated, while taking stock and making meaning of one's life through looking back are aspects of growth in late adulthood. Such different perspectives can create a generational gap in understanding each other.

Activity 10.2 THE GENERATION EFFECT

PROCESS

Consider the following brief life sketches.

Elizabeth Eden Elizabeth is 86 years old in the year 2004. She has lived through a series of major world crises. She was born in the period following World War I, when people were enjoying life to the full, believing that peace and prosperity were their birthright. These hopes were dashed by the Great Depression, which occurred when she was a teenager, and World

War II, which occurred when she was in her twenties. Like many others who lived through the Depression of the 1930s, Elizabeth suffered extreme economic privations. Her father was out of work. She managed to do some casual piecework, which was very poorly paid, but she was, nevertheless, grateful for it. She learned to scrimp and make the most of limited amounts of food and clothing, and to waste nothing. She married Tom when she was in her mid-twenties.

A few years later, World War II started. Tom, along with many other young husbands, went to war. Many soldiers' wives, including Elizabeth, were forced to work outside the home, taking on the work that the men had to leave. Elizabeth and Tom's first child was conceived during Tom's military leave. She had to manage the child virtually as a single working mother, while at the same time coping with her anxiety about Tom, who had been taken as a prisoner of war. Tom did not meet his child until he returned from a prisoner-of-war camp in 1945. After the war, their two other children were born.

After the war was over, Elizabeth gratefully retreated to the home to finish bringing up her children, and Tom returned to his former occupation. When the women's movement gained momentum in the 1970s, Elizabeth had little sympathy for the aim of equal employment opportunities for women and felt that women were better off not working outside the home.

Mark Yates Mark was born in 1952, during the postwar baby boom. His childhood was spent during a period of economic affluence and full employment. He took economic security for granted and expected to walk straight into a job when he completed his education.

In contrast to Elizabeth, whose life spanned a number of major world crises, Mark has been beset by a number of more indefinite concerns about the future of the world. The Cold War between the Soviet Union and the United States was at its peak during his youth and, as he grew up, Mark became increasingly aware of the possibility of the world being devastated by nuclear war. He was a teenager during the period of Australia's involvement in the Vietnam War and became accustomed to news reports of the suffering and devastation suffered by the Vietnamese. During his adolescence, there was increasing public discussion of the effects of overpopulation on the world and the environment. Drugs were rife in schools, and the crime rate was increasing at a rate that was causing public alarm. The revolution in sexual attitudes and freedom was well under way.

Many of his friends, having grown up with security, shunned the exhortations of their parents to get 'a steady job'. They were vocal in their cynicism about national and international leaders.

DISCUSSION

1 Divide into small groups and discuss how Elizabeth's and Mark's views of life might differ. List these differences on large sheets of paper and post them around the room.

2 In a large group, discuss how world events may have shaped the views of people who are now in their sixties and seventies. How might they be different from people who are now in their twenties and thirties?

3 What do you fear most about growing old? What do you look forward to most?

4 How can nurses reduce interaction difficulties with their patients that are due to a generation gap?

Losses associated with ageing

The process of ageing is associated with many losses, such as the death of loved ones and the realisation that one's own death is closer. These are social in nature. Some, such as the reduction in social roles and social status, are a direct result of negative social attitudes towards older people. Many older people face a decline in economic status as they retire from paid employment and become dependent on a government pension or superannuation.

The most obvious losses are sensory, with loss of vision and hearing being most pronounced. The loss of hearing has been shown to affect over 50% of middle-aged and older adults, and negatively affect their quality of life (Dalton et al 2003).

Activity 10.3 EXPERIENCING SENSORY DEFICITS

PROCESS

1 Find an old pair of sunglasses. Cut out a piece of clear contact adhesive (the kind that is used for covering books) and attach it to the lens of the glasses. This should have the effect of allowing in some light but reducing visual acuity. Wear a pair of thin cotton gloves to simulate loss of skin sensation. Wrap elastic bandages firmly around your knees and ankles to simulate a feeling of stiffness in your joints. Place cotton wool plugs in your ears.

2 Spend at least one hour trying to carry out your normal daily activities.

DISCUSSION

1 How difficult was it to carry out your usual activities with impaired sensory input and impaired mobility?

2 How much do you think the vagueness of old people could be attributed to difficulties in sensory perception?

Interacting with the person with a hearing impairment

There are a number of guidelines that can be applied to facilitate interactions with patients who experience hearing difficulties. Most people can lip read to some extent if they can see the speaker's mouth, so nurses should stand where the patient can see them. It is important to speak clearly, articulating the words well and refraining from shouting. If the patient does not understand, the nurse probably needs to try rephrasing sentences, using different words and shorter sentences. Soft-sounding consonants such as 'p' and 'f' are difficult to detect; therefore, using words that avoid these might be helpful. Nurses can be creative in using any means at their disposal to communicate meaning, such as using pictures, or gestures, or writing or drawing.

When nurses are interacting with patients who wear hearing aids, additional techniques are necessary to promote effective interaction. Hearing aids assist individuals with specific types of hearing impairments; they do not restore normal hearing. They are much more sensitive to background noise than natural hearing. When conversing with a patient with a hearing aid, nurses should try to find a quiet room where there are no other conversations going on in the background. Just hitting a glass on a table or clicking a pen can be a source of interference. Using hearing aids effectively requires perseverance on the part of the user and cooperation on the part of others.

Interacting with the person with a cognitive impairment

Cognitive impairment, such as poor attention and concentration and poor memory and retention of information, is often present in older adults. It is important that nurses do not expect all older people to be cognitively impaired, yet it is likely that they will care for people in this state. Impairment of this type affects the person's ability to communicate, as they are frequently confused. Cognitive impairment can be the result of dementia or delirium, and these are specific clinical conditions that require advanced skills and training. Nonetheless, there are a few approaches that all nurses need to know in the care of the cognitively impaired.

First, when communicating with people who are cognitively impaired, it is important to remember that the person has feelings and their affective self often stays intact. They are easily frightened and can become quite distressed when their confusion increases. Therefore, recognising their feelings (Ch 6) is often helpful in establishing interpersonal contact. Eye contact, a calm manner, addressing the person by name and speaking slowly are essential (Bulechek et al 2008) to making such contact.

It is also important to avoid frustrating the person by quizzing them, especially about their orientation to time and place, as this may increase their frustration. Likewise, their ability to retain new information is impaired, so nurses should not expect cognitively impaired persons to be able to easily recall events and conversations. They should never be confronted with their memory loss (e.g. by saying, 'I just told you that'). Most importantly, when a patient is confused, a nurse should never argue with the patient's faulty thinking. Rather, a nurse should listen to the underlying feeling being expressed. For example, if a patient says to a nurse, 'That doctor is out to get me', it might be tempting to counter this thought by saying, 'That is not so'. Rather, the nurse should reflect the feeling that is being expressed (e.g. by saying, 'That sounds really frightening').

Nurses need an enormous amount of patience when patients are cognitively impaired, especially when being asked the same questions over and over again. Answer the questions in a matter of fact manner and do not confront cognitively impaired people with their losses. It is far better to focus on their feelings and perceptions than to confront them with reality.

As much as possible, the nurses who care for cognitively impaired people should be consistent, as new people and faces only add to their frustration. Consistency in caregivers also aids in the ability to 'know the patient' and understand their unique life history. This makes family involvement essential when caring for cognitively impaired older people.

Consider the following story

Maria, an 86-year-old woman, was brought into the emergency department of a busy metropolitan hospital by her daughter and husband. Although diagnosed with dementia, her behaviour over the past day had become markedly different. She was more confused than usual, slurring her speech and dismantling all of her favourite flower arrangements in her home.

While in the emergency department, she was left alone on a stretcher in the hallway as she waited for diagnostic tests to be completed. Her daughter and husband were told to wait elsewhere. Maria perceived that she was left 'for hours' and that no one was there to assist her and she had to run up and down the corridor looking for help. She became quite anxious and agitated about this situation; her family members could have anticipated this reaction. They would have preferred to be able to remain with her in order to reassure and orient her, especially because she had not been left alone for a number of years. By the time they returned to her bedside, Maria was in a state of near panic. While her perceptions were not real, the associated emotions were very real, and avoidable in their opinion.

After the tests were completed, Maria was admitted to hospital with a suspected stroke. She was placed on routine neurological observations, which included questions about her orientation and recollection of facts such as her age and number of years married. Prior to her hospitalisation, she was having difficulty remembering these facts, thus rendering any findings of the mental status examinations invalid. Had there been an assessment of her baseline functioning (prior to hospitalisation) in the form of history taking from her family members, staff would have realised that routine testing in this would not yield accurate results.

The continuous neurological observations were anxiety provoking for Maria, as she realised that she was being 'tested' and was failing because she could not remember facts such as her age. She expressed her concerns to her family on numerous occasions, and became increasingly anxious about all the questions she was being asked. Had the nursing staff involved the family in Maria's care, they would have realised her fear of being alone. More importantly, they would have realised that the results of their neurological testing were invalid as Maria had not been able to remember her age, how many years she had been married, or the current date, for a number of years. Quizzing her in this manner not only produced invalid results, but added to her distress.

Relating to family members of older people

As with caring for children, when nurses are caring for older people they must consider the involvement of family members in that care, especially when a particular family member has been the primary carer for that person. Involving family members in care situates the patients within the broader context of their life, not just as an individual. Such involvement requires good communication skills and the development of a trusting relationship. Of utmost importance is the recognition of the uniqueness of the patient, and family members are often able to provide such insights.

In a recent systematic review of research, Haesler et al (2007) found that the evidence suggests that while nurses recognise that inclusion of families in care is important, their involvement remains problematic. Family members want to be involved, but are often reticent because they perceive nurses as unapproachable, and nurses are not always encouraging of such involvement. Issues embedded into the culture of care delivery, with nurses maintaining power and control, and organisational factors such as workload and staff turnover (see Ch 11) affected the level of involvement of families. Family members were expected to 'fit in' to the structure of the care, and nurses maintained control of that care because they felt responsible.

There are a number of communication skills that have been shown to produce productive relationships with families of older people (Haesler et al 2007). Initially, it is important that the nurse approach family members in an open, honest and caring manner. The skills of active listening (Ch 5) and understanding (Ch 6) were of particular relevance, as these encourage family members to express their needs. Of central importance is the provision of information and support (Ch 8), especially with the nurse initiating such provision and not waiting for family members to make the first move. Thus, the skills of this book are as relevant to the involvement of families as they are to the care of patients.

Organisational factors were shown to affect the quality of relationships with families. Workload, adherence to routines and a medical model of care were impediments to communication (Haesler et al 2007). Working collaboratively with families, and involving them in care, affected both the satisfaction with care and quality of care in organisations that used this approach.

CHAPTER SUMMARY

Challenges in helping people make transition through illness have been presented as difficulties that result in conflict within the social context of the patient–nurse relationship. Conflict has been reviewed and strategies for the successful resolution of conflict have been presented, with an emphasis placed on collaboration through negotiation. Skills necessary for collaboration have placed particular emphasis on assertion, as these have not been previously reviewed in other chapters.

The importance of adjusting communication, especially those of explanations about illness, to the age of the patient has been reviewed in light of developmental milestones throughout childhood. A brief review of some of the factors related to ageing that affect interactions has been undertaken. The importance of including family members and carers has been emphasised.

While these considerations may seem to complicate the process of learning how to interact effectively with patients, they also add richness to the experience. As nurses interact with patients, they come to appreciate and know the complexity and abundance of human experiences relating to crisis and illness.

REFERENCES

Bee H, Boyd D 2006 The developing child, 11th edn. Allyn & Bacon, Boston, MA

Bibace R, Walsh ME 1981 Children's conceptions of illness. In: Bibace R, Walsh ME (eds), Children's conceptions of health, illness and bodily functions, pp 31–48. Jossey-Bass, San Francisco, CA

Bulechek GM, Butcher HK, Dochterman JM 2008 Nursing interventions classification (NIC), 5th edn. Mosby Elsevier, St Louis

Burback DJ, Peterson L 1986 Children's concepts of physical illness. A review and critique of cognitive developmental literature. Health Psychology 5:307–325

Chang EML, Bidewell JW, Huntington AD, Daly J, Johnson A, Wilson H, Lambert VA, Lambert CE 2007 A survey of role stress, coping and health in Australian and New Zealand hospital nurses. International Journal of Nursing Studies 44:1354–1362

Corlett J, Twycross A 2006 Negotiation of parental roles within family-centred care: a review of the research. Journal of Clinical Nursing 15:1308–1316

Crisp J, Taylor C 2009 Potter & Perry's fundamentals of nursing, 3rd edn. Elsevier Australia, Sydney

Dalton DS, Cruikshank KJ, Klein EK, Wiley TL, Nondahl DM 2003 The impact of hearing loss on quality of life in older adults. The Gerontologist 43(5):661–669

Erikson EH 1963 Childhood and society, 2nd edn. Norton, New York

Haesler E, Bauer M, Nay R 2007 Staff–family relationships in the care of older people: a report on a systematic review. Research in Nursing and Health 30:385–398

Johnson DW 2009 Reaching out: interpersonal effectiveness and self actualization, 10th edn. Allyn and Bacon/Merrill, Boston, MA

Johnson M, Webb C 1995 Rediscovering unpopular patients: the concept of social judgement. Journal of Advanced Nursing 21:466–475

Jordan PJ, Troth AC 2007 Emotional intelligence and conflict resolution in nursing. Contemporary Nurse 13:94–100

Macdonald M 2007 Origins of difficulty in the nurse–patient encounter. Nursing Ethics 14(4):510–521

McCartan PJ, Hargie ODW 2004 Assertivesness and caring: are they compatible? Journal of Clinical Nursing 13:707–713

Neikrug SM 2003 Worrying about a frightening old age. Aging and Mental Health 7(5):326–333

Olsen DP 1997 When the patient is the problem: the effect of patient responsibility on the nurse–patient relationship. Journal of Advanced Nursing 26:515–522

Power N, Franck L 2008 Parent participation in the care of hospitalized children: a systematic review. Journal of Advanced Nursing 62(6):622–641

Russell S, Daly J, Hughes E, Op't Hoong C 2003 Nurses and 'difficult' patients: negotiating non-compliance. Journal of Advanced Nursing 43(3):281–287

Santamaria N 2000 The relationship between nurses' personality and stress levels reported when caring for interpersonally difficult patients. Australian Journal of Advanced Nursing 18(2):20–25

Santrock JW 2004 Child development, 10th edn. McGraw Hill, Boston, MA

Skjorshammer M 2001 Co-operation and conflict in hospital: interprofessional difference in perception and management of conflict. Journal of Interprofessional Care 15:7–18

Timmins F, McCabe C 2005 Nurses' and midwives' assertive behaviour in the workplace. Journal of Advanced Nursing 51(1):38–45

Vaillant G 1977 Adaptation to life. Little Brown, Boston, MA

Vaillant G 2002 Ageing well. Scribe Publications, Melbourne

Valentine PEB 2001 A gender perspective on conflict management strategies of nurses. Journal of Nursing Scholarship 33:69–74

Wolf ZR, Robinson-Smith G 2007 Strategies used by clinical nurse specialists in 'difficult' clinician–patient situations. Clinical Nurse Specialist 21(2):74–84

CHAPTER 11

Building a supportive workplace

INTRODUCTION

The central premise of this book is that effective communication and therapeutic relationships between patients and nurses are at the heart of good nursing care. This is because care can be personalised as a result of the process of 'knowing the patient' through communicating and relating. Delivery of personalised care is a long-held value in the nursing profession, and nurses recognise that interactional processes such as comforting, supporting and enabling patients are primary ways that nurses make a difference to patients.

Current workload task demands, such as administrative duties not directly related to nursing care, often prevent nurses from having time to interact meaningfully. When time spent with patients is in short supply, the quality of care suffers, and so do nurses. In the absence of a work environment that supports patient interaction as a central nursing activity, even the most interpersonally skilled nurses will find it difficult to 'know the patient'. Therefore, consideration must be given to the organisational environment of nursing care.

Organisational arrangements are in place for the smooth operation of complex systems, such as hospitals for acutely ill patients. Such arrangements may impact on patient–nurse relationships. For example, when nursing work is organised in such a way that the patient and nurse rarely see each other on more than one occasion in the course of a health event, then the depth of mutual understanding may be restricted by limited opportunity to get to know each other. The patient in this situation may need continuity of interaction with a nurse. For example, for a young woman attempting to cope with life after having a mastectomy, her needs would be best served by organisational arrangements that enable nurse and patient to get to know each other on more than a clinical level.

Not only might such arrangements impact on the capacity of the nurse to form therapeutic patient–nurse relationships, but there is mounting evidence that organisational arrangements may also impact, for better or worse, on the nurse's wellbeing and the quality of healthcare in general. The emphasis of this chapter is just such arrangements, with a focus on developing effective working relationships with colleagues in healthcare in an effort to support therapeutic relationships with patients. The development of good working relationships requires the use of the same skills as those of therapeutic interactions, especially those of listening, understanding and exploring.

Chapter overview

This chapter firstly explores nursing as a stressful occupation. It cites the main sources of job-related stress as being the work itself and the organisational environment of nursing work (e.g. conflicts with colleagues). Potential consequences of nurse stress are then reviewed, including burnout and job dissatisfaction. The importance of the organisational environment as it relates to job stress is then reviewed with evidence from 'magnet' hospital research to support an example of an 'ideal environment'. The interaction between nurse stress and professional relationships with colleagues is explained next, with an explanation of how such interactions are often conflicted. Nurse–doctor interaction is explored next, and includes a discussion of traditional doctor–nurse relationships. Dealing with workplace conflict is reviewed, especially in relation to the need for assertive skills (see Ch 10). Ways of coping with job-related stress are reviewed, with an emphasis on colleagues as an effective coping resource. Finally, there are suggestions of how to promote supportive colleague relationships through organisational arrangements. The importance of nursing leadership in developing and sustaining supportive colleague relationships is emphasised.

STRESS AND NURSING

Stress is a complex phenomenon that encompasses more than simply the factors that provide its stimulus (stressors). Stress is a transactional process involving a complex interplay between perceived demands of the environment and the perceived resources for meeting these demands (Lazarus & Folkman 1984). In this regard, there is always a degree of stress in living beings as they adjust and adapt to the demands of a dynamic environment. Stress becomes troublesome when a person perceives that a demand is potentially harmful, may result in personal loss, is threatening or challenging *and* that resources for meeting the demand are inadequate, unavailable, unusable or inappropriate in the situation.

Personal appraisal (perception) is critical in the experience of stress because it determines whether the demand is interpreted as harmful or threatening, and whether internal and external resources for coping are seen to be accessible and adequate. For example, a nurse working in a critical care area may be required to wean a patient off a mechanical ventilator (demand). An experienced critical care nurse, who has weaned many patients from ventilators, may perceive this situation as relatively benign (no distress). On the other hand, a nurse who has recently completed an advanced course in critical care nursing may view the same situation as a challenge and call on available coping resources such as knowledgeable problem solving and more experienced nurses. A newly graduated nurse, with little or no experience and education in critical care, may appraise the same situation as a threat for which there are no capabilities or resources. The same event results in three different responses according to how it is perceived. It is not an event itself (stressor), or the personal resources and coping capabilities alone that create stress, but rather their dynamic combination (see Ch 9 for a full discussion of coping).

Sources of nurse stress

The provision of nursing care is both physically and emotionally demanding; therefore, stress in nursing is accepted as part and parcel of the profession. Investigations into the main causes of nursing stress have revealed similar results over a number of years. The studies show that there are stress sources that relate directly to nursing work and those that relate to the work environment (Chang et al 2007, Lambert et al 2004, McVicar 2003, Bennett et al 2001, Stordeur et al 2001, Bratt et al 2000, Demerouti et al 2000, Hillhouse & Adler 1997, Kushner et al 1997, Dunn et al 1994). The main source of stress in nursing is related to demanding workloads, with nurses experiencing the pressure of too much to do in too little time.

Workload

Workload, as a source of stress in nursing, means that nurses experience the demands of having to do more and more for patients, with inadequate resources to meet the demands. Staff shortages and increasingly ill patients are part of this stressor (Laschinger et al 2003), and job satisfaction is associated with patient-to-nurse ratios (Aiken et al 2002b). A demanding workload can result in nurses being torn between that which is most important in a professional sense and that which is most urgent and pressing in an organisational sense. For example, nurses on a busy surgical unit might find themselves transporting patients to and from the operating theatre instead of teaching patients and their families how to care for themselves postoperatively. Transporting patients is an organisational demand, while teaching and counselling patients are professional demands. When these demands come into conflict, the organisational demands often take precedence. Nurses report being stressed by management tasks that take them away from the bedside (Aiken et al 2001). Job-related stress results because nurses are not able to fulfil their professional role and uphold the values and standards of the profession.

Lack of time to fulfil a professional role has been termed 'moral stress' (Lutzen et al 2003, Sundin-Huard & Fahy 1999). This type of stress results from internal conflicts experienced by nurses when institutional constraints prevent nurses from acting in what they believe is the best interest of patients.

Work environment

Stress in nursing is not only generated from the work itself, including workload, but also from factors related to the work environment. Sources of stress other than workload include: dealing with death and dying; lack of professional autonomy and control; conflict relationships with colleagues; lack of leadership support; and poor group cohesion in the workplace (Chang et al 2007, Lambert et al 2004, McVicar 2003, Bennett et al 2001, Stordeur et al 2001, Bratt et al 2000, Demerouti et al 2000, Hillhouse & Adler 1997, Kushner et al 1997, Dunn et al 1994). Organisational factors that contribute to nurse satisfaction are primarily related to less than supportive professional interactions with colleagues, as well as a lack of professional autonomy. That is, interpersonal relationships in the workplace contribute to nurse stress, and these include relationships with nursing colleagues as well as other professionals.

Coping with work stress

As reviewed in Chapter 9, there are two types of coping efforts to deal with stress. There are efforts aimed at meeting or altering the demands of the situation through problem-focused coping, and efforts designed to minimise the impact of stress through emotion-focused coping (Lazarus & Folkman 1984). Coping efforts that are problem-focused include creative problem solving and reappraisal of the situation. For example, seeking informational support from more experienced colleagues, or locating research evidence to support clinical decision making in situations that are ambiguous and challenging, are effective problem-focused coping efforts. When situations are stressful but cannot be altered (e.g. an untimely death of a young person in a preventable accident), emotion-focused coping may serve best. Emotion-focused efforts, aimed at keeping anxiety in check, include distancing, denial and avoidance.

While both types of coping may be effective in dealing with job stress in nursing, there is research evidence to suggest that problem-focused coping is associated with better mental health and job satisfaction (Chang et al 2007, Lambert et al 2004, Healy & McKay 2000, Santamaria 2000). Seeking advice and support and 'talking it over with someone who could do something' are both active coping strategies that have been shown to lower stress in situations of moral distress (McDonald 1999) and in cases of bullying (Quine 2001).

Consequences of work stress

One reason for the continued interest in work stress in nursing is that stress is associated with job satisfaction; higher levels of stress are linked with lower levels of satisfaction and job turnover (Zangaro & Soeken 2007, Irvine & Evans 1996, Blegen 1993). Workload stress, along with disempowering leadership, poor colleague relationships and lack of autonomy have all been implicated in poor job satisfaction and subsequent turnover in nursing staff (Coomber & Barriball 2007, Hayes et al 2006). In a recent survey, 40% of hospital-based nurses indicated that they were dissatisfied with their work (Aiken et al 2001).

Current structural arrangements in many healthcare facilities can be at odds with nursing values of patient-centred care, placing the true meaning of 'caring' in nursing (see Ch 1) at risk. In a recent guest editorial, Corbin (2008) addresses this risk by asking, 'Is caring a lost art in nursing?', and concludes that caring, while not lost, is 'an art that is at odds with many of the conditions under which nurses are working today' (p 163). Such conditions generate discontent among nurses, as the delivery of quality patient-centred care has been shown to be an enduring value in professional nursing and a major contributor to job satisfaction (Schmalenberg & Kramer 2008, Smith et al 2005). When workloads are such that nurses are unable to deliver the kind of care they deem of high quality, they experience stress.

Burnout is a term used to describe an accumulation of work stress over time. It is a phenomenon that is particularly relevant to people in a service profession such as nursing. In nursing, burnout is often due to the demanding and emotional nature of the relationships between nurses and their patients (Maslach & Schaufeli 1993). People who hold high ideals and standards are at most risk of burning out because they may never be able to achieve the standards that they set for themselves. Once burnout occurs, nurses feel as if there is 'nothing left to give', and this is described as emotional exhaustion. In addition, nurses who are burnt out treat patients like objects, not because they are being deliberately uncaring, but rather because they are protecting themselves from further stress through acknowledging patients' subjective realities and needs. They can tend to the tasks without making reference to the idiosyncratic ways of individual patients. That is, they function in a disengaged manner as a way of protecting themselves from further stress. Finally, burnout is characterised by a loss of job satisfaction. Burnout and dissatisfaction have been shown to be predictors of nurses' intention to leave their jobs (Aiken et al 2002b).

Nurses who experience a high degree of job-related stress over a period of time are at risk of being lost to the profession through burnout. This is sad, as these are the very nurses who uphold the highest standards of care for their patients. There is an irony that, in the midst of a worldwide shortage of nurses, those who would do their best to embody the values of the nursing profession are at most risk of leaving it behind.

Demerouti and colleagues (2000) have described a 'breeding ground' for burnout as being circumstances in which there are increasing job demands, insufficient resources, lack of colleague support and performance feedback, and limited participation in decision making (control/influence). As such, burnout, as a consequence of nurse stress, is as much an organisational matter as it is an individual nurse problem. In a meta-analysis of research studies to investigate the relationship between job satisfaction and nurses leaving their jobs, Irvine and Evans (1995) found that individual differences in nurses were not as influential as organisational or work environment variables in predicting job dissatisfaction and turnover in nursing staff. In another meta-analysis, Blegen (1993) identified a relationship between job satisfaction and organisational attributes such as adequate information and support from supervisors. While nurses need to develop their individual coping strategies (e.g. through stress management courses), there is equal evidence to suggest that organisational attributes and arrangements also affect nurse stress (Bennett et al 2001).

PRODUCTIVE NURSING ENVIRONMENTS

Workload, as the primary source of nurse stress in hospitals, is directly related to nurse staffing levels. Individual nurses may be unable to cope with work stress under circumstances that are impossible to manage (e.g. when there are inadequate numbers of nurses to competently care for their assigned patients). Adequate patient-to-nurse staff ratios have been shown not only to promote job satisfaction and reduce burnout in nurses (perceived stress), but also to improve patient outcomes (Aiken et al 2002a). In addition to ratios, there are other characteristics of the organisational environment that are associated with reduced stress in nurses and better patient outcomes. The relationship between organisational characteristics and nurse retention has been investigated over a number of years in institutions that are known as 'magnet' hospitals.

The magnet hospital story

A crisis of nurse recruitment and retention in the 1980s sparked an interesting investigation into the problem. Rather than focusing on further description of the difficulty, which had already been subjected to lengthy analyses, the

American Academy of Nursing commissioned an investigation into those hospitals with nursing shortages that were less acute than others. That is, the study investigated hospitals to which nurses were attracted (recruited) and in which they remained employed (retained). They became known as 'magnet hospitals' for these reasons.

The original investigations into the magnet hospitals revealed striking similarities in their organisational arrangements and operations (Kramer & Schmalenberg 1988a, 1988b, McClure et al 1983). In addition to adequacy of staffing, there were other features of the work environment that typified these institutions. One organisational feature was the professional autonomy of nurses in assuming responsibility for quality patient care. The care was based on a nursing philosophy of holistic and individualised care (i.e. care that is based on patient-centred values).

Management structures and attributes of nursing leaders were also similar in the original magnet hospitals. Organisational structures were conducive to participatory decision making and nursing self-governance, with decision making at a local level. Nursing leaders in these organisations were highly visible and accessible to nursing staff. They demonstrated enthusiasm and commitment to nurses and nursing, and conveyed a vision and value system for the profession. These structures and leader attributes, originally observed in the magnet hospitals, have continued to be associated with high nursing job satisfaction and quality nursing care (Schmalenberg & Kramer 2008).

Ongoing investigations into magnet hospitals have produced results that go beyond this description of organisational distinctiveness. There is also evidence that these institutions do not just attract and retain nurses; they also provide a higher standard of care and better patient outcomes than those institutions without magnet characteristics (Laschinger & Leiter 2006, Kazanjian et al 2005, Aiken et al 1994, Aiken et al 2002b). The evidence 'suggests that outcomes are better when nurses are able to render professional judgments about patients' needs and to act on the basis of those professional judgments' (Aiken et al 1998 p 222). That is, patients and nurses are better off when nurses are able to practise their profession to the full scope of their knowledge and ability.

Three key attributes have emerged supporting nursing practice at this level and have become defining organisational characteristics of magnet hospitals. They are professional autonomy, control over nursing practice and good collegial relationships between nurses and doctors.

Professional autonomy

The first characteristic is professional autonomy of the nursing staff. This means that nurses can practise nursing in a way that they judge best (i.e. they have authority in relation to clinical decisions about patient care). With autonomy comes the freedom to be self-defining and self-governing—characteristics associated with professional status. In describing autonomy, nurses working in magnet hospitals refer to clinical decision making and action that is free from bureaucratic constraints that have little to do with patient care. In addition to such freedom, nurses need to be clinically competent and knowledgeable in order to practise in an autonomous fashion (Kramer & Schmalenberg 2003a).

Control over nursing practice

Related to professional autonomy, which is at an individual clinical decision-making level, control over nursing practice involves participation in decision making at an organisational level. Control over practice involves the responsibility to set standards for nursing care, and having commensurate authority to meet those standards. Such control is not possible unless organisational structures include nurses at the highest decision-making level (i.e. when nurses have legitimate authority, status and recognition). Organisations that are structured in such ways engender a culture in which nurses take pride in themselves as a professional group (Kramer & Schmalenberg 2003b).

Collaboration with doctors

The third characteristic of the magnet hospitals is good collaboration between nurses and doctors. Such collaboration is marked by shared decision making and mutual respect for each other's contribution to clinical problem solving. An unequal power distribution between nurses and doctors hampers collaboration, as equality of contribution is implied. Nurses in magnet hospitals do not see themselves as subservient to the power of doctors and willingly cooperate with each other. There is recognition that both nursing and medical knowledge are needed in making sound decisions about patient care (Kramer & Schmalenberg 2003c).

The evidence that shared decision making between nurses and doctors is positively linked to patient outcomes extends beyond the magnet hospital investigations. In a frequently cited national survey of intensive care units (ICUs), Knaus et al (1986) reported that better patient outcomes, as measured by readmission to ICU and mortality within 24 hours of discharge from the ICU, were evident in organisational systems that included shared clinical decision making between nurses and doctors. Further investigations into nurse–doctor collaboration in ICUs have supported these findings, demonstrating better patient outcomes when nurses and doctors engage in mutual decision making (Mitchell & Shortell 1997, Shortell et al 1994, Baggs et al 1992).

Implications of magnet hospital research

The body of research into magnet hospitals does indicate that work environments supportive of professional nursing practice are associated with better nursing and patient outcomes. This support includes manageable nursing workloads in the form of adequate nurse-to-patient ratios (i.e. nurses cannot cope without adequate resources to meet the demands of nursing work). Adequate staffing is a critical variable to the success of the magnet hospital story (Aiken et al 2002a). Other characteristics of magnet hospitals relate to this variable. For example, control over nursing practice involves influencing decisions about nurse staffing levels. That is, the organisational characteristics that distinguish magnet hospitals are interrelated.

The characteristics are interrelated in other ways. For example, leaders in magnet hospitals were able to provide learning resources and opportunities for nurses to develop their clinical competence, a necessary requisite for clinical autonomy. Rafferty et al (2001) have shown that control over resources is associated with clinical autonomy and, more importantly, autonomous practice is synergistic with teamwork. Even when able to practise autonomously, there was a great deal of group cohesion in magnet hospitals. Building supportive colleague relationships is an aspect of the magnet hospital research that relates directly to the interpersonal work environment.

Nursing leadership

There are numerous implications about nursing leadership embedded into the magnet hospital organisations. Nursing leaders demonstrated pride in their profession and projected a 'positive professional identity', both critical aspects of reversing oppression (Roberts 2000). Magnet hospital leaders remained visible and accessible to the nursing staff. Focusing on mistakes, referred to as 'management by exception' (i.e. when things go wrong), is associated with increased nursing stress (Stourdeur et al 2001). Magnet hospital leaders were available, offering feedback not only when things went wrong, but also when they went well.

By understanding and articulating a nursing perspective on healthcare and providing strong advocacy for nursing, magnet hospital leaders were able to assist in the clarification of work roles and to reduce role conflicts. Such role clarity is associated with reduced nursing stress (Stordeur et al 2001, Demerouti et al 2000). Leaders in the magnet hospitals are pivotal in promoting a positive practice environment for nurses (Upenieks 2003). They not only profess the value of caring in nursing practice, they are also able to live these values in their interactions with colleagues.

COLLEAGUE INTERACTION AND WORK STRESS

The relationship between colleague interaction and stress in nursing is complex because co-workers function both as a resource for handling or modifying this stress *and* as a source of stress (e.g. conflict with colleagues and lack of performance feedback). Relationships with colleagues, in that they both add to and diminish work stress, can be considered flip sides of the same coin. Supportive interactions and relationships with colleagues have potentially positive effects; colleague interactions and relationships that lack support can add to work stress, creating negative effects.

Nurse–nurse interaction

Strained relationships and open conflict add stress to any working environment, but it is an absence of support, especially from nursing leaders (Bennett et al 2001), rather than the presence of conflict, that often creates strain in colleague relationships in nursing. More often than not, it is that which is missing in colleague relationships that contribute to stress in nursing. Lack of support from supervisors, lack of feedback, withheld information, lack of understanding in response to mistakes and lack of peer cohesion are all reported as factors that positively correlate to stress in nursing (Stordeur et al 2001, Hillhouse & Adler 1997, Dunn et al 1994). Nurses create stress for other nurses largely by failing to provide support when it is needed.

The sad irony is that work-related stress is exacerbated when colleague support is absent, and colleague support is lacking when it is needed most—during times of increased stress. What is most disturbing is that colleague relationships add to stress, not necessarily by creating overt conflict but by failing to provide needed support.

The following story, told by a recent graduate, highlights this lack of support:

I chose theatre nursing because of the challenge of working in a high-tech environment, an interest in anatomy and physiology, and the order and structure of the day's work. I also take my responsibility to patients very seriously. Their protection, privacy and safety are foremost in my mind as I work. In the year I worked in the operating theatre, I became fairly competent. I enjoyed my work there, except when working with one particular surgeon.

This was not because of his skills as a surgeon, but because of the way he treated nursing staff. He could be flirtatious and sometimes made lewd comments to women. Although uncomfortable, I tried to ignore the conversation. I never made eye contact with him in response to his inappropriate sexual comments. I just ignored his behaviour and got on with the work at hand.

Being a fairly private person, I never said much about my discomfort in working with this particular surgeon. That was, until the day he crossed the line. I was preparing for a case and scrubbing my hands when this surgeon came up to me, from behind, and placed his hands on my breasts. I resisted my impulse to slap his face, and instead firmly asked him to remove his hands from my body. Although quiet and reserved most of the time, I can be quite assertive. He mumbled something about my sense of humour and walked away. The case for which we were preparing proceeded as planned.

Just as well that the surgical procedure went quickly, as I could not wait to get out of the operating room with that surgeon. Once I knew the patient was safely on his way, I went straight to my nursing supervisor to report, in detail, the incident with the surgeon. I calmly told her what happened, expressed my anger at the situation and requested to not be rostered to work with that surgeon again.

It was my supervisor's reaction that really got to me. She calmly stated that she had a very busy operating theatre to run and that requests such as mine could not be accommodated. When I became visibly upset by her response, she suggested that I calm down. 'After all,' she told me, 'you certainly must be aware that this sort of thing has always occurred in the operating theatres. You will figure out your own way of dealing with it—like we all have. That is how you survive in this environment. You are still young. You will learn.'

I was appalled by what she said, yet helpless to take any further action. The surgeon in question was a powerful force in the organisation of the hospital. Although I knew that my supervisor's response was in direct violation of hospital policy in relation to workplace behaviour, I was also not going to take that issue further. She was known for her vindictive streak if you crossed her. Instead, I resigned and found an environment where I knew I would feel safe coming to work.

I never really told anybody the reasons I left that job. My friends thought I was happy there and were surprised to hear I took a position in the theatres of another hospital, which was further from my home. I told them I thought it was a good career move. In hindsight it was, as I have not looked back. I knew my personal survival was of most importance and chose to leave the incident behind in that hospital.

This situation illustrates the potentially disastrous effects of an environment that is lacking support for other nurses. This nurse coped with the situation by altering the immediate situation (through change in work location), but avoided the main cause of the problem. Not only did the supervisor in this situation fail to support this newly graduated nurse, but also she violated workplace policies that mandate reporting the surgeon's behaviour as it amounts to harassment. Most workplaces have policies that require supervisors to report such instances. Not only should the instance have been reported, but the nursing supervisor also lacked understanding of the new graduate's distress.

The lack of colleague support between nurses raises questions about why and how this happens in a caring profession. Nurses risk losing their credibility as caring persons when caring for other nurses is not apparent and active in their work environment. Nurses should be able to demonstrate support for colleagues and cultivate a nourishing work environment. Sadly, there are aspects of nursing culture that work exactly against the creation of such environments.

Culture of horizontal violence

A potential explanation of how colleague interaction is troubled in nursing is the phenomenon termed 'oppressed group behaviour'. Observed in nursing many years ago (Roberts 1983), this interpersonal dynamic continues to receive research interest in studies that have been conducted across a variety of cultural contexts (Curtis et al 2007, Longo 2007, McKenna et al 2003, Jackson et al 2002, Lee & Saeed 2001, Taylor 2001). Sometimes termed 'horizontal violence', members of oppressed groups are often unsupportive and in conflict with their peers. Horizontal violence creates a climate of divisiveness within nursing groups and pits nurses against each other, thus destroying camaraderie and esprit de corps. As such, it can create a breeding ground for interpersonal conflict among nurses. Understanding the dynamics of groups that are oppressed is essential if this negative phenomenon is to be reversed in nursing.

Behaviours of oppression often stem from feeling powerless against a dominant force. Nurses often perceive themselves as powerless against a system that dominates them, shouldering great responsibility within healthcare organisations, without a commensurate degree of authority. The dominant culture reveres technology and devalues caring (Benner & Wrubel 1989) and places curing as superior to caring. This oppression results in feelings of inferiority and creates the myth that the dominant group's value system and culture is 'right' and superior. In oppression, there is an internalisation of the dominant group's view of the world and a tendency within the oppressed group towards self-blame and rejection of their own values and culture as inferior (McCall 1996). This leads to the development of a collective poor self-esteem within the group and has the potential to result in poor peer relationships (McKenna et al 2003, Jackson et al 2002, Randle 2003, Taylor 2001).

There are frustrations and complaints about the oppressor and the oppression, yet no direct action is taken. Frustrations are directed at each other because the 'system' excludes nurses and silences their voice. The anger that builds as a result of oppression is released on members of the group, rather than on the oppressor, because there is less risk of consequences in fighting each other than there is in fighting the dominant group. The lateral violence within the group keeps the group divided, prevents cohesion and maintains the status quo (Roberts 1983).

Examples of horizontal violence include withholding information, undermining, back-stabbing and snide remarks. Blaming and scapegoating other nurses are also evidence of the behaviour of oppression in nursing work environments. As long as blame can be found, and it usually is found within the oppressed group, real issues are not addressed because the culprit, another nurse, has been targeted, and there is no need to delve further into what is behind the cause of the problem.

Often horizontal violence is levelled at the most junior of nursing staff. This includes students of nursing (Curtis et al 2007, Longo 2007) who experience being discredited and put down, as well as feeling humiliated in the presence of others. Termed 'eating our young', this phenomenon of lack of support for those new to the profession is one form of horizontal violence that pervades many nursing cultures.

Bullying, perhaps the most extreme example of horizontal violence in nursing, is a matter of increasing concern (Lewis 2006, Randle 2003, Jackson et al 2002, Taylor 2001). Bullying involves persistent and negative acts towards an individual or group in which there is a power imbalance between the perpetrator and the victim (Salin 2003). The presence of such acts creates hostility and conflict within the work environment. Perhaps most importantly for nursing is the evidence that bullying is a learnt behaviour in the work environment and not related to personality factors (Lewis 2006).

In a recent investigation into professional relationships, Duddle and Broughton (2007) found that conflicted and difficult interactions between nurses were prominent and included forms of horizontal violence and bullying behaviour. They also described how the participants in the study did manage to deal with such interactions in a resilient manner by learning how to seek help from their colleagues, thus reducing their stress.

Nursing colleagues as a coping resource

Seeking support from colleagues is an active coping endeavour that can assist in problem solving through practical assistance and advice. That is, colleague support can support problem-focused coping. Likewise, seeking colleague support can also be an emotion-focused coping effort when used to minimise the impact of a devastating situation. For example, using another person as an emotional sounding board for the expression of feelings helps to reduce tension.

Colleague support has the potential to alter positively the experience of stress in two identifiable ways. Firstly, support from colleagues can have the direct effect of reducing or preventing stress itself (e.g. by encouraging a reappraisal of the situation). An appraisal of death as a natural and expected part of life lessens the likelihood that death will be viewed as a failure. The realisation that nurses are not personally responsible for a patient death from cancer, for example, is achievable through open, honest interaction with other nurses. The reappraisal of the situation creates a new perception that directly alters the experience of stress.

Secondly, colleague support can buffer the negative effects of stress in that colleague support reduces the negative effects and consequences of stress. Talking to a trusted colleague, whether through formal or informal channels, can offset a sense of isolation. More than likely, other nurses are experiencing or have experienced similar feelings and reactions, but sometimes a 'conspiracy of silence' prevents these experiences from being shared. Keeping feelings hidden, especially fears, places nurses in the position of worrying alone and perpetuates the fallacy that, 'I am the only one who feels this way' or 'There must be something wrong with me'. There is comfort in knowing one is not alone, and not the only one with fears, worries and negative reactions.

Effective working relationships with colleagues are a necessity in nursing because of the need for collaboration and team effort in most work situations. The interdependence created by this need to pull together has potential to strain colleague relationships and lead to interpersonal conflict with colleagues.

Colleague support has been shown to be correlated with less job stress and strain and is therefore beneficial to nurses' wellbeing (Shirvey 2004, Hillhouse & Adler 1997, Lee & Henderson 1996). Such support is helpful to nurses for the same reasons social support helps patients (see Ch 9). Colleagues provide direct aid, assistance and access to useful and relevant information, in addition to personal affirmation and emotional support. Such relationships are reflective of an organisational culture and point to the importance of environmental factors in nurse stress. Healthcare organisational structures and work practices contribute to lack of cohesion and staff conflict (Farrell 2001). Effective coping is not simply a matter for an individual nurse; the whole of the nursing work environment comes into play.

Reversing the culture of horizontal violence

Nurses can easily remain victims of oppression and horizontal violence if they continually focus on negative characteristics within the culture of nursing. Raising awareness of horizontal violence provides an opportunity for nurses to reverse its negative effects.

Oppressed groups such as nurses often remain submissive to those who dominate them because members of the group are unaware of their behaviour. As a result, horizontal violence stifles the development of support between nurses in an insidious manner. Nurses often unconsciously collude in their own subordination (e.g. by unknowingly diminishing the importance of nursing knowledge) (Jackson et al 2002, Freshwater 2000, Roberts 2000). In reversing the culture of oppression, Roberts (2000) suggests that nurses challenge internal beliefs that nursing is less valuable than others' contributions to patient wellbeing.

Instead of identifying with the dominant authority, one characteristic of leaders who emerge from oppressed groups (Roberts 1983), leaders of the magnet hospitals were able to articulate a nursing perspective on patient care and provide strong advocacy for nursing practice. In the magnet hospitals, nursing knowledge assumed authority, as nurses were able to practise their profession in an autonomous, yet collaborative, fashion. Aiken et al (1998) speculate that the underlying reason for the magnet hospital outcomes of better job satisfaction for nurses and better outcomes for patients is the professional status of nursing. Having recognised professional status enables nurses to engage in interprofessional decision making.

Nurse–doctor interaction

The dominance of medical authority and concomitant nurse subservience, as observed in nurse–doctor interaction, has been cited as evidence of one reason that nurses feel oppressed and powerless (McCall 1996). In what is now a classic article on the subject of nurse–doctor interaction, Stein (1967) describes a system of communication between nurses and doctors that he termed 'the doctor–nurse game'. When abiding by the rules of the 'game', nurses are only able to express their own ideas and judgments about patient care when they appear *not* to have an opinion of their own. For example, rather than directly requesting a change in analgesic medication, the nurse playing the game would suggest that the doctor may want to consider reviewing the patient's medications. This is because the doctor has to appear all-knowing, at all times. More importantly, the approach used in the game avoids any possibility of conflict between nurse and doctor.

Not only did the game perpetuate a myth of the omnipotent doctor, but also it stifled nursing knowledge from finding direct expression about patient care. Twenty-three years after the original article, Stein et al (1990) claimed that the 'game' was played to a lesser extent than originally observed because of the increasing professional status of nurses. Nevertheless, the idea of the doctor–nurse game retained attention in the literature over a number of years (Farrell 1997). The amount of nursing literature on nurse–doctor communication indicates that the subject receives more attention from nurses than doctors (Corser 1998, McMahan et al 1994).

Analysis of the 'game' that supported medical dominance and nursing subservience was often based on gender, as nursing is a female-dominated profession. Hughes (1988) demonstrated that more than gender was at play, as the rules of the game changed when 'senior' female nurses interacted with 'junior' male doctors in the highly charged atmosphere of an emergency department. Seniority had more influence than gender in these instances because experienced nurses had more knowledge of how to run emergency services than did junior, inexperienced doctors. Likewise, Porter (1991) reported that aspects of the game existed when female doctors interacted with male nurses, suggesting the need for analysis of this complex interpersonal dynamic that extends beyond gender. The continued focus on gender in doctor–nurse interaction has led to a claim of rigid thinking and inaction (May & Fleming 1997), and the need for an analysis that extends beyond gender alone (Keenan et al 1998, McMahan et al 1994).

Analyses of conflicts that arise from ethical dilemmas in healthcare provide one such example of understanding of nurse–doctor interaction. Ethical conflicts often arise under circumstances in which continuing medical treatment is thought by nurses to be contributing to patient suffering. Analyses of such conflicts demonstrate that nurses and doctors use different information to arrive at a clinical judgment, a considered opinion about what 'should' be done in relation to the patient (Stein-Parbury & Liaschenko 2007, Shannon 1997, Karlawish 1996, Anspach 1987). In formulating their judgments, nurses are likely to use what is termed 'subjective' information about the patient's circumstances, while doctors rely on what are considered to be 'objective' facts and figures. Doctors rely on standardised knowledge (e.g. selecting an intervention that has been shown to be effective in the majority of cases). Nurses take into consideration that which is idiosyncratic and specific to a particular patient (e.g. through coming to 'know the patient' as an individual). Conflicting perspectives may arise under such circumstances.

Rather than working towards a mutually acceptable decision, medical knowledge and authority often supercedes other types of knowledge as a way of resolving the conflict. True collaboration occurs when there is mutual respect for differences in clinical perspective, not when one perspective dominates and silences other ways of viewing the situation. In effect, nurses' tendency to avoid open conflict with doctors silences their views on ethical dilemmas in patient care. Doctors make the decisions about continuing or discontinuing care and nurses live with the outcome (Oberle & Hughes 2001).

Poor collaboration with doctors is a source of stress for nurses because this can reduce nurses' capacity to influence patient care to the best of their knowledge and ability. There is evidence to suggest that interprofessional conflict is more stressful to nurses than intraprofessional conflict (Hillhouse & Adler 1997). Moreover, there is evidence to suggest that interactions with doctors not only influences nurses' job satisfaction, but also patient outcomes (Zangaro & Soeken 2007, Rosenstein 2002, Chaboyer et al 2001, Baggs et al 1999, Gleason Scott et al 1999, Mitchell & Shortell 1997, Shortell et al 1994, Knaus et al 1993).

Interprofessional decision making

Nurses need to be mindful not to play the 'doctor–nurse game' (Stein 1967), which prevents collaboration due to inequality of status and authority. Nurses who 'play the game' unwittingly stifle and oppress the voice of nursing. Stein et al (1990) claim that the game was played less than originally observed in 1967, as nurses achieved professional status. However, they also point out that freeing the oppressed will free the oppressor from the destructive discourse of the doctor–nurse game. The 'perceived' omnipotence of medical authority, embodied in the form of the 'doctor knows best' (i.e. the doctor–nurse game), can be a burden for doctors who are then expected, sometimes by patients, to have all of the answers. When no answers are forthcoming or immediately obvious, doctors may turn to nurses for information about the best course of action to follow in relation to patient wellbeing.

However, interprofessional decision making is difficult to achieve without organisational structures to support the process. Nurses need to be involved in decision making at every level from the patient bedside to the executive boardroom. However, simply changing arrangements alone may not result in shared decision making between doctors and nurses. Manias and Street (2001) found that information offered by nurses was not central to clinical decisions about patient care, despite an attempt to have this information offered by including nurses in medical ward rounds in critical care units. Nursing voices remained marginalised, with a lack of acknowledgment by doctors of nursing knowledge and patient assessment. Simply involving nurses in medical ward rounds did not change clinical decision making.

EFFECTIVE CONFLICT RESOLUTION

Conflict is considered a natural part of social life, and interpersonal conflicts in the workplace are not unique to the nursing environment. This is because nurses work closely with other people with whom there is a high degree of interdependence (i.e. the need to work together towards mutual goals). Differences of opinions and perspectives are inevitable when people work in this interdependent way. Rather than try to avoid conflicts, it is more important to develop skills in their management and resolution.

In Chapter 10, the management of conflict was introduced in relation to interpersonal interactions with patients; in all likelihood, conflicts with colleagues will be encountered more frequently in the workplace. The causes of conflict include: differences in perspectives about patient care; differences in values and opinions; poor or incompetent communication; workload stress; unclear expectations; and incompatible priorities. Successful resolution of conflicts can bring people closer and adds to satisfaction and creativity in the workplace; when handled poorly, conflicts can create extra strain and tension.

As in managing conflicts with patients, nurses need to be skilled in the processes of negotiation and collaboration. These processes rely on the use of skills of assertion and responsiveness because they get the job done (task focus), while maintaining working relationships based on mutual respect (relationship focus). While the same skills and processes are used in conflicts with patients, the nature of colleague relationships is not the same as therapeutic ones.

In therapeutic relationships, the focus is always on supporting and helping the patient, and maintaining the helpful nature of the relationship is paramount. Responsibility lies with the nurse to initiate the resolution of the conflict in these relationships. In colleague relationships, the responsibility is shared, although often one person will make the first step in finding a resolution.

With patients, it is more likely that conflict will be experienced in an individual interaction or episode, and the relationship will not be ongoing. In colleague relationships, the conflict may be ongoing, as working relationships last much longer than therapeutic relationships with patients.

In working relationships, the importance of achieving the task may take precedence to focusing on the relationship. While maintaining harmonious working relationships is important, handling conflicts with colleagues requires a focus on the goal or task and doing so assertively does run the risk of disrupting the relationship (Rakos 2006). For example, advocating for a patient's right to participate in decision making regarding care may cause friction with other members of the healthcare team. The focus on the task of advocacy may disrupt the working relationships because the task protecting the patient's right is more important. This is not to suggest that treating other members of the team with disrespect is warranted; it means that defending a patient's right may take precedence over the desire to keep colleague relationships running smoothly.

The usual ways of handling interpersonal conflict through withdrawing, forcing, smoothing, compromising and negotiating (reviewed in Ch 10) can be used when resolving workplace conflict. Nonetheless, compromising and negotiating are best suited to working with colleagues in a collaborative manner. Compromising may need to be used when there is little time available for discussion and negotiation. But compromising can lead to less than ideal solutions that leave many of those involved less than satisfied with the solution. Negotiating and collaborating, while more time consuming, often leads to mutually agreed solutions. Collaboration is characterised by open dialogue about the problem, thus bringing the conflict actively into the open (McCabe & Timmins 2006).

Nurses are likely to meet conflict in the workplace in a passive manner, with avoidance and giving in (withdrawing and smoothing), rather than with active and assertive attempts to negotiate and collaborate (Valentine 2001, Healy & McKay 2000). People who use passive strategies, often designed to 'keep the peace', are seen as more likeable (Rakos 2006), and this may be one reason nurses behave this way. Because they are caring and compassionate towards patients, nurses may suffer under what Street (1992) has termed the 'tyranny of niceness'. That is, they may think that active assertion, which is required for successful negotiation, is not compatible with being a caring person (McCartan & Hargie 2004).

Passive strategies, such as avoiding and giving in, are not always successful in resolving the conflict; and, more importantly, they are associated with increased stress and decreased mental wellbeing in nurses (Chang et al 2007,

Lambert et al 2004, Healy & McKay 2000, Santamaria 2000). Therefore, it is important that nurses learn how to deal with workplace conflict through the use of assertive skills. When used deliberately, compromising and acquiescing can be assertive in their own right; however, more active assertion is often required when dealing with workplace conflict.

Assertiveness in the workplace

Nurses who behave assertively in the workplace are able to express their own thoughts, feelings and needs to colleagues, while simultaneously maintaining good working relationships. The use of assertive skills in the workplace is based on the right to be heard and treated with respect. Assertive skills are often viewed as midway between passive and domineering communication. While sometimes confused with assertiveness, domineering or aggressive communication violates the rights of others to be treated with respect. Conversely, people who are usually passive and overly accommodating in their communication violate their own rights to be heard.

Nurses who are assertive are able to state their own thoughts in a clear manner, often through the use of 'I' statements (see Ch 10). Such statements are best accompanied by an empathic statement that recognises the obligation to maintain good working relationships. Simply stating a personal view, especially when in conflict with another's view, without acknowledging the perspective of the other person, is likely to be seen as aggressive (Rakos 2006). While early definitions of assertiveness emphasised the notion of 'rights', there is now recognition that the assertion of rights carries with it the obligation to others (Rakos 2006). When being assertive, it is vital that nurses take time and try to understand the perspective of the other person or people involved in the conflict.

Although most of the research into assertiveness has focused on conflict and negative encounters, behaving assertively also includes giving and receiving compliments, initiating and maintaining relationships, and expressing positive feelings (Rakos 2006). A study by Timmins and McCabe (2005) found that nurses were better at being assertive in positive situations, such as complimenting or thanking a colleague, than they were at expressing their own opinion or to make requests. When they are assertive, it is triggered by a sense of responsibility for the patient (Timmins & McCabe 2005). That is, nurses could be assertive in showing care for others, but were less likely to act on their own behalf.

Assertiveness involves expressing an opinion that may be different from others and even one that is unpopular. Requesting behavioural change in another person, and asking for help, are also examples of assertive behaviour. Asking for help involves the admission of one's own limitations, which is in itself an assertive act.

Making requests and asking for help are assertive skills that are particularly relevant to the novice nurse. Colleague support, through the provision of information and opportunities for professional development, is an expectation of professional practice (ANMC 2005); therefore, new nurses should be confident in seeking such support from more experienced colleagues. It is their professional right.

New nurses are often reluctant to ask for help because of the manner in which they have been treated in the workplace (Duddle & Broughton 2007).

Recognising it and talking about it is helpful; however, developing skills in assertion helps to build coping and resilience.

Here is an example of using assertive skills in the context of colleague interaction. An inexperienced nurse might say to a more experienced nurse (who does not appear busy at present): 'Can you please help me with this procedure, as I don't have much experience with doing it?' (this is being assertive by asking for help). Responses from the more experienced nurse might include:

- 'Don't they teach you anything in university?' (attack that is off the issue)
- 'I did learn about it, but I do not have much experience actually doing it and I need help.' (asserting needs and sticking to the issue)
- 'That's the trouble with nursing education today—not enough real-world experience, if you ask me.' (continues to focus on another issue)
- 'It very well may be true that there is not enough clinical in basic nursing education, but I still need help with this procedure. Can you help me? If not, I will find somebody else.' (fogging over a potential sidetrack issue).

As this example demonstrates, it is important to clearly identify the issue at hand and to stay focused on it when dealing with conflicts in the workplace. Staying focused on the issue and separating the person from the problem are essential to successful conflict resolution and assertion. This means not getting sidetracked onto other matters, especially those laden with emotions. In order to do so, it is essential that emotional responses are contained and managed.

Controlling the expression of emotions in this way is an aspect of emotional intelligence (EI). It has been shown that nurses with high EI tend to use collaborative approaches (Jordan & Troth 2007) in their response to conflict. Collaboration can lead to true negotiation, which is perhaps the best approach for use in work settings.

The skills of assertion are learnt behaviours and must therefore be rehearsed and practised in the workplace in order to be developed and refined. In practising and using the skills, it is important to be selective about time and place. An assertive confrontation of a co-worker in front of other co-workers is not usually a suitable context, as it is better to choose a place where there is privacy. There are also times when nurses will choose not to be assertive, either because they do not have the emotional energy to do so or the situation does not warrant such an approach. Perceiving the right time to be assertive is a skill in itself. However, lack of assertion should not be because nurses lack the skills. Like all interpersonal skills, they must be tried and used in order to be effective in resolving conflict.

CLINICAL SUPERVISION

Clinical supervision is a formalised way for nurses to receive support in the workplace. It is a process of professional support and learning in which nurses are assisted in developing their practice through regular discussion time with more experienced and knowledgeable colleagues (Bond & Holland 1998, Fowler 1996). The purpose of clinical supervision is to improve nursing practice and therefore it needs to be focused on nurse–patient interaction (van Ooijen 2000). During clinical supervision, nurses employ the processes of reflection (Ch 3) in order to identify and meet needs for professional development.

The term 'supervision' is associated with management functions and an industrial model in which supervisors are present to spot and rectify worker mistakes (Titchen & Binnie 1995). This association is unfortunate because clinical supervision is designed as a process for leadership support and the professional development of nurses (Butterworth & Faugier 1992). With an emphasis on learning, clinical supervision has the capacity to enable individual nurses to develop their knowledge and competence.

Clinical supervision has been shown to be effective in reducing stress in nursing (Brunero & Stein-Parbury 2008, Williamson & Dodds 1999, Severinsson & Hallberg 1996), and therefore can be considered an effective coping resource. In addition to support for nurses, clinical supervision has been shown to affect the quality of care by helping to both improve and maintain professional standards of nursing care (Hyrkäs et al 2003, Bowles & Young 1999) and aid in the professional development of nurses (Brunero & Stein-Parbury 2008). That is, nursing practice in general can be improved through the process of clinical supervision.

The interpersonal interaction of clinical supervision can occur in either one-to-one arrangements (individual supervision), or in a work group (group supervision). Individual supervision is more suited to nurses who practise independently (e.g. community mental health nurses who function as case managers for chronically ill people). Group supervision may be more appropriate in hospital settings where nurses function daily as members of a work team. Team clinical supervision offers opportunities for nurses to engage in mutual problem solving for particularly challenging clinical situations.

Clinical supervision is therefore an example of how nurses can provide support to each other, especially when clinical situations are emotionally demanding. Other nurses provide a special and unique insider perspective that can challenge unrealistic fears and expectations, and also allow coping options to be explored and developed. For example, if fears of incompetence and inadequacy stem from lack of knowledge, then this could be addressed through an informal sharing of knowledge or more formalised staff development programs such as clinical supervision.

Clinical supervision can pave a path by which nurses can actively share their concerns and emotions generated by the job, and be heard and understood by other nurses. Acknowledging another's perceptions through attentive listening can be helpful in and of itself. Colleague support can be requested and received. Another nurse is in a prime position to respond to a need for support. Other nurses already know colleagues, and the nursing work context is familiar. Empathy is easy to demonstrate under these circumstances because colleagues have shared experiences and meanings. Colleagues are also able to provide practical advice and solutions for managing clinical situations that are taxing for an individual nurse.

Reflective listening clarifies these difficulties and emotions, and promotes mutual understanding, but understanding alone may not be sufficient in providing effective colleague support. Challenging (Ch 8) is sometimes necessary because of the need to develop new ways of approaching clinical situations. Challenging offers new perspectives, reframes existing perspectives, spurs nurses on to improve their work, and helps to overcome obstacles to meeting goals. Challenging can only be effective in a general climate of trust and openness. Trust is promoted between nurses when individual differences are tolerated, and feedback is given directly and honestly. Conflict is not absent within this climate, but these conditions establish a climate in which effective resolution of conflict can occur.

In order to be effective as a supportive strategy for nursing, clinical supervision must be embedded into organisational structures. When nurses are burdened by workload, 'finding' time for supervision may seem impossible. Clinical nursing leaders need to provide both time and structure if clinical supervision is to be successful as a practice development activity. There must also be organisational clarity about how clinical supervision differs from other types of developmental activities, such as educational programs.

CHAPTER SUMMARY

All of the skills described in this book will effectively promote supportive relationships with colleagues because these skills are not exclusive to patient–nurse interactions. Being attentive, responsive, encouraging, understanding and challenging are not skills that can be switched on and off at will, and enactment of these skills on a daily basis in the work environment creates a supportive environment. A necessary backdrop to supportive colleague interaction is an interpersonal work climate that acknowledges and validates nurses as people, and is responsive to nurses' reactions, feelings, anxieties and confusions. Nurses cannot be expected to give of themselves without such support, from other nurses and the healthcare organisation that employs them, because work-related stress is best dealt with in the work environment.

However, colleague support is often lacking in nursing work environments. Reasons for this lack of support have been discussed in relation to the behaviour of oppressed groups and historical subservience of nursing to medicine. The characteristics of magnet hospitals have been described as 'ideal' in creating support for nurses and nursing practice. These characteristics, clinical autonomy, control over nursing practice and collaborative relationships with doctors, support not only nurses but aid in the development of nursing practice. Most importantly, they are associated with good patient outcomes.

Clinical autonomy, one of the characteristics of magnet hospitals, is evident in patient–nurse relationships. Although levels of involvement between nurse and patient are mutually negotiated (Ch 2), it is within nurses' independent professional domain to develop therapeutically meaningful relationships with patients. Doing so may cause nurses to become stressed. Reflective practice, especially with colleague support, can be effective in dealing with that stress through problem solving and action, or simply a new understanding or perspective on the situation. Clinical supervision has been presented as a formalised process for such reflection.

REFERENCES

Aiken LH, Clarke SP, Sloane DM 2002a Hospital staffing, organisation, and quality of care: cross-national findings. International Journal for Quality in Health Care 14(1):5–13

Aiken LH, Clarke SP, Sloane DM, Sochalski J 2002b Hospital nurse staffing and patient mortality, nurse burnout, and job dissatisfaction. Journal of the American Medical Association 288(16):1987–1993

Aiken LH, Clarke SP, Sloane DM, Sochalski J, Busse R, Clarke H, Giovannetti P, Hunt J, Rafferty AM, Shamian J 2001 Nurses' reports on hospital care in five countries. Health Affairs 20(3):43–53

Aiken LH, Sloane DM, Sochalski J 1998 Hospital organisation and outcomes. Quality in Health Care 7:222–226

Aiken LH, Smith HL, Lake ET 1994 Lower medicare mortality among a set of hospitals known for good nursing care. Medical Care 32:771–787

Anspach RR 1987 Prognostic conflict in life-and-death decisions: the organization as an ecology of knowledge. Journal of Health and Social Behavior 28:215–231

Australian Nursing and Midwifery Council (ANMC) 2005 National Competency Standards for the Registered Nurse. ANMC, Canberra

Baggs JG, Ryan SA, Phelps CE, Richeson JF, Johnson JE 1992 The association between interdisciplinary collaboration and patient outcomes in a medical intensive care unit. Heart and Lung 21:18–24

Baggs JG, Schmitt MH, Muslin AI, Mitchell PH, Eldredge DH, Oakes D, Hutson AD 1999 Association between nurse–physician collaboration and patient outcomes in three intensive care units. Critical Care Medicine 27:1991–1998

Benner P, Wrubel J 1989 The primacy of caring: stress and coping in health and illness. Addison-Wesley, Menlo Park, CA

Bennett P, Lowe R, Matthews V, Dourale M, Tattersall A 2001 Stress in nurses: coping, managerial support and work demand. Stress and Health 17:55–63

Blegen MA 1993 Nurses' job satisfaction: a meta-analysis of related variable. Nursing Research 42:36–41

Bond M, Holland S 1998 Clinical supervision for nurses: a practical guide for supervisees, clinical supervisors and managers. Open University Press, Buckingham.

Bowles N, Young C 1999 An evaluative study of clinical supervision based on Proctor's three function interactive model. Journal of Advanced Nursing 30(4):958–964

Bratt MM, Broome M, Delber S, Lostocco L 2000 Influence of stress and nursing leadership on job satisfaction of pediatric intensive care unit nurses. American Journal of Critical Care 9:307–317

Brunero S, Stein-Parbury J 2008 The effectiveness of clinical supervision: an evidenced based literature review. Australian Journal of Advanced Nursing 25(3):86–94

Butterworth T, Faugier J 1992 Clinical supervision and mentorship in nursing. Chapman & Hall, London

Chaboyer W, Najman J, Dunn S 2001 Factors influencing job valuation: a comparative study of critical care and non-critical care nurses. International Journal of Nursing Studies 38:153–161

Chang EML, Bidewell JW, Huntington AD, Daly J, Johnson A, Wilson H, Lambert VA, Lambert CE 2007 A survey of role stress, coping and health in Australian and New Zealand hospital nurses. International Journal of Nursing Studies 44:1354–1362

Coomber B, Barriball L 2007 Impact of job satisfaction components on intent to leave and turnover for hospital-based nurses: a review of the research literature. International Journal of Nursing Studies 44:297–314

Corbin J 2008 Is caring a lost art in nursing? International Journal of Nursing Studies 45:163–165

Corser WD 1998 A conceptual model of collaborative nurse–physician interactions: the management of traditional influences and person tendencies. Scholarly Inquiry for Nursing Practice 12(4):325–346

Curtis J, Bowen I, Reid A 2007 You have no credibility: nursing students' experiences of horizontal violence. Nurse Education in Practice 7:156–163

Demerouti E, Bakker AB, Nachreiner R, Schaufeli WB 2000 A model of burnout and life satisfaction amongst nurses. Journal of Advanced Nursing 32(2):454–464

Duddle M, Broughton M 2007 Intraprofessional relations in nursing. Journal of Advanced Nursing 59(1):29–37

Dunn LA, Rout U, Carson J, Ritter SA 1994 Occupational stress amongst care staff working in nursing homes: an empirical investigation. Journal of Clinical Nursing 3:177–183

Farrell GA 1997 Aggression in clinical settings: nurses' views. Journal of Advanced Nursing 25:501–508

Farrell GA 2001 From tall poppies to squashed weeds: why don't nurses pull together more? Journal of Advanced Nursing 35(1):26–33

Fowler J 1996 The organization of clinical supervision within the nursing profession: a review of the literature. Journal of Advanced Nursing 23:471–478

Freshwater D 2000 Crosscurrents: against cultural narration in nursing. Journal of Advanced Nursing 32(2):481–484

Gleason Scott JG, Sochalski J, Aiken L 1999 Review of magnet hospital research. Journal of Nursing Administration 29(1):9–19

Hayes LJ, O'Brien-Pallas L, Duffield C, Shamian J, Buchan J, Hughes F, Laschinger HKS, North N, Stone PW 2006 Nurse turnover: a literature review. International Journal of Nursing Studies 43:237–263

Healy CM, McKay MF 2000 Nursing stress: the effects of coping strategies and job satisfaction in a sample of Australian nurses. Journal of Advanced Nursing 31(3):681–688

Hillhouse J, Adler CM 1997 Investigating stress effect patterns in hospital staff nurses: results of a cluster analysis. Social Science and Medicine 45(12):1781–1788

Hughes D 1988 When nurse knows best: some aspects of nurse–doctor interaction in a hospital casualty department. Sociology of Health and Illness 10:1–22

Hyrkäs K, Koivula M, Lehti K, Paunonen-Ilmonen M 2003 Nurse managers' conceptions of quality management as promoted by peer supervision. Journal of Nursing Management 11:48–58

Irvine DM, Evans MG 1995 Job satisfaction and turnover among nurses: integrating research findings across studies. Nursing Research 44(4):246–253

Jackson D, Clare J, Mannix J 2002 Who would want to be a nurse? Violence in the workplace— a factor in recruitment and retention. Journal of Nursing Management 10:13–40

Jordan PJ, Troth AC 2007 Emotional intelligence and conflict resolution in nursing. Contemporary Nurse 13:94–100

Karlawish JHT 1996 Shared decision making in critical care: a clinical reality and an ethical necessity. American Journal of Critical Care 5:391–396

Kazanjian A, Green C, Wong J, Reid R 2005 Effect of the hospital nursing environment on patient mortality: a systematic review. Journal of Health Services Research and Policy 10(2):111–117

Keenan GM, Cooke R, Hollis SL 1998 Norms and nurse management of conflicts: keys to understanding nurse–physician collaboration. Research in Nursing and Health 21:59–72

Knaus WA, Draper EA, Wagner DP, Zimmerman JE 1986 An evaluation of outcomes from intensive care in major medical centers. Annals of Internal Medicine 10:410–418

Knaus WA, Wagner DP, Zimmerman JE, Draper EA 1993 Variation in mortality and length of stay in intensive care units. Annals of Internal Medicine 118:753–761

Kramer M, Schmalenberg C 1988a Magnet hospitals: part I: institutions of excellence. Journal of Nursing Administration 18(1):13–24

Kramer M, Schmalenberg C 1988b Magnet hospitals: part II: institutions of excellence. Journal of Nursing Administration 18(2):1–19

Kramer M, Schmalenberg C 2003a Magnet hospital staff nurses describe clinical autonomy. Nursing Outlook 51:13–19

Kramer M, Schmalenberg C 2003b Magnet hospital staff nurses describe control over practice. Western Journal of Nursing Research 25(4):432–452

Kramer M, Schmalenberg C 2003c Securing 'good' nurse–physician relationships. Nursing Management 34(7):34–38

Kushner T, Rabin S, Azulai S 1997 A descriptive study of stress management in a group of pediatric oncology nurses. Cancer Nursing 20:414–421

Lambert V, Lambert CE, Itano J, Inouye J, Kim S, Kuniviktikul W, Sitthimongkol Y, Pongthavornkamol K, Gasemgitvattana S, Ito M 2004 Cross-cultural comparison of workplace stressors, ways of coping and demographic characteristics as predictors of physical and mental health among hospital nurses in Japan, Thailand, South Korea and the USA (Hawaii). International Journal of Nursing Studies 41:671–684

Laschinger HK, Almost J, Tuer-Hodes D 2003 Workplace empowerment and magnet hospital characteristics: making the link. Journal of Nursing Administration 33(7/8):410–422

Laschinger HK, Leiter MP 2006 The impact of nursing work environments on patient safety outcomes. Journal of Nursing Administration 36(5):259–267

Lazarus RS, Folkman S 1984 Stress, appraisal and coping. Springer, New York

Lee MB, Saeed I 2001 Oppression and horizontal violence: the case of nurses in Pakistan. Nursing Forum 36(1):15–24

Lee V, Henderson MC 1996 Occupational stress and organizational commitment in nurse administrators. Journal of Nursing Administration 26(5):21–28

Lewis MA 2006 Nurse bullying: organizational considerations in the maintenance and perpetration of health care bullying cultures. Journal of Nurse Management 14:52–58

Longo J 2007 Horizontal violence among nursing students. Archives of Psychiatric Nursing 21(3):177–178

Lutzen K, Cronqvist A, Magnusson A, Lars A 2003 Moral stress: synthesis of a concept. Nursing Ethics 10(3):312–322

Manias E, Street A 2001 Nurse doctor interactions during critical care ward rounds. Journal of Clinical Nursing 10 (4):442–450

Maslach C, Schaufeli WB 1993 Historical and conceptual development of burnout. In: Schaufeli WB, Maslach C, Marek T (eds), Professional burnout: recent developments in theory and research, pp 1–16. Taylor and Francis, Washington DC

May C, Fleming C 1997 The professional imagination: narrative and symbolic boundaries between medicine and nursing. Journal of Advanced Nursing 25:1094–1100

McCabe C, Timmins F 2006 Communication skills for nursing practice. Palgrave Macmillan, Hampshire

McCall E 1996 Horizontal violence in nursing. The Lamp 53(3):28–29, 31

McCartan PJ, Hargie ODW 2004 Assertiveness and caring: are they compatible? Journal of Advanced Nursing 13:707–713

McClure M, Poulin M, Sovie M, Wandelt M 1983 Magnet hospitals: attraction and retention of professional nurses. American Academy of Nursing Task Force on Nursing Practice in Hospitals. American Nurses Association, Kansas City, MO

McDonald S 1999 Whistleblowing: effective and ineffective coping responses. Nursing Forum 34(4):5–13

McKenna BG, Smith NA, Poole SJ, Coverdale JH 2003 Horizontal violence: experiences of registered nurses in their first year of practice. Journal of Advanced Nursing 42(1):90–96

McMahan EM, Hoffman K, McGee GW 1994 Physician–nurse relationships in clinical settings: a review and critique of the literature, 1966–1992. Medical Care Review 51(1):83–112

McMahon R 1990 Power and collegial relations among nurses on wards adopting primary nursing and hierarchical ward management structures. Journal of Advanced Nursing 15: 232–239

McVicar A 2003 Workplace stress in nursing: a literature review. Journal of Advanced Nursing 44(6):633–642

Mitchell PH, Shortell SM 1997 Adverse outcomes and variations in organization of care delivery. Medical Care 35:NS19–NS32

Oberle K, Hughes D 2001 Doctors' and nurses' perceptions of ethical problems in end-of-life decision. Journal of Advanced Nursing 33(6):707–715

Porter S 1991 A participant observation study of power relations between nurses and doctors in a general hospital. Journal of Advanced Nursing 17:720–726

Quine L 2001 Workplace bullying in nurses. Journal of Health Psychology 6(1):73–85

Rafferty AM, Ball J, Aiken LH 2001 Are teamwork and professional autonomy compatible, and do they result in improved hospital care? Quality in Health Care 10(4):32–38

Rakos RF 2006 Asserting and confronting. In: O Hargie (ed.), The handbook of communication skills, 3rd edn. pp 345–381. Routledge, London

Randle J 2003 Bullying in the nursing profession. Journal of Advanced Nursing 43(4):395–401

Roberts SJ 1983 Oppressed group behavior: implications for nursing. Advances in Nursing Science 5:21–31

Roberts SJ 2000 Development of a positive professional identity: liberating oneself from the oppressor within. Advances in Nursing Science 22(4):71–82

Rosenstein AH 2002 Nurse–physician relationships: impact on nursing satisfaction and retention. American Journal of Nursing 102(1):9–19

Salin D 2003 Ways of explaining workplace bullying: a review of enabling, motivating and precipitating structures and processes in the work environment. Human Relations 56(10):1213–1232

Santamaria N 2000 The relationship between nurses' personality and stress levels reported when caring for interpersonally difficult patients. Australian Journal of Advanced Nursing 18(2):20–26

Schmalenberg C, Kramer M 2008 Essentials of a productive nurse work environment. Nursing Research 57(1):2–13

Severinsson E, Hallberg I 1996 Clinical supervisors' views of their leadership role in the clinical supervision process within nursing care. Journal of Advanced Nursing 24(1):151–161

Shannon SE 1997 The roots of interdisciplinary conflict around ethical issues. Critical Care Nursing Clinics of North America 9(1):13–28

Shirvey MR 2004 Social support in the workplace: nurse leader implications. Nursing Economics 22(6):313–319

Shortell SM, Zimmerman JE, Rousseau DM, Gillies R, Wagner DP, Draper EA, Knaus WA, Duffy J 1994 The performance of intensive care units: does good management make a difference? Medical Care 32(5):508–525

Smith HL, Hood JN, Waldman JD, Smith VL 2005 Creating a favorable practice environment for nurses. Journal of Nursing Administration 35(12):525–532

Stein LI 1967 The doctor–nurse game. Archives of General Psychiatry 16:699–703

Stein LI, Watts DT, Howell T 1990 The doctor–nurse game revisited. New England Journal of Medicine 322(8):546–549

Stordeur S, D'hoore W, Vandenberghe C 2001 Leadership, organizational stress, and emotional exhaustion among hospital nursing staff. Journal of Advanced Nursing 35(4):533–542

Street AF 1992 Inside nursing. State University of New York Press, New York

Summer J, Townsend-Rocchiccioli J 2003 Why are nurses leaving nursing? Nursing Administration Quarterly 27(2):164–172

Sundin-Huard D, Fahy K 1999 Moral distress, advocacy and burnout: theorising the relationship. International Journal of Nursing Practice 5:8–13

Stein-Parbury J, Liaschenko J 2007 Understanding collaboration between doctors and physicians as knowledge at work. American Journal of Critical Care 16(5):470–477

Taylor B 2001 Identifying and transforming dysfunctional nurse–nurse relationships through reflective practice and action research. International Journal of Nursing Practice 7:406–413

Timmins F, McCabe C 2005 Nurses' and midwives' assertive behaviour in the workplace. Journal of Advanced Nursing 51(3):38–45

Titchen A, Binnie A 1995 The art of clinical supervision. Journal of Clinical Nursing 4(5): 327–334

Upenieks V 2003 What constitutes effective leadership? Perceptions of magnet and nonmagnet leaders. Journal of Nursing Administration 33(9):456–467

Valentine PE 2001 A gender perspective on conflict management strategies of nurses. Journal of Nursing Scholarship 33(1):69–74

van Ooijen E 2000 Clinical supervision: a practical guide. Churchill Livingstone, Edinburgh

Williamson GR, Dodds S 1999 The effectiveness of a group approach to clinical supervision in reducing stress: a review of the literature. Journal of Clinical Nursing 8:338–344

Zangaro GA, Soeken KL 2007 A meta-analysis of studies of nurses' job satisfaction. Research in Nursing and Health 30:445–458

APPENDIX

Notes on the use of activities

INTRODUCTION

The information in this appendix supports the book's learning activities by presenting guidelines and suggestions about conducting the activities in a learning group. As such, it is primarily for the benefit of those people who are promoting learning through the use of activities. These people are referred to as 'facilitators' rather than teachers, because this term more accurately reflects the nature of 'teaching' through the use of experiential activities.

The appendix begins with a brief overview of experiential learning, with specific reference to how the skills can actually be used to facilitate this method of learning. Figure A.1 illustrates the relationship between experiential learning and the skills presented in this book.

Included in this section are some suggestions for facilitators who are using experience-based learning approaches. General guidelines for employing 'role play' as an experiential learning form of activity follow; and, finally, discussion and material specific to a number of the book's various activities are presented. (Note: each activity referred to in this final section of the appendix is highlighted in its respective chapter by the symbol ➡.)

EXPERIENTIAL LEARNING

The activities in this book are designed to stimulate learning of interpersonal skills in nursing and consolidate the theory presented in the text. Some activities trigger learners to reflect on previous experiences, considering theoretical concepts in a 'there-and-then' manner. Other activities enable learners to put into practice interpersonal skills in a 'here-and-now' manner. All are designed to produce meaningful learning experiences by actively involving participants in understanding the concepts described in the text.

Learning through experience is one of the most effective ways to integrate interpersonal skills into professional behaviour. While a theoretical comprehension of the skills is essential, they are most effectively understood by participating in experiences that make them 'come to life'. By putting the skills to use in some

FIGURE A.1 The relationship of processing (outer circle) and experiential learning (inner circle)

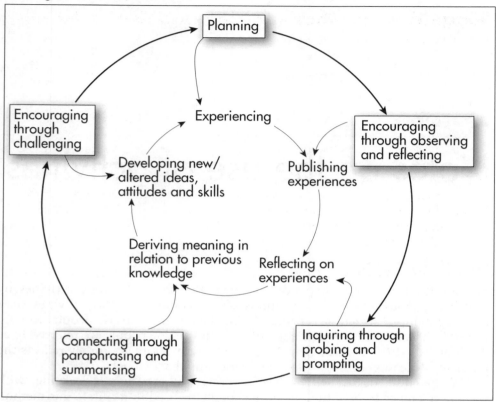

Source: Stein-Parbury J 1992 Processing skills: enhancing experiential learning. In: Members of the 1991 Teaching Enhancement Team, Quality of Teaching Matters at UTS, Centre for Learning and Teaching, University of Technology, Sydney.

way through experiential activities, theoretical understanding is developed in conjunction with the technical know-how of employing them.

The majority of the activities are most effective when they are conducted in a learning group led by a knowledgeable and sensitive guide. This guide, the learning facilitator, is a person who not only understands the concepts illustrated in the activity, but who is also able to help participants discuss the experience in a meaningful manner.

The majority of the activities include a discussion section that focuses on processing the learning experiences. Processing refers to that aspect of experiential learning that enables learners to derive personalised meaning from their experiences. In processing learning experiences, facilitators respond rather than direct, pull ideas together rather than prescribe what they should be, and encourage reflection rather than expect automatic reactions.

When interacting with learners, facilitators who demonstrate the attitudes, skills and knowledge embedded in this book will be most effective if they use an experience-based approach to learning. In addition, facilitators of the method of learning through experience are most productive when they are knowledgeable about experiential learning.

Suggestions for facilitators of experiential learning

Sometimes, experiential learning activities produce lively responses from participants. At other times, experiences designed to facilitate learning may fall flat. Here are some general suggestions for handling some of the more common difficulties that may surface when using experience-based learning:

1 Because the meaning derived from an experience is personalised, it is difficult to be pedantic about the 'right' or correct way to respond to an experience. This may be uncomfortable for facilitators who are accustomed to presenting material in a step-wise procedural manner. Facilitators of learning through experience need to refrain from using procedural approaches when teaching interpersonal skills, to allow learners to derive personally relevant meaning from their experiences, and to function as a guide on a journey, rather than an expert who demonstrates how it 'should' be done. They should be 'the guide on the side', rather than the 'sage on the stage'.

2 When activities are conducted in a traditional classroom, it is sometimes tempting to leave the room while participants engage in an activity. As a general rule, this is not a good idea, because participants often need further guidance and assistance during the activity. It is helpful to 'float' around the room, making sure that instructions for the activity are understood. This is also a useful opportunity to discuss the associated concepts with participants.

3 Sometimes, activities are ineffectual, producing a 'so what?' experience— that is, they fail to enhance participants' learning because no meaning can be constructed from it. An indication that this may be happening occurs when participants do not have much to say in response to the items in the discussion section of the activity. When an activity or its discussion seems to be 'going nowhere', it is often useful to ask a general question such as, 'What's happening here?' or 'What's going on?' When facilitators ask questions such as these, they may be surprised to learn that participants are responding to events other than the presented activity. At other times, there is 'nothing happening', and at this point the activity should be abandoned. Nevertheless, when the 'so what?' experience happens once, it is not enough reason to abandon an activity altogether. Try it again with another group of participants. It may trigger significant learning in another context.

4 When participants seem hesitant to engage in an activity, make sure they understand the instructions. Most often, reluctance is a result of failure to comprehend what is expected. Do not assume that hesitancy is a result of lack of interest or motivation. Always assume the participants' goodwill. It helps to establish trust.

5 It is often beneficial to begin formal classes that use an experience-based approach to learning with a 'warm-up' activity. These activities enable participants to get their minds in gear, ready to learn in an active, involved manner. Some suggestions for warm-up activities include:
   • **Word association**. Have participants say the first word that comes to their mind in response to the theme of the session (e.g. old age).

- **Brainstorm**. Generate as many ideas as possible about a given topic (e.g. reassurance).
- **Touch base**. Have each participant state how they are feeling at the moment.
- **Tell a story**. Begin the session by sharing a personal anecdote about the topic of the session (e.g. 'the time I became overinvolved with a patient').
- **Show a picture**. Display a picture that depicts something of relevance to the session (e.g. a patient who is crying).

These warm-up activities need to be short and snappy in order to be effective. As a general rule, they should consume no more than 10 minutes of a given session.

Guidelines for role play

Role playing is one of the most commonly used experiential learning methods. Role playing is a process of acting 'as if' the situation is real. While it does not require formal drama skills, the participants' willingness to behave in ways that may be unfamiliar is essential if the action is to proceed.

Throughout this book, various activities rely on this method. Whenever it is used, it is crucial that the following guidelines be presented to participants (on a whiteboard or butcher's paper, or circulate copies) who are enacting the role play. *Remember* that the onus is on the facilitator to present this information to the learners each time a role play exercise is introduced.

Before the action

1 Assume the role. Try not to let personal thoughts and feelings about the role interfere with your ability to adopt the role; accept it for what it is—an act designed to enhance learning. Take a few minutes before the role play to 'put yourself' into the role.
2 Do not be concerned if you think you cannot enact the role because you are not good at dramatising and performing. The purpose of role playing is to act naturally, although you may be required to adopt a stance that feels different from your usual way of interacting with others.
3 Once you have assumed the role, let the action flow naturally. Do not overact or exaggerate your actions in an effort to be a good role player.
4 During the role play, invent needed information, about yourself or specific details of the situation. Do not let the role play stop or flounder because you think you should know something; simply make it up in an effort to keep the action going.
5 It is acceptable, sometimes desirable, to change your ideas and attitudes during the role play. Even if your role prescribes certain attitudes and feelings, these may change as a result of the progress of the action. When this happens, let it flow naturally; do not cling to your original script.

After the action

1 Remain in the role and take a few minutes to discuss how you responded to the role and how it felt playing the role.
2 Make sure you clarify any information or detail that was fabricated in an effort to keep the action going.

3 Discuss any concerns you have about what others who participated in the role play may think or feel about you as a result of the role you have just assumed.
4 When the time comes, state aloud that you are no longer in the role and are returning to who you really are.

ADDITIONAL MATERIAL FOR ACTIVITIES
Chapter 3 Nurse as therapeutic agent

Activity 3.1 WHAT DO I HAVE TO OFFER PATIENTS?

This activity can be threatening and frightening to participants if they think they will be expected to reveal their responses. For this reason, it is essential to stress that participants will not be required to disclose the answers to the questions posed in the process section. Participants should be seated in a manner that allows their papers to remain in their own view only. The discussion centres on how it felt to complete the activity, not on the answers to personal questions asked during the process.

Activity 3.4 BELIEFS ABOUT HELPING IN NURSING PRACTICE

The questionnaire used in this activity is designed to trigger thoughts about assumptions of personal responsibility for problems and how these assumptions affect approaches to helping. Participants may take issue with some of the items on the questionnaire, especially if their results are not in accordance with what they believe, want to believe, or think they 'should' believe. Much time and effort could go into discussing the items, and this may detract from the purpose of the activity. Individual participant's results are therefore not the major issue, and this should be stressed during the discussion of the activity.

It is equally important to emphasise that a mismatch between how patients view their responsibility and how nurses view personal responsibility can create problems in the relationship. For this reason, participants should be encouraged to develop awareness of patients' orientation to helping as well as of their own orientation.

Activity 3.11 SELF-ASSESSMENT OF SPECIFIC SKILLS

This activity can be attempted only after participants have been engaged in learning specific skills.

Chapter 4 Considering culture

Activity 4.2 WORKING WITH AN INTERPRETER

See 'Guidelines for role play' on page 300.

Activity 4.3 COMMUNICATING WITHOUT LANGUAGE

See 'Guidelines for role play' on page 300.

Chapter 5 Encouraging interaction: listening

Activity 5.4 PHYSICAL ATTENDING

INSTRUCTIONS TO A

You are going to speak to person B for about 5 minutes on a topic of your choosing. About 2 minutes into the conversation, inform B that you are going to share a secret with them. Make sure you say that it is a secret, and then proceed to share it with B. You will need to fabricate this 'secret', so prepare yourself by thinking of something really interesting to share.

INSTRUCTIONS TO B

Seat yourself comfortably and place a seat facing you for person A. Person A is going to talk to you for about 5 minutes. Act naturally during the conversation, while you listen to what A has to say.

INSTRUCTIONS TO C

Person A and person B are going to have a conversation lasting about 5 minutes. You are to observe and note person B's non-verbal behaviour during the conversation. You do not need to actually hear what A and B are discussing. Pay particular attention to body posture, eye contact and other behaviours that indicate B's level of interest in the conversation. Note especially any change in B's non-verbal behaviour about 2 minutes into the conversation.

See 'Guidelines for role play' on page 300.

Activity 5.5 ATTENDING AND NON-ATTENDING

See 'Guidelines for role play' on page 300.

Activity 5.7 LISTENING FOR CONTENT

Participants often request to have stories read more than once. Facilitators need to emphasise that doing so would interfere with the purpose of the activity. While nurses may request patients to repeat what they have said (e.g. when nurses cannot hear what has been said, or the patient's speech is garbled), such requests may be interpreted as a failure to listen in the first place.

Participants' responses (the who, what, when and where content) should be reviewed after each story is read, rather than reading all stories, then reviewing the responses. As each story is reviewed, participants become more skilled at listening for content (i.e. the learning is immediate).

In answering the 'who, what, when and where' of each story, participants often become frustrated if the facilitator is pedantic about the 'correct' answers. Rather than giving the impression of right and wrong answers, it is better to focus discussion on reasons for discrepancies between participants, and between participants' answers and the ones provided at the end of the chapter. The purpose of the activity is to discover the process of listening, not to 'get' the right answers. This may need to be continually reinforced.

Activity 5.8 LISTENING FOR FEELINGS

Participants' responses should be reviewed after each patient statement is read, rather than reading all the statements and then reviewing the responses. There is often great variety between participants in their interpretation of feelings. Because answers are provided at the end of the chapter, these may be perceived as 'correct' and any other answers as 'incorrect'. Take care not to give the impression that responses that are different from those presented at the end of the chapter are 'incorrect'. Rather, focus discussion on why the interpretations differ between participants. Some of the reasons for these differences include cultural variance, role expectations, personal needs, values and beliefs. Emphasise the importance of self-understanding within the context of listening for feelings.

This activity often highlights problems with the language used to describe feelings; participants sometimes find it difficult to 'find the words' to express emotions. A general discussion about the role of language in discussing feelings is useful and timely in the discussion phase of this activity. It is also beneficial to follow this activity with Activity 6.5 Building a feeling-word vocabulary.

Activity 5.9 LISTENING FOR THEMES

See 'Guidelines for role play' on page 300.

Activity 5.11 RESPONSES THAT INDICATE LISTENING

Do not become overly concerned if there is a discrepancy between participants' answers and the ones provided at the end of the chapter. Sometimes, such discrepancies indicate different interpretations of the words used in the responses; at other times, different meanings are constructed. Sometimes, participants want to argue about the answers in an effort to determine the correct one and this can become counterproductive to learning. Rather than arguing, participants should be encouraged to reflect on their interpretation of the given responses, and compare these with other participants' interpretations. As a result of this type of discussion, participants are better able to understand that meanings are in people, not words.

Chapter 6 Building meaning: understanding

Activity 6.2 RECOGNITION OF THE TYPES OF RESPONSES

Participants often experience difficulty differentiating an analysing and interpreting response (A) from a paraphrasing and understanding response (U). It should be explained that an A response 'adds' to what the patient has expressed. When such additions are an accurate reflection of what a patient is experiencing, this is referred to as 'advanced empathy'. Advanced empathy delves into feelings and meanings that are beneath the surface. When such additions are inaccurate, they are often a reflection of the nurse's personal value judgments. A U response remains on the surface and does not delve more deeply into hidden and obscured meaning.

Activity 6.4 PARAPHRASING: HAVE I GOT IT RIGHT?

See 'Guidelines for role play' on page 300.

Activity 6.7 CONNECTING THOUGHTS AND FEELINGS

Sometimes, participants are frustrated by using the format, 'You feel … when …' When this happens, encourage them to use their own style of expression, as long as the connection between thoughts and feelings is made. Emphasise that the suggested format is a useful mental aid; it is not a prescription for connecting feelings and thoughts. When adhered to rigidly, the suggested format interferes with the development of a personal style.

Chapter 7 Collecting information: exploring

Activity 7.2 WAYS OF EXPLORING: QUESTIONS VERSUS STATEMENTS

See 'Guidelines for role play' on page 300.

Activity 7.3 CONVERTING PROBES INTO PROMPTS

Some participants may find it difficult to develop exploratory statements (prompts) because they are accustomed to exploring through the use of questions (probes). If this happens, it is useful to find participants who are not having difficulty converting probes to prompts and encourage these participants to assist those who are experiencing difficulty. Emphasise that the activity is not a 'test' of ability, rather a method of enhancing learning.

Activity 7.5 EFFECTS OF 'WHY?' QUESTIONS

See 'Guidelines for role play' on page 300.

Activity 7.7 RECOGNISING TYPES OF QUESTIONS

Some participants may not be able to perceive the disguised 'why?' question and further explanation may be necessary to complete the process. 'Why?' questions are often hidden behind statements such as, 'What made you feel that way?', 'What are your reasons for thinking this way?' and 'How come?' If the word 'why' can be substituted for a word or phrase in the question without destroying its meaning, then there is a good chance that a disguised 'why?' question has been asked.

Activity 7.9 CUES AND INFERENCES

Some of the inferences presented in this activity could actually be cues. For example, item 2 would be a cue if the patient directly stated that they were uninterested in the interview. This point should be brought out during the discussion phase of the activity.

It should be stressed that inferences can be valid interpretations of cues. Sometimes, participants may form the impression that inferences should be avoided at all costs. The discussion phase of this activity provides a useful opportunity to clarify this incorrect impression.

Finally, nurses must take care in supporting inferences with the cues on which they are based. In recording patient data in a chart, for example, it is essential that inferences are not stated, unless their supporting cues are also stated. On the other hand, cues can be recorded on their own—that is, they do not require an interpretation (inference).

Activity 7.11 PATIENT INTERVIEW

See 'Guidelines for role play' on page 300.

Chapter 8 Intervening: comforting, supporting and enabling

Activity 8.4 SHARING INFORMATION

This activity is conducted over two sessions. In the first session, participants are given scenarios for sharing information (developed in steps 1 and 2 of the process). In doing so, they have the opportunity to familiarise themselves with the information that they will be sharing. They can come to the next session prepared to share information. Without this opportunity, participants may be caught 'off guard' and feel unable to share information because they do not know enough about a given topic.

See 'Guidelines for role play' on page 300 and 'Guide for sharing information' (below).

GUIDE FOR SHARING INFORMATION

Did the nurse ...

1 Identify what the patient wants to know?
Yes No
How?

2 Clarify what the patient already understands?
Yes No
How?

3 Assess the accuracy of the patient's current information?
Yes No
How?

4 Determine the patient's readiness to receive the information?
Yes No
How?

5 Limit the amount of information shared (about two items at a time)?
Yes No
How?

6 Use understandable language?
Yes No
How?

7 Present information clearly?
Yes No
How?

8 Assess the patient's comprehension?
Yes No
How?

9 Request feedback from the patient?
Yes No
How?

10 Discuss the patient's reaction to the information?
Yes No
How?

Index